CLASSICS IN GROUP PSYCHOTHERAPY

CLASSICS
in
Group Psychotherapy

K. Roy MacKenzie, M.D.
Editor

A Publication of
the American Group Psychotherapy Association

THE GUILFORD PRESS
New York   London

© 1992 The Guilford Press
A Division of Guilford Publications, Inc.
72 Spring Street, New York, N. Y. 10012

Printed in the United States of America

This book is printed on acid-free paper

Last digit is print number: 9 8 7 6 5 4 3 2 1

Library of Congress Cataloging-in-Publication Data

Classics in group psychotherapy /   edited by K. Roy MacKenzie
    p.   cm.
Consists of articles reprinted from various sources from
1905–1981.
Includes bibliographic references and index.
ISBN 0-89862-799-0
1. Group psychotherapy.   I. MacKenzie, K. Roy, 1937–
[DNLM: 1. Psychotherapy. Group— collected works.   WM 430 C614]
  RC488.C53   1992
  616.89'152—dc20
  DNLM/DLC   91-35412
  for Library of Congress   CIP

Foreword

Humans are social creatures. Our personalities are largely shaped by the family group into which we are born and thereafter by the groups we join, voluntarily or otherwise. We form our values and attitudes and guide our behavior by continually checking the validity of our perceptions and feelings against other members of these groups. Consequently our "reference groups" exert powerful psychological forces to maintain or change our view of ourselves and the world. Group psychotherapies seek to mobilize these forces to combat the maladaptive attitudes that contribute to the distress and disability of all illness.

Throughout history and in every culture sufferers have sought relief through group rituals led by healers. The healers were believed to have special access to supernatural healing forces whose benevolent intervention was elicited by the rituals. In most pre-industrial cultures, the group healing rituals characteristically involved members of the sufferer's extended family. In some cultures, however, as in the temples of Aesculapius of the Greeks, participants in the rituals were fellow sufferers who were unacquainted with each other.

In the Western world, with the advances of science, secular healers and rituals under the name of medical treatments eventually dispensed with appeals to supernatural forces, and group healing was overshadowed by therapy of individuals in the physician's private office. At the same time, somatic and psychological illness became more sharply distinguished, with medical and surgical methods considered the treatments of choice for the former and psychotherapies for the latter.

Today interactions between body and mind in the causes and cures of illness are being rediscovered and described at increasingly sophisticated levels, as is the healing potential of groups of strangers or family members. That the healing potentials of group forces are being rediscovered in today's socially fragmented industrial civilizations is not surprising. What should cause astonishment is that group psychotherapies have taken so long to come to prominence.

In Europe and America psychotherapy as a self-defined discipline, distinguished from medical healing on the one hand and faith healing on the other, may be said to have originated with the writings of Freud and Janet, among others, in the last decade of the 19th century. Yet the first paper calling attention to the power of group healing forces in this well chosen selection did not appear until 1907. Interestingly enough, it was written by a general practitioner and concerned the treatment of tuberculosis, a chronic medical disease. The next two papers that the editors found to be worthy of inclusion did not appear until some 20 and 30 years later.

This lag in acceptance of the therapeutic powers of groups may have been related to the emphasis on individual autonomy in Western societies as expressed in the medical model of treatment, an emphasis reinforced by Freud's view of psychoanalysis as a strictly private affair between the individual patient and the analyst, a relationship distinctly removed from the patient's daily life. Lending plausibility to this speculation is the fact that the overwhelming majority of the papers in this volume are psychoanalytic in orientation.

Whatever the reasons, group approaches to the treatment of clinical populations did not become popular until the shortage of psychotherapists in World War II necessitated group treatment of psychiatric casualties. The results were so gratifying that since then group psychotherapies have steadily expanded in number and variety. This postwar growth is reflected in this volume by the fact that out of 26 contributions chosen as particularly influential, 19 appeared after 1940.

In the half-century since that watershed group methods have permeated the entire realm of efforts to change the behavior and attitudes of troubled individuals. Such persons range far beyond conventional psychiatric inpatients and outpatients and their families, who are the concerns of most of the writers in this collection, to include those at the mercy of their drives, such as addicts and sexual deviates, as well as those with chronic nonpsychiatric illness, including the terminally ill.

Today participants in groups also include persons who are not physically or psychologically ill. Some seek simply to enrich their lives through so-called encounter groups, while disadvantaged or oppressed members of society, including women, racial minorities and prisoners, band together in consciousness-raising groups to enhance their power.

Corresponding to the spread in the variety of members of groups has been a spread of qualifications of group leaders. Originally physicians, typically psychiatrists, they have been joined and even superseded by psychologists, social workers and members of other healing professions, as well as the clergy, self-designated healers of healing cults such as EST, and fellow-sufferers in what have been termed peer self-help psychotherapy groups.

Concomitantly the settings of group therapies have overflowed from psychiatric hospitals and outpatient departments to business and factory offices as well as settings created especially for these activities such as personal growth centers. This expansion and differentiation of the practice of group psychotherapies has been accompanied and guided by a parallel expansion of their conceptual underpinnings.

While appropriately reflecting the dominance of concepts derived from psychoanalysis in the formative years of group psychotherapy, the selection in this book also include other seminal contributions that have extended the range of group therapies. One, that of Adler, which may be inferred from the paper by Dreikurs, is in the psychoanalytic spectrum, but with a salutary shift from intrapsychic determinants toward interpersonal ones.

The concepts and therapeutic procedures of psychodrama, created by Moreno, have been extremely influential, as have those of Carl Rogers. The paper of Bion, although in the psychoanalytic spectrum, marks a further development—the beginning of a shift in focus from individuals in groups to emergent properties of groups themselves as they affect individual members, an orientation also exemplified by Frank. A natural extension of this trend has been interest in dynamics of small groups largely independent of the properties of their individual members, as seen in the papers of Lewin and Rioch. This perspective, while relevant to group psychotherapy, has facilitated the extension of group concepts and methods far beyond treatment of individuals in distress to such areas as increasing the efficiency and job satisfaction of members of dysfunctional organizations.

Returning, in conclusion, to the therapeutic focus of this book, I venture to prophesy that the powerful therapeutic properties of group methods, coupled with their relative economy, will eventually lead them to become treatments of choice for most persons suffering from psychologically caused distress and disability. Individual therapy will be reserved for those few for whom it has specific advantages.

Regardless of how valid this prophecy proves to be, this well chosen sampling of trail-breaking papers on group therapy is highly recommended as providing an illuminating introduction to this exciting field.

Jerome D. Frank, Ph.D., M.D.
Professor Emeritus of Psychiatry
Johns Hopkins University School of Medicine

Preface

This book is a celebration of the 50th Anniversary of the founding of the American Group Psychotherapy Association. Over these fifty years, AGPA has provided the principal forum in North America for group clinicians, teachers, and researchers, and the *International Journal of Group Psychotherapy*, its publication, has reflected the changing priorities and interests of successive generations of group therapists. It seemed a fitting tribute to AGPA on this occasion to publish a selection of classic articles from the literature, articles that are often referenced but not easy to find in the original version. This provides a double benefit: access to seminal articles and a way to honor people who have made an important contribution to the field. The AGPA Board of Directors eagerly supported the recommendation from the Publications Committee to sponsor such a book.

It has been a great pleasure as Editor to work with a prestigious group of Editorial Advisors. I have particularly appreciated their willingness to put personally chosen articles aside in favor of the majority opinion, not an easy task when each in his or her own right has an extensive knowledge of the literature. We are honored that Dr. Jerome Frank agreed to write the Foreword. Dr. Frank has been a pioneer in psychotherapy teaching and research, whose career has spanned close to five decades, beginning with his association with Kurt Lewin. I am also grateful to Dr. Saul Scheidlinger and Mr. Gerald Schamess for the historical chapter that begins the book. Saul's involvement in the group psychotherapy field began in the early years of AGPA, so he brings a unique personal perspective to the task. The necessity for summarizing history into a limited space has been a challenging one.

Initially the task of developing such a book sounded relatively straightforward—to compile a list of some 25 to 30 core articles. However, an early collection of recommended articles expanded to well over 300. Everyone, it seemed, had his or her own absolutely indispensable list of references. The Editorial Advisors exchanged innumerable phone calls and faxes to pare down the list, and a set of principles was developed. We would exclude all references after the 1970s and include only those written by authors who were no longer active in the current literature (my apologies to the small number who are still very much active). Preference would be given to journal articles over book chapters unless there was a compelling reason to do otherwise. We would try to avoid articles that were printed in other anthologies such as Scheidlinger's *Psychoanalytic Group Dynamics,* which is still in print, and Rosenbaum and Berger's *Group Psychotherapy and Group Function,* which is now out of print but widely distributed. We would select for the person first and the article second, that is, we wanted to feature people who had made important contributions to the field, and gave preference to earlier works that represented an emerging area of contribution. It was important to provide a reasonable survey of various theoretical orientations.

It will become apparent to the reader that the book does not cover the application of group psychotherapy to special patient populations. In part, this may be explained by the fact that the early literature tended to deal primarily with general group phenomena. In addition, it seemed impossible to do justice to this general literature and at the same time to give adequate representation to all the specific uses that are being made of group techniques. The book therefore does not include articles concerning groups for children and adolescents (with one exception), for the elderly, for the longer term maintenance of the chronically ill, for alcohol and substance abusers, for inpatient units, for various medical disorders, and the many targeted groups that have emerged over the years. Perhaps these are topics for future *Classics* publications.

A secondary goal of this book was to highlight, and to some extent address, splits that have occurred in the field of group psychotherapy. An attempt has been made to include representative articles that might help to mediate across these divisions. Several have been addressed. (1) The issues surrounding the tension between those espousing concepts derived from individual analytic approaches versus those who advocate group-as-a-whole ideas are well laid out in this volume. Several of the articles in the final section represent a synthesis of these two traditions. (2) The early split between psychodrama and psychoanalysis resulted in two parallel organizations and journals that continue to this day. A number of articles are included that deal with the more "action oriented" techniques that are in wide use but not well represented within more orthodox group psychotherapeutic circles. (3) Attention to the empirical study of the social psychology of small groups that was common in the 1950s and 1960s is not well represented in the later literature. Some articles come from that period as well as more recent ones. (4) In the early literature, there was a sense of excitement about group psychotherapy as a means of revolutionizing clinical care and influencing the norms of society. The original enthusiasm associated with these social goals is evident in several articles. The table illustrates the organization of the content of the book by time period and by major focus of the authors.

Book Subdivision		Authors Organized by Major Orientation			
		Analytic	Group-as-a-Whole	Action Oriented	Empirical
The Formative Years	1907				Pratt
	1928	****	****		Burrow
	1936	Wender			
	1940			Moreno	****
	1943	****	Bion		
	1947		****	****	Lewin
	1948			Jones	
	1951		****	****	Dreikurs
Years of Theoretical Expansion	1952	****	Ezriel		
	1955			****	Corsini
	1957	****	Foulkes		
	1957				Frank
	1957	Slavson			
	1957	Durkin	****		
	1958	****		Berne	
	1958		Stock		****
	1963	Redl	****		****
	1967			Rogers	****
Years of Consolidation	1968	****	****		Parloff
	1970	****	Rioch		
	1971				Yalom
	1974	Scheidlinger	****		
	1977	Schiffer			
	1977	****	Horwitz		
	1978	Glatzer			
	1981	Stein	****		

Note. Asterisks indicate significant cross-linkage between areas of interest.

One divergence that has not been adequately addressed is that between psychodynamically influenced approaches and behavioral and cognitive-behavioral theories and techniques. Given our cutoff date of the 1970s there were few articles to choose from that addressed the specific application of these techniques in groups, even though many of them are applied in that format. However, cognitive-behavioral methods have been used in group work for a long time without specific acknowledgment of their origins. I have tried to highlight such material in the introduction to each article.

Because of space constraints, sections of some of the articles have been deleted. These deletions consist of additional clinical examples, detailed statistical results, or diversions from the main theme of the article. In a few instances, particularly in the case of book chapters, more extensive editing has been performed in an effort to maintain a focus on the principal issue under discussion. This has been noted in the Editor's introduction to those selections. The original list of references has been retained for each selection even though they may not all be cited because of deletions to the text.

It has been a personally rewarding experience to have undergone this renewed exposure to the length and breadth of the group psychotherapy literature. Several impressions come to mind. The vigorous confronting debates that characterized the early literature have been stilled. By contrast, the present literature seems uncontroversial and somewhat pedestrian. At the same time, it is disturbing to look back at the manner in which some creative thinkers were excluded from the main stream. A number of authors represented here would, in their time, have taken sharp exception to some of their companions in this book's Table of Contents. At the moment the field appears to be more open to integration and consideration of new ideas, while at the same time, the forces of orthodoxy express concern that standards be maintained. Little attention is still paid to empirical findings that might help to resolve at least some of these issues. It is always a shock to appreciate how few ideas are really new—you will find concepts and applications that sound very contemporary in many of the early articles.

The use of group psychotherapy has always reflected general social trends. It would seem that the current focus on effective and efficient treatment methods should herald a renewed interest in the use of group modalities. Certainly current outcome studies indicate that group treatment is every bit as effective as individual therapy. Perhaps a volume of classic reprints on the occasion of AGPA's 100th Anniversary in the year 2042 will find that 1992 was a critical turning point in the use of group psychotherapy.

The Editorial Advisors and myself are reconciled to the fact that the present selections will satisfy no one entirely. As the limitations of space pressed ever tighter, it was with a degree of anguish that many senior names were dropped from the book, but we believe that the articles chosen should make stimulating and absorbing reading for today's group therapist. I hope that you enjoy this volume and that you will murmur a "Happy Anniversary" to AGPA as you open the cover.

Vancouver, British Columbia   **K. Roy MacKenzie, M.D.**
September 1991   Chairman
          American Group Psychotherapy
            Association
          Publications Committee

Acknowledgments

Permission to reprint the following (in order of their appearance in this volume) is gratefully acknowledged:

The Class Method of Treating Consumption in the Homes of the Poor, by *Joseph H. Pratt.* © 1907 American Medical Association.

The Basis of Group-Analysis, or the Analysis of the Reactions of Normal and Neurotic Individuals, by *Trigant Burrow.* © 1928 British Psychological Society.

The Dynamics of Group Psychotherapy and Its Application, by *Louis Wender.* © 1936 Williams & Wilkins.

Psychodrama, by *J. L. Moreno.* © 1940, 1966 American Society of Group Psychotherapy and Psychodrama.

Frontiers in Group Dynamics: Concept, Method and Reality in Social Science; Social Equilibria and Social Change, by *Kurt Lewin.* © 1947 Plenum Publishing Corporation.

Emotional Catharsis and Re-Education in the Neuroses with the Help of Group Methods, by *Maxwell Jones.* © 1948 British Psychological Society.

The Unique Social Climate Experienced in Group Psychotherapy, by *Rudolph Dreikurs.* © 1951 American Society of Group Psychotherapy and Psychodrama.

Notes on Psychoanalytic Group Therapy: II. Interpretation and Research, by *Henry Ezriel.* © 1952 Washington School of Psychiatry.

Group-Analytic Dynamics with Specific Reference to Psychoanalytic Concepts, by *S. H. Foulkes.* © 1957 American Group Psychotherapy Association.

The Deviant Member in Therapy Groups, by *Dorothy Stock, Roy M. Whitman, and Morton A. Lieberman.* © 1958 Plenum Publishing Corporation.

Mechanisms of Group Psychotherapy: Processes and Dynamics, by *Raymond J. Corsini and Bina Rosenberg.* © 1955 American Psychological Association.

Contents

YEARS OF CONSOLIDATION, 1968–1981

CLASSICS IN GROUP PSYCHOTHERAPY

Fifty Years of AGPA 1942–1992: An Overview

SAUL SCHEIDLINGER, PH.D.
Albert Einstein College of Medicine, Bronx, NY
GERALD SCHAMESS, M.S.S.
Smith College of Social Work, Northampton, MA

A history of the first 50 years of the American Group Psychotherapy Association must be seen in the light of the growth of group psychotherapy as well as the social context in which this occurred. In his 25-year history of our Association, Pattison (1970) concluded that "The story of the AGPA is not the story of group psychotherapy, but each has been a large part of the other" (p. 21). Given the perspectives of an additional 25 years, we would add that the AGPA has also been a part of a broader post-World War II world as reflected in the human services in general and those in mental health in particular.

The Beginnings (1942–1952)

The logo with its emblazoned year 1942 notwithstanding, available evidence suggests that the first two meetings preceding the AGPA's founding actually occurred in 1943. These were held in conjunction with two sessions on group therapy, featured at the annual meeting of the American Orthopsychiatric Association in February of 1943 in New York. This Special Section on Group Therapy was chaired by Dr. Lawson G. Lowrey, the then Editor of the American Journal of Orthopsychiatry. Mr. Samuel R. Slavson, Dr. Nathan W. Ackerman, Dr. Harris B. Peck, and two clinical social workers, Helen Glauber and Dorothy Spiker, participated. In his Introduction to the Section, Lowrey (1943) referred to his Jewish Board of Guardians' study of over 100 children treated by activity group therapy stating ". . . it is obvious that here is a technique which is as effective as individual therapy" (p. 650).

Following these sessions, S.R. Slavson convened an informal luncheon of people interested in this new modality. At a follow-up meeting held at New York's Jewish Board of Guardians where Slavson worked, he was asked to head a Steering Committee of five, charged to draft a provisional constitution for the new organization. As described below, the composition of that Steering Committee foreshadowed the ideological differences that would soon shake the foundations of the young organization. Four of the members were psychiatrists, among them Nathan Ackerman, the subsequent founder of family therapy and Harris Peck, a future Editor of the *International Journal of Group Psychotherapy*. Only one, Saul Bernstein, was a social group worker.

At the next meeting in November of the same year, also held at Slavson's office, about one-half of the 20 participants were from the Jewish Board of Guardians. The enacted constitution delineated the mission of the then-named American Group Therapy Association, it became the American Group Psychotherapy Association in 1952, as being designed to ". . . promote interest in group therapy and coordinate and clarify the efforts of those involved in its practice and theory" (Durkin et al., 1971, p. 412). Membership was restricted to psychiatrists, psychologists, and psychiatric case workers who had at least three years of postgraduate supervised practice in psychotherapy. Persons without these educational credentials had to have five years of psychotherapy experience ". . . under approved supervision with psychiatrists participating" (Pattison, 1968, pp. 10–11). Slavson was elected the first President of AGTA, but the subsequent 12 Presidents were all psychiatrists. This stress on psychiatric dominance is significant and reflects, in our view, Slavson's desire to associate this new, interdisciplinary organization with what he perceived as the prestige of psychiatry. In this connection, a special invitation to join the AGTA was sent to all members of the American Psychiatric Association. History must be repeating itself; AGPA today is once more seeking to attract more psychiatrists to the Association.

Slavson's insistence that AGTA membership be restricted to clinicians trained in psychotherapy precipitated a number of organizational conflicts during the 1945 and 1946 annual meetings. These culminated in the precipitous 1947 resignation of Dr. Temple Burling, a psychiatrist and AGTA President who believed that all people working with groups should be included. In his hastily drawn resignation note he said: "It is the group dynamics that does the therapy—not the skilled use of psychotherapy" (Durkin, 1949). This issue, which he perceived as a dichotomy of group dynamics versus group psychotherapy was to haunt Slavson throughout his career and will be discussed later.

When the AGTA was founded, America was embroiled in an all-out global war and its economy had been converted to a war basis. At the 1942 annual meeting of the American Orthopsychiatric Association, ". . . the ominous shadow of a world in a struggle to avoid an all-embracing eclipse hung more heavily . . . than was anticipated" (*American Journal of Orthopsychiatry*, 1942, p. 175). That meeting carried many programs devoted to the war effort.

The contributions of group therapy to military psychiatry were also referred to at meetings of the AGTA, particularly the fact that many of the group field's leaders (and later AGPA members) were experimenting with group methods while in the armed forces. Among these leaders were S. H.

Foulkes and W. R. Bion in England as well as Samuel Hadden, Alexander Wolf, Irving Berger, and Donald Shaskan in the United States (Berger, 1978; Shaskan, 1978). It is noteworthy here that W. C. Menninger, America's Chief of Military Psychiatry, considered the use of group therapy during the war as one of the three major contributions to civilian psychiatry (Menninger, 1946). Following the war's end, the AGTA approached the American Red Cross offering its services in helping veterans to obtain group therapy.

The AGTA's beginnings were unquestionably the product of Slavson's untiring and zealous efforts. He was aided at first by a few loyal associates at the Jewish Board of Guardians, among them George Holland, the organization's first Secretary-Treasurer, Charles G. McCormick, Mortimer Schiffer, and later Hyman Spotnitz. After his term as President, Slavson continued in 1944 as chairman of the influential Administrative Committee for 10 years and edited a Bulletin until the founding of the *International Journal of Group Psychotherapy* in 1951. He continued as its de facto Editor until 1961. Furthermore, Slavson's Jewish Board of Guardians office served as the Association's headquarters until his retirement in 1955. The move to new offices enabled the first step toward the founder's relinquishing some of his earlier control of the organization.

Slavson never disguised his strong preference for a group therapy rooted in Freudian psychoanalysis. This held true for his children's activity group therapy begun in 1934 as well as for activity-interview groups initiated by Betty Gabriel in 1937, and for therapy groups designed for adults. For more than two decades, his strict guardianship of the Association's psychiatric–psychoanalytic identity served to isolate AGPA from alternative group treatment models.

Years of Expansion and Conflict
(1952–1962)

In 1952, the organization was incorporated under the laws of the State of New York and its name changed to the American Group Psychotherapy Association. This followed the initial publication of the *International Journal of Group Psychotherapy* in April 1951 under the editorship of Lewis Loeser. In the Journal's first issue, the AGPA was described as an interest group comprising ". . . professional persons in a cooperative effort to study, interpret and encourage sound practices and training in the field of group psychotherapy. Its membership comprises practitioners in the fields of psychiatry, psychiatric casework and clinical psychology." The quest to become a competency organization was to emerge later.

Meanwhile, the AGPA had grown by 1952 to 318 members from a mere 60 members in 1944. The Journal began with 300 paid subscribers. In his continuing effort to attract more psychiatrists to the organization,

Slavson persuaded the Board of Directors in 1953 to make psychiatrists eligible for membership without the requirement for supervised experience expected of psychologists and of social workers (Durkin, 1949).

The years following AGPA's move in 1955 to new headquarters, with a paid Executive Secretary, were marked by much internal dissent. The conflicts arose as younger, more autonomy-minded new Presidents refused to follow Slavson's dictates. Personality and ideological clashes pervaded the Board meetings; democratic procedures were frequently violated. Durkin (1949) observed: "As the younger members began to become of age and aspire to leadership, they espoused some new views, and rebelled against the conservatism and control of the founders" (p. 7).

Despite Slavson's initial qualms lest standards be compromised, a separate training institute, attended by 200 registrants, was added to the 1957 annual conference under the direction of Milton Berger and Maurice Linden. Over the years, these institutes have grown in quality, diversity, and, especially prestige. Experienced professionals began to compete so vigorously for the small number of voluntary instructor positions that these assignments had to be apportioned (Christ, 1977). At present, the institute has come to be generally considered as the high point of the annual conferences.

Another source of conflict during the late 1950s pertained to the quest of the local affiliate and regional societies for greater autonomy and power. In 1956, the newly formed Affiliate Local and Regional Society Committee recognized the Delaware Valley, Eastern, Louisiana, New Jersey, and Tristate Societies and by January of 1959 those in Maine, Northern California, and the South-West. In a special memorandum addressed to the AGPA Board of Directors, Slavson (1959) called for increased scrutiny of the activities of these societies, including an examination of their constitutions so as to assure their conformity with the national By-Laws. This memorandum also called for an evaluation of the institutes, which Slavson still distrusted. Slavson's influence, though diminished, was still formidable. The Board voted him ". . . life membership . . . with full powers and privileges, including voting" (Durkin, 1949, p. 21).

With AGPA's increasingly popular publications and training endeavors came the wish to extend this recognition to the international sphere. Slavson had already lectured in a number of foreign countries and maintained an active correspondence with professionals abroad. Not to be outdone by J. L. Moreno's far flung international activities, Slavson had already named the AGPA's *national* organ, the *International Journal of Group Psychotherapy*. He and Wilfred Hulse arranged in 1953 to have the Association join the World Federation of Mental Health. A planned International Conference of Group Psychotherapy in conjunction with the World Mental Health Congress in Toronto in 1954 failed to materialize because of irreconcilable differences between Slavson and Moreno. In

1954, AGPA established a new Committee on the International Aspects of Group Psychotherapy which served as a liaison with the growing number of foreign affiliate societies. The Journal also began to carry news items about group therapy abroad including special reports from France (Lebovici, 1958) and Holland (Spanjaard, 1958).

The 1952–1962 decade of AGPA's "growing pains" coincided with the years of Eisenhower's presidency (1953–1961) also fraught with many conflicts: the Korean War, the McCarthy hearings, desegregation struggles, and political scandals. The 1950's have also been termed the years of conformity, with America categorized as "a case of the bland leading the bland." It was the land of *The Lonely Crowd* (Riesman et al., 1953), *The Man in the Grey Flannel Suit* (Wilson, 1955), and of *The Organization Man* (Whyte, 1956).

During that same period the mental health field was beset by unprecedented squabbles between competing schools of thought and claims for hegemony which held true for group therapy as well. In the words of Newell (1951), "By defending hypotheses with a dogmatic, almost religious zeal, by resisting demonstration and investigation, and by clothing our thoughts in jargon, we retard the progress of science and knowledge in our field" (p. 449). Within the AGPA these ideological struggles revolved around two basic camps: (1) adherents of the orthodox Freudian position championed by Slavson, and (2) practitioners of neo-Freudian, Existentialist, and Transactional Analysis, some of whom managed to attain positions as officers of the association. Such questions as whether the group therapist should disclose anything about his/her own feelings to the group, or whether one should ever touch a patient physically caused vituperative debates.

The Years of New Visions and of Maturation (1962–1972)

This decade encompassed the Kennedy years of new hope too soon overshadowed by the dark experiences of Vietnam and Watergate. In the early 1960's the Kennedy brothers managed, not unlike F.D.R., to capture the attention of America's young, reflecting an image of courage and of concern for the poor and for Blacks. The New Frontier and Great Society legislation which included Medicare and Medicaid, as well as the Community Mental Health Center Act of 1963, had profound influences on the human services.

The new Comprehensive Community Mental Health Center model was so boldly innovative in theory, practice, and scope that it was at times connoted as a "Third Mental Health Revolution," purporting to supplant the one initiated by Freud. This program called for hundreds of federally funded community-based mental health services all over America to meet the needs of all citizens, young and old. Not unlike the public health model, emphasis was divided among prevention, treatment of pathology, and maintenance of positive mental health.

The profound effect of these developments on the group field in general and on the AGPA in particular is evident when one realizes that most of the Community Mental Health Center's services had to rely heavily on group therapy and on allied group techniques. The accumulated knowledge and experience of group therapists in outpatient, day hospital, inpatient, and even preventive contexts was now in great demand. In the absence of the urgently needed cadres of skilled group practitioners, harassed administrators began to resort to rash and risky solutions, among them the assignment of individual therapists and auxiliary professionals to work with groups. Moreover, an earlier trend to employ paraprofessionals in the mental health services was extended as well to the group field.

As might be expected, these rapid developments in a sphere already beset by professional role conflicts and confusing terminology refueled the fiery issues of boundaries, of methodologies, and of differential treatment goals. Many workers began to demand that the traditional aims of uncovering unconscious conflicts and of character reconstruction be replaced with less ambitious expectations focused on enhanced ego functioning, social competence, and symptom removal. The AGPA's annual conferences and the Journal reflected this marked ferment. But the agenda of the conferences, especially, broadened to provide additional training opportunities for beginning group practitioners. The training programs of the affiliate societies responded in tandem.

During this period, clinical group therapy practice issues were also consolidated. For example, combined therapy (Aronson, 1964) was delineated with considerable clarity as were group approaches geared to the "hard-to-reach," namely, substance abusers, delinquents, and the chronically ill. Modified ways in which group modalities could be employed with socially disadvantaged minorities who populated urban ghettoes were also included (Peck & Scheidlinger, 1968).

Efforts to solidify theories of group therapy continued during the 1960's. Slavson's Textbook in Analytic Group Psychotherapy (1964) distilled 50 years of his work. Other significant works also appeared, e.g., by Wolf and Schwartz (1962) and by Foulkes (1964). Interestingly, the first two volumes, though espousing differing technical ways of treatment, share an underlying belief in the primacy of the individual-focused approach in group therapy. Foulkes, in contrast, espoused a more group-centered position reflecting an earlier assertion of his: "Take care of the group and the individual will take care of himself." Beyond this issue there lay more complex questions under dispute such as, "Are there group dynamics in therapy groups?" Or even, "Are group dynamic manifestations anti-therapeutic?" The more extreme positions of such British "Object Relations" practitioners as Ezriel (1950) and Bion (1959), who asserted that the group therapist's task resides essentially in confronting the group-as-a-whole with its shared unconscious fantasy themes, evoked much controversy among some American group therapists.

Given the relative newness of group psychotherapy and the complexity of the task of theory-building, some theoreticians, among them Arsenian, Semrad, and Shapiro (1962), Durkin (1964), and Scheidlinger (1968), considered any broad generalizations or fixed dichotomies as premature. While allowing for the presence of certain generic elements characteristic of all psychotherapy, they advocated instead a continued objective scrutiny of how these cardinal factors appear in the therapy group with its multipersonal character and group dynamic processes.

Under the 1968 leadership of its new President, Clifford Sager, a family and community psychiatrist, AGPA became more energetic in altering its earlier exclusionary stance moving to an active interchange with the broader human services in the community. By this time the organization had experienced a further impressive expansion in numbers and in prestige. With a membership of about 2000 people and annual meeting attendance of about 1000 registrants, it became a force to be reckoned with, inviting the increased interest of many allied professionals. These conferences, formerly held in New York City only, were now rotating among a number of U.S. cities with the large affiliate societies serving as hosts.

In 1970, Emanuel Hallowitz, a social worker, became AGPA's first nonmedical President since Slavson. His election served to reinforce the interdisciplinary character of the organization. An expert in organizational dynamics, he also became the permanent architect of AGPA's modernized By-Laws. He had earlier served as a peacemaker in the factional disputes during the 1960's.

As they acquired strength and influence, the presidents of the local societies were encouraged in the early 1960's to participate in the meetings of the Board of Directors "with voice but no vote." Their power was enhanced further via the creation of an Affiliate Societies' Committee which met annually with the national Association's President. After many heated debates, the Board of Directors decreed in 1963 that only people with qualifications for national AGPA membership could be members of local societies. This move served to assure the protection of quality requirements for membership, and led to AGPA's defining itself officially in 1968 as a competency organization.

While there had been a token Research Committee since its founding, it was not until the 1960's that truly sophisticated research, including statistical designs, became a part of the Committee's concerns (Dies, 1979). In addition, the annual institute inaugurated a Research Section whose findings appeared in the pages of the Journal.

Unlike the meetings of other professional organizations in mental health, AGPA's conferences escaped the open expression of youth revolts spawned by the Vietnam War and the sense of alienation and helplessness following the assassinations of Martin Luther King, Jr. and of Robert Kennedy. In this connection, even the 1969 annual meeting of the American Orthopsychiatric Association, which was known for its liberal stance on social issues, suffered disruption by a group of radical young mental health professionals.

The so-called Encounter Group Movement which attracted much public and media attention, even producing a best seller by one of the movement's proponents (Schutz, 1967), both challenged and embarrassed the AGPA because many people began to equate these controversial group enterprises with group therapy. That they did so was not surprising since a senior psychologist and clinician, Carl Rogers, had gone so far as to claim that the intensive encounter group was ". . . perhaps the most significant social invention of this century" (1968, p. 268). It is to AGPA's credit that it approached this sensitive issue in an open and responsible fashion. Relevant symposia at its annual conferences and its publications began to place encounter groups in proper perspective within the human services, stressing their being *affective-educational endeavors* designed for the general public, and not for the *treatment of the sick*. Furthermore, in a seminal paper by Parloff (1970), group therapists were asked to warn against ". . . the dangers of indiscriminate application of these procedures by undisciplined leaders to the psychologically unstable" (p. 301). Soon, other professional organizations spoke out as well, enjoining the sponsors of encounter groups to apply a series of safeguards in their operations, including the screening of participants, the employment of informed consent, and, above all, the use of trained leaders.

Elitism, Differentiation, and Competency (1972–1982)

With the morale of the country weakened by the Vietnam War and by Nixon's resignation, there ensued in the United States an era of self-questioning aggravated by President Carter's uncertain leadership and a distraught economy. The quickening pace of technological and of societal change spawned the Women's Movement in the early 1970s, together with a dawning ecological crisis. Social and moral confusion, frustration, fear, and violence all made Ronald Reagan's presidential victory a virtual certainty.

Within the AGPA, the Encounter Group Movement and the multiplicity of groups operating under trained and untrained leadership in the many Community Mental Health Centers (763 in 1982) made urgent the need for some kind of differentiation among "people helping groups" and for the careful surveillance and training of group practitioners. What soon emerged was a general consensus that clinical psychotherapy groups with their primary focus on the "repair" of personality pathology differed from "therapeutic" group modalities in mental health, as well as from the varied personal growth, training, and support–self-help groups in the community (Scheidlinger, 1982). As for training, a suggested *Guidelines for the Training of Group Psychotherapists* was developed in 1970, seeking to standardize the mushrooming training programs sponsored by the affiliate societies. A few years later, the Board of Directors decided in principle that AGPA accreditation be made available to all group therapy training institutions. In addition, the 1974 annual conference was the first interdisciplinary program approved to offer Continuing Education credits for physicians, a procedure which has by now been standardized at our conferences for other professions as well.

Echoing the call from the universal Women's Movement, a "grass roots" group of AGPA women members demanded the creation of a Women's Issues Task Force to foster a greater recognition of women's contributions to the organization and to facilitate their obtaining more influential roles in governance. While Henriette Glatzer had been elected the first woman President of AGPA in 1976, her contributions to the organization and to group therapy had long since received deserved recognition. More than the appreciation of one woman's worth was needed and demanded. Alonso and Rutan's article, "Women in Group Therapy" (1979), stood as part of this new Zeitgeist which also served to enhance a tangible increase in "power roles" for women in both the educational and "political" areas of the AGPA.

An "Umbrella" Organization in Pursuit of Excellence (1982–1992)

Despite the economic reverses in the United States during the late 1970s, which resulted in a substantial loss of paid AGPA memberships, the organization had by now become an effective functioning body with a sophisticated internal structure, newly purchased headquarters, and skilled administrative leadership. At a time when some other professional mental health organizations floundered in the weakened national economy and diminished funding for the human services, AGPA's cadre of dedicated leaders managed to maintain a flexible stance, prepared to adapt imaginatively to the recurring external challenges. Thus, when member-ship declined sharply, AGPA restructured its base, during Norman Neiberg's presidency, along pluralistic lines. After decades of being a predominantly elite, psychoanalytic movement, the Association opened its doors to all responsible mental health professionals who worked with groups. Needless to say, an equally compelling factor in this expansion was the realization that the earlier, counterproductive ideological parochialism had gone out of date. As was noted in another context (Scheidlinger,

1991), there was a growing awareness among the senior practitioners of all the major therapeutic models that: (1) single system ideologies and techniques had distinct clinical limitations; (2) research had shown that experienced workers from divergent theoretical camps tended to get similar outcomes; (3) the commonalities in all forms of psychotherapy were more impressive than was generally acknowledged; and (4) most seasoned American psychotherapists had come to view themselves as eclectics.

With all major systems of group therapy enjoying equal status, the organization's programs and publications have begun to reflect this new diversity. A variety of ideologies, intervention measures, contexts, and patient populations, featured at the recent AGPA conferences under strict quality controls, have served to draw ever-increasing numbers of human services' professionals to these events. Another example of the new flexibility and openness resides in markedly streamlined membership application procedures. Student and associate membership levels allowing for early entry are a part of this new system.

In the mid-1980s, Leonard Horwitz, AGPA President, spearheaded a novel, individualized, intra-organizational training program to encompass those practitioners lacking access to training sites which are usually located in large cities. This program combined didactic input from annual conference offerings with supervised clinical practice in the "home" communities, under the guidance of AGPA mentors.

As for publications, aside from the phenomenal growth of the *International Journal of Group Psychotherapy*, to be covered separately, the Association produced a series of highly regarded monographs dealing with research (Dies & MacKenzie, 1983), bibliography (Lubin & Lubin, 1986), the group treatment of children (Riester & Kraft, 1986), of adolescents (Azima & Richmond, 1989), of the elderly (MacLennan et al. 1987), of difficult patients (Roth et al. 1989), and with psychoanalytic group theory and therapy (Tuttman, 1991)—a total of seven monographs to date.

The Influence of Group Therapy's Pioneers

The history of group psychotherapy as a treatment modality which includes its precursors and pioneers lies outside the scope of this chapter, devoted as it is to the history of the AGPA. The broader history of the field is available elsewhere (Rosenbaum & Berger, 1963; Anthony, 1971; Sadock & Kaplan, 1983).

What is of relevance here is the extent to which AGPA's founders had been influenced by these historical figures. To begin with, Slavson, except for some brief references to Joseph H. Pratt as the first practitioner of modern group treatment in 1905, and to Trigant Burrow as the first person to use the term "group analysis," had little to say about his predecessors other than Freud (Slavson, 1951). This is somewhat surprising since he had known about the work of Paul Schilder (1936) and Louis Wender in New York. As for the latter, Slavson served as a Discussant (together with Alexander Wolf and Jacob Moreno) of a major paper presented by Wender at the 1951 meeting of the Association for the Advancement of Psychotherapy (Wender, 1951).

Alexander Wolf, in contrast, credited his reading of Schilder and of Wender's works as having encouraged him to try group treatment in his private practice. While Jacob Moreno's prolific writings, beginning in 1910, dealt with important themes in group psychology such as spontaneity, role-play, and sociometry, followed by his writing on psychodrama in the 1920s, his direct influence on the early members of the AGPA was minimal. In part this was probably due to Moreno's (1953) disdain for psychoanalysis. More significant, perhaps, was the extreme personal competitiveness and animosity between Slavson and Moreno throughout their lives. Besides Slavson, Moreno was personally known to Wilfred Hulse, Samuel Hadden, and Saul Scheidlinger through contacts at professional meetings. Hadden, an early collaborator of Slavson's, contributed a chapter to a book which Moreno had edited in 1945. At a later point, Hadden (1955) wrote about having been influenced in his early group work by Pratt (1922), a personal acquaintance of his, as well as by Marsh (1935) and Lazell (1921), two other group pioneers.

In their original work designed to study the process of group psychotherapy, Powdermaker and Frank (1953) utilized an eclectic psychoanalytic approach, borrowing from what they considered to be the most desirable aspects of the various contemporary models of group psychotherapy. To quote them: "Our approach to group therapy with neurotic patients had points in common with that of Foulkes, Ackerman, Slavson, and Wolf, and we were influenced in our thinking by Schilder's analytic concept and Trigant Burrow's emphasis on the study of group interaction" (p. 4).

During the 1950s and 1960s there was a cohesive subgroup of Adlerian group therapists active in the AGPA, among them Helene Papanek (1954). They spoke and wrote frequently about Alfred Adler's and Rudolf Dreikurs' pioneering group work in Vienna with children and with groups of parents. This program, begun in 1921, was termed "collective therapy." According to Dreikurs (1959), this collective therapy was a mere by-product of the general group-centered orientation which characterized these early child guidance clinics. After his emigration to the United States, Dreikurs became well-known for his group work in the Chicago school system.

Pinney (1978) visited Boston's Emanuel Church and reviewed the 1905 records of Dr. Pratt's and the Rev. Worcester's groups with medical patients. Pinney (1978) also delved into Schilder's early work with groups at New York's Bellevue Hospital, concluding that Schilder's reliance on transference manifestations and on the interpretation of dreams entitled

him to be considered the first analytic group therapist. Donald Shaskan, an
early AGPA President, had been a student of Schilder's and wrote a book
about him (Shaskan & Roller, 1985).

Aaron Stein, another former AGPA President, who had trained a
generation of psychiatrists at New York's Mount Sinai Hospital, was a
student of Wender's. He had worked under Wender at Hillside Hospital
in New York where Stein subsequently became the Director of Group
Therapy. Stein co-authored some papers with Wender, in which they
proposed a parallel between Freud's group psychology and the dynamics of
group psychotherapy (Kibel, 1989).

The Journal

The *International Journal of Group Psychotherapy* is the official organ of the
AGPA. Founded in April 1951, it represents, in a sense, the Association's
window to the group world outside, insofar as contributors do not have to
be members of the AGPA. The editor, whose tenure cannot exceed two
consecutive five-year terms, is appointed by the Board of Directors of the
Association. He wields almost complete autonomy in the selection of his
Editorial Board and in the designing of the Journal's contents.

In the formative years of the AGPA, a number of basic themes
characterized the Journal's content. The first of these centered on the
applicability and clinical efficacy of group therapy as a treatment
modality. A large number of practitioners reported on their creative and
energetic efforts to establish group programs in a wide range of practice
settings including mental hospitals, outpatient clinics, general hospitals,
rehabilitation programs, as well as correctional institutions. The patient
populations were far-ranging: from children and adolescents to adults with
varied psychiatric disturbances, to patients with psychosomatic problems,
to homosexuals, and to the mentally retarded and sexual offenders. These
contributions demonstrated the wide applicability of group treatment and
the enthusiasm of the practitioners in this relatively new field.

The second theme reflected the need to establish the efficacy of group
psychotherapy as a valid form of treatment, consonant with the basic tenets
of psychoanalysis. This was especially important since Freudian psychoanalysts of the day were generally intolerant of any approach which was at
variance with the dyadic treatment situation with its focus on the probing
of intrapsychic conflicts. The issue was formally joined in the Journal in
1958 when Lawrence Kubie, a liberal among the Freudian analysts,
questioned whether group psychotherapy could engender as profound an
insight into unconscious processes as individual psychoanalysis. He
suggested that group treatment might best serve as a "vitalizing
antechamber" to the deeper individual analysis. In responding to this
article, Foulkes (1958) asserted that the group therapy verbalizations were

equivalent to free associations and subject to appropriate individual and group level interpretations. Slavson (1958) believed that while group treatment might well be less "intensive" than psychoanalysis, it was uniquely suited to patients with problems in ego functioning. Kubie (1958) was troubled by these discussions, saying in a Rejoinder ". . . that my questions have been taken up in a defensive and resentful spirit . . ." (p. 361). A few years later, Fried (1961) demonstrated group therapy's potential to go "beyond insight" in repairing ego-related pathologies. It is ironic that these apologetic-sounding discussions have given way in recent years to a plethora of papers in the Journal devoted to the unique value of the "here and now" experiential aspects of group therapy in reaching "preoedipal" levels of narcissistic and borderline disturbances of patients with arrested emotional development. Glatzer (1962) was among the earliest workers to employ group therapy with narcissistic patients.

Another theme articulated in the Journal during the 1960's pertained to the adaptation of core psychoanalytic concepts to the group psychotherapy situation. The titles, too many for listing, ranged from transference and countertransference, resistance, acting-out, working-through to identification and regression. Hand-in-hand with such theoretical productions went other articles dealing with the "how-to" aspects of group therapy: differential criteria for suitability; homogeneous versus heterogeneous groups; the handling of absences, and of dropouts as well as combined and conjoint treatment.

As might be expected, the newly emerging contributions from the so-called British School of Object Relations comprising such group therapy writers as Ezriel (1950), Bion (1959), and Foulkes (1975) found resonance in the pages of the Journal beginning with the 1960s and continuing to the present. They promoted renewed discussions of theoretical issues pertaining to the focus on the group-as-a-whole as well as clinical considerations of the earlier-noted treatment of patients with preoedipal pathology.

As AGPA moved toward enhancing competency and consistency in the training of group practitioners, the *International Journal of Group Psychotherapy* also showed impressive growth in quality and in the quantity of its readership. By 1975 the Journal boasted 5000 subscribers.

The Journal's 25th Anniversary issue of April 1975 constituted a high point in the transition from its beginning as a provincial publication in April 1951 to a journal recognized internationally for the most sophisticated reporting of the major developments in group therapy theory, practice, and research. In his "Reflections upon the Anniversary," Foulkes (1975) lauded the Journal's ". . . leading position internationally" (p. 171).

In the same Anniversary issue, Peck (1975), a former Editor, identified two major challenges facing the group psychotherapy movement in the future. The first foresaw a role for group therapy in the promotion of social and institutional changes in the community in conjunction with the community mental health center model and with the therapists' need to help the patient adapt to his institutions. The second challenge concerned the expansion of group therapy's theoretical framework to make place for the newly emerging group intervention modalities such as family therapy, as well as Gestalt and Transactional Analysis. In line with general systems theory he proposed: "When a patient changes his characteristic mode of behavior in the group, it almost inevitably alters the group's shape and character . . . involving the individual members, the group leader and the group as a whole in a circular process wherein change in any part of the system affects every other part, as well as every other group in which each individual participates" (p. 156).

Peck's first challenge disappeared with the early demise of the community mental health center movement. What survived from it in the Journal was a body of theory which tries to integrate psychoanalytic concepts with those of organizational dynamics (Kernberg, 1978, 1984). These formulations highlighted the personality problems of organizational leaders (i.e., narcissistic and paranoid) as they attempt to provide "rational" leadership.

As for Peck's prediction about the need to open AGPA's boundaries to neo-analytic and non-analytic contributions, he proved to be right on the mark. As we noted earlier, a broadening of ideological perspectives and a loosening of earlier rigidities occurred not only via more diverse publications in the Journal but also at the organization's scientific meetings and in its monographs. While most articles in the Journal still reflected the predominant psychoanalytical model of practice, contributions from the perspectives of transactional, existential, behavioral, and Gestalt groups were included as well.

Despite the field's original reliance on traditional drive theory and ego psychology, group therapists' sights have shifted to include considerations of object relations theory and of self-psychology. This is reflected in the Journal's recent symposia dealing with such themes as Group Treatment of Borderline and Narcissistic Patients, The Group-as-a-Whole Approach, as well as Therapeutic Ingredients-of-Change in Group Psychotherapy. As might be expected, there are still some honest areas of basic disagreement among group therapy practitioners. An example is Scheidlinger's (1987) contention that, given the complex and sensitive function of interpretation in group psychotherapy, it best be reserved for the experienced and trained professional group therapist. Napolitani (1987), in contrast, believes in an egalitarian approach in which the group therapist helps the patients and the group to take over all therapeutic functions including those of interpretation.

In addition to psychoanalytically oriented discussions, the Journal contained a number of articles which were an outgrowth of AGPA s Task Force on General Systems Theory. Thus, Durkin (1981) presented systems theory as a "superordinate" framework for group therapy practice. Within this framework, systems theory is believed to address in a more satisfactory manner the complex, circular interrelationships which encompass the group's effect on individuals, on subgroups, and on the therapist. The individual's effect on the group-as-a-whole and on the therapist as well as the latter's effect on each individual and on the group. Other contributions with a general system's perspective were Beck's and Peter's on leadership roles, MacKenzie's (1979) on group norms, and Slife and Lanyon's (1991) on the power of the "here and now" in group therapy.

In a series of three articles (1982, 1987, and 1990) Grunebaum and Solomon reviewed the relevant literature pertaining to the role of peer relationships throughout the life cycle. They offered cogent ideas about the usefulness of a peer group "history" in evaluating prospective patients for group treatment as well as in the viewing of group therapy as a corrective peer group experience.

As might be expected, since its beginning, the Journal has been a prime medium for the elaboration of Slavson's activity group therapy for children stressing its application to different patient populations and to different settings. In the 1960s and 1970s a growing number of publications began to question the primacy of the original nonverbal, action-oriented approach and introduced treatment models emphasizing verbal therapist interventions and planned group discussions (Epstein & Altman, 1972). Some of these new models were adapted to the unique needs of the growing numbers of children with socially and emotionally deprived backgrounds including impulse-ridden and psychotic ones (MacLennan, 1977). A comprehensive overview of the theory and practice of child group therapy was published by Schamess in 1976.

As for the group treatment of adolescents—often considered the treatment of choice for this age group—there appeared a similar overview paper by Kraft (1968). Prior to that, Ackerman (1957) had described a successful experience with a co-educational group of adolescents. This paper represented a kind of technical "breakthrough" insofar as group practitioners had heretofore worked with separate gender groups, in the fear that mixed groups would promote excessive sexual acting out.

Many of the early writings in the Journal dealt with therapy groups for delinquent adolescents, who were especially hard to reach in one-to-one treatment encounters. One of these papers was co-authored by Slavson (Altman & Slavson, 1962). In the same year, Feder (1962) wrote about short-term groups for delinquent boys in a residential setting. Most of the authors stressed the need for structure in all group work with adolescents, lest too much anxiety render these groups as unworkable. As might be expected, the papers on work with adolescents almost invariably touched on issues of countertransference, an ever-present phenomenon, because adolescents tend to turn their therapists into allies against their parents and other authority figures. In addition, the adolescent's characteristic openly provocative and "testing" behavior is bound to abrade adult sensitivities and to evoke emotional reactions. For this reason, some otherwise competent group therapists were found to be simply unsuited to working with adolescent groups.

The Legacy of S. R. Slavson

On the occasion of Slavson's 80th birthday, the October 1971 issue of the *International Journal of Group Psychotherapy* was dedicated to him, including a special Tribute by Hyman Spotnitz (1971). Having ceased to be involved in AGPA's governance, Slavson had by that time become President Emeritus and Consulting Editor of the Journal, for life. During his rare appearances at major organizational functions he seemed to relish his role of elder statesman.

Slavson died at the ripe age of 90 on August 5, 1981 and was appropriately memorialized by his disciple and long-time collaborator, Schiffer (1983). We believe that there probably would not have been an AGPA without this man's evangelical zeal, drive, and persistence. In the words of Anthony (1971) ". . . he has instigated group therapy's development as a profession, its recognition as a scientific discipline, and its acceptance as an arena of worthwhile research by behavioral scientists" (p. 24). His tight control of AGPA's direction during its beginning years assured its location in the psychiatric–psychoanalytic realm with stress on solid educational and clinical requirements for membership. His seminal contributions to the development of group therapy for children and to the group guidance of parents (Slavson, 1950) are unquestioned.

There is disagreement, however, regarding Slavson's lasting contributions to the general theory of group psychotherapy, his prolific writings on the subject notwithstanding. Anthony (1971) for example, thought that ". . . as a theoretician he is more categorical than creative and there is a positiveness about his position that the state of the art hardly merits" (p. 24).

In our view, Slavson lost credibility because of his tenacious, lifelong denial of any connection between group dynamics and group psychotherapy. It is truly puzzling that this brilliant man and astute clinician, while describing a variety of group processes in therapy groups (using his own terminology), failed to see that many of these processes can occur in all small groups. One wonders here whether his "missing of the boat" (Anthony, 1975) might have been related to more subjective factors. It seems paradoxical that prior to his discovery of the therapeutic potential in children's groups, Slavson was a progressive educator and social group worker, had written a number of books in these fields (1937, 1939), and had even edited a group work journal! Might it be that his excessively emphatic repudiation of these professional roots in group dynamics was essential to protect and insulate his later hard-earned and self-taught role as psychoanalyst–clinician–therapist?

Thus, when Lawson Lowrey (1943) referred in public to Slavson's new activity group method as being rooted in ". . . group work, progressive education and psychoanalysis" (p. 650), he might unwittingly have touched on an issue uniquely sensitive to S.R. Slavson whose covert task might have been to deny the first two of these roots. Interestingly, the above-noted comment of Lowrey's occurred at the very same Special Section on Group Therapy at the 1943 meeting of the American Orthopsychiatric Association, which gave rise to Slavson's convening of AGPA's "founding" luncheon.

A Glimpse at the Future

At a time when other interdisciplinary organizations in mental health are in trouble, it is gratifying to report that AGPA has managed to reach its 50th Anniversary in fine health, with a stable membership and with uniquely successful annual conferences and publications. Its next immediate objectives are within reach: to develop a credentialing system for trained group practitioners and perhaps also to establish a much needed set of Guidelines for the Training of Child and Adolescent Group Therapists to parallel the existing Guidelines for the Group Therapy of Adults.

Given the continued unprecedented expansion of the broader "Group Helping Field," the need for trained group practitioners is bound to grow. Contemporary trends point to an emphasis on homogeneous, short-term, and open-ended groups for people who share similar symptoms or handicaps as in substance abuse, eating disorders, phobias, and chronic disabilities. AGPA members might also find roles, perhaps as consultants and trainers, in the mushrooming area of indigenous self-help and support groups operative all over America. Lieberman (1990) estimated that from 9 to 12 million people regularly rely on some kind of support group.

As for existing paths, the intensive outpatient and inpatient group treatment of patients with impaired early development (i.e., borderline and narcissistic disorders) including schizophrenia, is bound to continue. Renewed focus will be required on the increased need of group modalities for children and adolescents, especially in schools, for medical patients and for the elderly.

As noted by Dies (1992), given the economic realities of our times, calls for pragmatism, integration, and clarification will be the order of the day. Reimbursable clinical practice will move toward greater professional specialization, codification, specificity, cost-effectiveness, and employment of combined therapies, including pharmacology. Long-term group therapy will be reserved for patients in the more affluent private sector, with emphasis on character reorganization, problems of living, and existential concerns. Spurred by the anxieties and alienations of a society caught up in an unprecedented rate of social change, the AGPA and its members will be productively occupied—and preoccupied—for at least the next fifty years.

References

Ackerman, N. W. (1957). Group psychotherapy with a mixed group of adolescents. *International Journal of Group Psychotherapy, 2*, 249–260.
Alonso, A. & Rutan, J. S. (1979). Women in group therapy. *International Journal of Group Psychotherapy, 29*, 481–491.
American Journal of Orthopsychiatry (1942). Association News. 13, 175.
Anthony, E. J. (1971). The history of group psychotherapy. In H. D. Kaplan & B. J. Sadock (Eds.), *Comprehensive group psychotherapy.* Baltimore, MD: Williams & Wilkins.
Anthony, E. J. (1975). There and then and here and now. *International Journal of Group Psychotherapy, 25*, 163–167.
Aronson, M. L. (1964). Technical problems in combined therapy. *International Journal of Group Psychotherapy, 14*, 403–412.
Arsenian, J., Semrad, E. V. & Shapiro, D. (1962). An analysis of integral functions in small groups. *International Journal of Group Psychotherapy, 12*, 421–434.
Azima, F. J. C,. & Richmond, L. H. (1989). *Adolescent group psychotherapy.* Madison, CT: International Universities Press.
Beck, A. P., & Peters, L. (1981). The research evidence for distributed leadership in therapy groups. *International Journal of Group Psychotherapy, 31*, 43–71.
Berger, J.L. (1978). *Development of group psychotherapy in the military and the Veteran's Administration, 1942–1949.* New York: American Group Psychotherapy Association (mimeographed).
Bion, W. R. (1959). *Experiences in groups.* New York: Basic Books.
Burrow, T. B. (1927). The group method of analysis. *Psychoanalytic Review, 14*, 268–280.
Christ, J. (1977). *History of the Institute of the AGPA, 1957–1977.* New York: American Group Psychotherapy Association (mimeographed).
Dies, R. R. (1979). Group psychotherapy: Reflections on three decades of research. *Journal of Applied Behavioral Science, 15*, 361–374.
Dies, R. R. (1992). The future of group therapy. *Psychotherapy* (in press).
Dies, R. R,. & MacKenzie, K. R. (1983). *Advances in group psychotherapy: integrating research and practice. Madison, CT: International Universities Press.*
Dreikurs, R. (1959). Early experiments with group psychotherapy. A historical review. *American Journal of Psychotherapy, 13*, 882–891.
Durkin, H. E. (1949). *Summary of the Board of Directors Minutes, 1943–1949.* New York: American Group Psychotherapy Association (mimeographed).
Durkin, H. E. (1964). *The group in depth.* New York: International Universities Press.
Durkin, H. E. et al. (1971). A brief history of the AGPA, 1943–1968. *International Journal of Group Psychotherapy, 21*, 406–435.
Durkin, H. E. (1981). *Living groups: group psychotherapy and general systems theory.* New York: Brunner-Mazel.

Durkin, H. E. (1982). Change in group psychotherapy: Therapy and practice. A system's perspective. *International Journal of Group Psychotherapy, 32*, 431–439.

Editorial (1969). Confrontation at Ortho. *American Journal of Orthopsychiatry, 39*, 720–721.

Epstein, N., & Altman, S. (1972). Experiences in converting an activity group into verbal group therapy. *International Journal of Group Psychotherapy, 22*, 93–102.

Epstein, N., & Slavson, S.R. (1962). Further observations on group therapy with adolescent delinquent boys. *International Journal of Group Psychotherapy, 12*, 199–210.

Ezriel, H. (1950). A psychoanalytic approach to group treatment. *British Journal of Medical Psychology, 23*, 59–74.

Feder, B. (1962). Limited goals in short-term group psychotherapy with institutionalized delinquent boys. *International Journal of Group Psychotherapy, 12*, 503–518.

Foulkes, S. H. (1958). Discussion. *International Journal of Group Psychotherapy, 8*, 20–25.

Foulkes, S. H. (1964). *Therapeutic group analysis.* New York: International Universities Press.

Frank, M. (1983). Modified activity group therapy with ego impoverished children. In E. S. Buchholz & J.M. Mishne (Eds.), *Ego and self psychology.* New York: Aronson.

Fried, E. (1961). Techniques of group psychotherapy going beyond insight. International Journal of Group Psychotherapy, 11, 297–304.

Glatzer, H. T. (1962). Narcissistic problems in group psychotherapy. *International Journal of Group Psychotherapy, 12*, 448–455.

Grunebaum, H., & Solomon, L. (1982). Toward a theory of peer relationships. II. On the stages of social development and their relationship to group psychotherapy. *International Journal of Group Psychotherapy, 32*, 283–307.

Grunebaum, H., & Solomon, L. (1987). Peer relationships, self-esteem and the self. *International Journal of Group Psychotherapy, 37*, 475–513.

Grunebaum, H., & Solomon, L. (1990). Toward a peer theory of group psychotherapy. International Journal of Group Psychotherapy, 30, 23–49.

Hadden, S. B. (1945). Group psychotherapy. In E.J. Moreno (Ed.), *Group psychotherapy: a symposium.* Beacon, NY: Beacon Press.

Hadden, S. B. (1955). Historic background of group psychotherapy. *International Journal of Group Psychotherapy, 5*, 162–168.

Kaplan, H. I,. & Sadock, B. T. (1983). History of group psychotherapy. In H. D. Kaplan & B. J. Sadock (Eds.), *Comprehensive group psychotherapy (2nd ed.). Baltimore, MD: Williams & Wilkins.*

Kernberg, O. F. (1978). Leadership and organizational functioning: Organizational regression. *International Journal of Group Psychotherapy, 28*, 3–25.

Kernberg, O. F. (1984). The couch at sea: The psychoanalysis of organizations. *International Journal of Group Psychotherapy, 34*, 5–23.

Kibel, H. D. (1989). A historical memoir on group psychotherapy. In D.A. Halperin (Ed.), *Group psychodynamics. New paradigms and perspectives.* Chicago: Year Book Medical.

Kraft, I. A. (1968). An overview of group therapy with adolescents. *International Journal of Group Psychotherapy, 4*, 461–480.

Kubie, L. S. (1958). Some theoretical concepts underlying the relationship between individual and group psychotherapies. *International Journal of Group Psychotherapy, 8,* 3–19.

Kubie, L. S. (1958). Rejoinder. *International Journal of Group Psychotherapy, 8,* 359–362.

Lazell, E. W. (1921). The group treatment of dementia praecox. *Psychoanalytic Review, 8,* 168–179.

Lebovici, S. (1958). Group psychotherapy in France. *International Journal of Group Psychotherapy, 8,* 471–472.

Lieberman, M. A. (1990). A group therapist perspective on self-help groups. *International Journal of Group Psychotherapy, 40,* 251–278.

Lowrey, L. G. (1943). Special section meeting on group therapy. American Journal of Orthopsychiatry, 13, 648–690.

Lubin, B., & Lubin, A. W. (1986). *Comprehensive index of group psychotherapy writings.* Madison, CT: International Universities Press.

MacKenzie, K. R. (1979). Group norms: Importance and measurement. *International Journal of Group Psychotherapy, 29,* 471–480.

MacLennan, B. W., Saul, S., & Weiner, M. B. (1987). *Group psychotherapies for the elderly.* Madison, CT: International Universities Press.

Marsh, L. C. (1935). Group therapy in the psychiatric clinic. *Journal of Nervous and Mental Disease, 82,* 381–392.

Menninger, W. C. (1946). Lessons from military psychiatry for civilian psychiatry. *Mental Hygiene, 30,* 571–580.

Moreno, J. L. (1953). *Who shall survive?* New York: Beacon House.

Napolitani, F. (1987). Commentary on Scheidlinger's paper on interpretation. *International Journal of Group Psychotherapy, 37,* 361–365.

Newell, H. W. (1951). Fulfilling our purposes. *American Journal of Orthopsychiatry, 21,* 445–451.

Papanek, H. (1954). Combined group and individual therapy in private practice. *International Journal of Group Psychotherapy, 8,* 679–686.

Parloff, M. B. (1968). Group psychotherapy. In J. Marmor (Ed.), *Modern psychoanalysis: new directions and perspectives.* New York: Basic Books.

Parloff, M. B. (1970). Group therapy and the small group field. An encounter. *International Journal of Group Psychotherapy, 20,* 267–303.

Pattison, E. M. (1970). *A brief history of the American Group Psychotherapy Association. The first twenty-five years: 1943–1968.* New York: American Group Psychotherapy Association (pamphlet).

Peck, H. B. (1975). Reflections on 25 years of the *International Journal of Group Psychotherapy. International Journal of Group Psychotherapy, 25,* 153–158.

Peck, H. B., & Scheidlinger, S. (1968). Group therapy with the socially disadvantaged. In J.H. Masserman (Ed.), *Current psychiatric therapies.* New York: Grune & Stratton.

Pinney, E. L. (1978). The beginning of group psychotherapy: Joseph Henry Pratt, M.D. and the Reverend Dr. Elwood Worcester. *International Journal of Group Psychotherapy, 28,* 109–114.

Pinney, E. L. (1978). Paul Schilder and group psychotherapy: The development of psychoanalytic group psychotherapy. Psychiatric Quarterly, 50, 133–143.

Powdermaker, F., & Frank, J. D. (1953). *Group psychotherapy.* Cambridge, MA: Harvard University Press.

Pratt, J. H. (1922). The principles of class treatment and their application to various chronic diseases. *Hospital Social Services, 6,* 401–417.

Riester, A. E., & Kraft, I. A. (1986). *Child group psychotherapy: future tense.* Madison, CT: International Universities Press.

Riesman, D. et al. (1953). *The lonely crowd. A study of the changing American character.* New York: Doubleday.

Rogers, C. (1968). Interpersonal relationships. *Journal of Applied Behavioral Science, 4,* 3–19

Rosenbaum, M., & Berger. M. (1963). *Group psychotherapy and group function: selected readings.* New York: Basic Books.

Roth, B. E., Stone, W. N., & Kibel, H. D. (1989). *The difficult patient in group.* Madison, CT: International Universities Press.

Sadock, B. J., & Kaplan, H. I. (1983). History of group psychotherapy. In H. I. Kaplan & B. J. Sadock (Eds.), *Comprehensive group psychotherapy* (2nd ed.). Baltimore, MD: Williams & Wilkins.

Schamess, G. S. (1976). Group treatment modalities for latency-age children. *International Journal of Group Psychotherapy, 26,* 455–474.

Scheidlinger, S. (1965). Three group approaches with socially deprived latency age children. *International Journal of Group Psychotherapy, 15,* 434–445.

Scheidlinger, S. (1987). On interpretation in group psychotherapy. The need for refinement. *International Journal of Group Psychotherapy, 37,* 339–352.

Scheidlinger, S. (1982). *Focus on group psychotherapy. Clinical essays.* New York: International Universities Press.

Scheidlinger, S. (1991). Conceptual pluralism: AGPA's shift from orthodoxy to an "umbrella" organization. *International Journal of Group Psychotherapy, 41,* 217–226.

Schiffer, M. (1983). S.R. Slavson (1890–1981). *International Journal of Group Psychotherapy, 33,* 131–150.

Schilder, P. (1936). The analysis of ideologies as a psychotherapeutic method. *American Journal of Psychiatry, 93,* 601–614.

Schutz, W. C. (1967). *Joy. Expanding human awareness.* New York: Grove Press.

Shaskan, D. (1978). *History of group psychotherapy in World War II.* New York: American Group Psychotherapy Association (mimeographed).

Shaskan, D., & Roller, W. L. (1985). *Paul Schilder - mind explorer.* New York: Human Sciences Press.

Slavson, S. R. (1937). *Creative group education.* New York: Association Press.

Slavson, S. R. (1939). *Character education in a democracy.* New York: Association Press.

Slavson, S. R. (1950). *Child centered group guidance of parents.* New York: International Universities Press.

Slavson, S. R. (1951). Current trends in group therapy. *International Journal of Group Psychotherapy, 1,* 7–15.

Slavson, S. R. (1958). Discussion. *International Journal of Group Psychotherapy, 8,* 36–43.

Slavson, S. R. (1959). *Memorandum to AGPA Board of Directors.* New York: American Group Psychotherapy Association (mimeographed).

Slavson, S. R. (1964). *A textbook in analytic group psychotherapy.* New York: International Universities Press.

Slife, B. D., & Lanyon, J. (1991). Accounting for the power of the here and now. A theoretical revolution. *International Journal of Group Psychotherapy, 41,* 145–184.

Spanjaard, J. (1958). News from the Netherlands. *International Journal of Group*

Psychotherapy, 8, 473.

Spotnitz, H. (1971). In tribute to S.R. Slavson. *International Journal of Group Psychotherapy, 21*, 402–405.

Symposium: Therapeutic ingredients of change in group psychotherapy (1982). *International Journal of Group Psychotherapy, 32*, 411–444.

Tuttman, S. (1991). *Psychoanalytic group theory and practice. Essays in honor of Saul Scheidlinger.* Madison, CT: International Universities Press.

Wender, L. (1940). Group psychotherapy: A study of its application. *Psychiatric Quarterly, 14*, 708–719.

Wender, L. (1951). Current trends in group therapy. *American Journal of Psychotherapy, 5*, 381–404.

Wilson, S. (1955). *Man in the grey flannel suit.* New York: Simon and Schuster.

Wolf, A., & Schwartz, E. K. (1962). *Psychoanalysis in groups.* New York: Grune & Stratton.

Whyte, W.H. (1956). *Organization men.* New York: Simon & Schuster.

THE FORMATIVE YEARS
1905–1951

The Class Method of Treating Consumption in the Homes of the Poor

JOSEPH H. PRATT, M.D.
Physician to Out-Patients,
Massachusetts General Hospital, Boston

This is the beginning. Joseph Hersey Pratt (1872–1956) began treating patients suffering from severe tuberculosis with a group approach on July 1, 1905. He is credited with the first use of groups in a specifically therapeutic manner. As an internist, Pratt continued his work in psychosomatic medicine at the Boston Dispensary instituting what he termed "thought-control" classes for functional nervous disorders. He reported in a 1953 paper that over 3,000 patients had been referred to his classes and that half continued for more than 5 sessions. He described his approach as "emotional reeducation and persuasion."

Pratt's use of groups was motivated by his concern for lower class patients who lived in wretched conditions. He concluded that a demoralized state contributed to their ability to follow through on rehabilitation programs. He began his groups with an educational intent, to teach his patients how to best care for themselves and their illness. He incorporated a number of behavioral techniques such as diary keeping, and recording weight gains publicly in the group. Gradually he came to realize that the group process itself appeared to have a therapeutic effect. His early descriptions mention some of what we now know as "group therapeutic factors."

There is a very contemporary quality to Pratt's descriptions of his community and volunteer based activities. Current programs for persons with AIDS embody many of the same principles for an illness for which, like TB at the turn of the century, there is at present limited treatment and high mortality. The alignment of group therapy with social consciousness has been a continuing theme over the years. Many prominent group theorists have spoken of group as a method for supporting the individual in the face of anonymous social pressures and control. —Editor

Pratt JH: The class method of treating consumption in the homes of the poor. *Journal of the American Medical Association* 49:755–759, 1907.

In the great outpatient department of the Massachusetts General Hospital several hundred consumptives seek advice and treatment every year. In my own clinic in that institution I have frequently seen two or three new cases in a single morning. In some of the favorable ones the patients are able to enter the state sanatorium at Rutland. But there are many more who have families depending on their weekly wages and no money in the bank.

need is some medicine to stop the cough or a good tonic to brace them up. Others too ill to work and yet with a good fighting chance for recovery under sanatorium treatment can not pay even the small weekly charge at Rutland. There is still another group, eager to get well, willing to spend their scanty savings if their life can be saved, and sometimes with kind friends and relatives who are willing to lend them money, who are refused admission to the sanatorium because the disease is too far advanced.

One day I found among the new patients two sisters sitting side by side in the examining room. The elder presented the typical picture of advanced phthisis. In the other girl the disease was just beginning. I called the younger sister aside and explained the nature of her illness, but assured her that if she went to Rutland for a few months in all probability she would recover. If she continued to work, I said, the disease would surely progress and her life would be the penalty. I told her frankly that her sister's lungs were so extensively diseased that I could not hold out to her any hope of cure.

She paused a few minutes before speaking and then told her story. Her parents were old and feeble and entirely dependent on her scanty earnings. With no outward sign of the inward struggle, she quickly made her final decision and said: "Before there was sister and I to work for father and mother, now I am the only one. I can not leave them."

There was no answer I could make. They left the room and I have never seen them since. Doubtless there were many people who would have been glad to help this unfortunate family, but I did not know where to find them and there was no organization to which application could be made, as they lived beyond the city limits and could not look for help to the Boston Society for the Relief and Control of Tuberculosis or to the Associated Charities. Furthermore, this, unhappily, was no isolated case. Every physician working in a large dispensary has had similar experiences. Thousands of men and women make this same renunciation. A few months of treatment would have restored the girl to health. Yet to meet the conditions in that family, home treatment, not sanatorium treatment, was indicated. The problem, as in this case, is often more complex than providing free treatment in sanatoria. There was the family to be supported and the sick sister needed nursing and medical attention.

Thanks to the Rev. Elwood Worcester, the rector of Emmanuel Church, such tragedies are fortunately a thing of the past at the Massachu- setts General Hospital. If the two sisters had come to the same clinic a year later they would have been referred to the Emmanuel Church Tuberculosis Class and I could have assured the younger sister that those in charge of the class would find some way to solve the financial difficulties so that she could give up her work and take the rest treatment at home. She would have also been told that the results obtained in the class even with have also been told that the results obtained in the class even with advanced cases had been so encouraging that some hope of recovery might be held out to her sister. The two girls would have gone home cheered and hopeful.

On the following day the friendly visitor would have called and explained to them and the rest of the family more about the class, the nature of the disease, the manner of its spread, the methods of disinfection, and how to get well by taking the treatment. Plans would have been made at once for erecting a balcony so that both girls could sleep out of doors. The friendly visitor would have begun at once the search for a housekeeper if the mother was found to be too feeble to do the work properly and to care for the sick ones. The financial problem would have been attacked at the same time. The employer of the sick girl would have been visited and his aid solicited, the friendly visitor would have called on the priest or minister and I am sure that his aid would have been secured, for we have never yet appealed in vain to Protestant, Catholic or Jewish organizations or to charitable or fraternal societies. If all other channels of relief were closed, and if a volunteer visitor of the class were unable to secure loans or gifts, then the actual necessities of the family would have been paid out of the class treasury until the girl was able to work again.

What the Emmanuel Church Tuberculosis Class has been to its members and what happiness it had brought into their lives is indicated by the numerous letters sent by its members who are now working, after years of illness and inactivity. The class was organized in July, 1905. In an article published in *The Journal of the Outdoor Life* the following September the plan for treating poor consumptives by sanatoria methods in their own homes was outlined. The first report was published February, 1906, in the *Boston Medical and Surgical Journal* and the class method explained more fully. Recently a report was issued by Dr. Hawes and Dr. Floyd of the work done in the Suburban Tuberculosis Class which was formed in January, 1906. This organization is designed for those consumptives who live too far from the city to be visited by the paid nurse of the Emmanuel Church Tuberculosis Class. In the suburban class the visiting is done by volunteers in the various towns and cities where the members live.

The admirable paper of Hawes and Floyd describes in detail the class system. It is important that the class should be small, as the doctor and the friendly visitor must establish close personal relations with each member. In the Emmanuel Church Tuberculosis Class the limit of membership is twenty-five. For the greater part of the time we have had from fifteen to twenty members. If more than twenty-five consumptive are to be treated an additional class should be formed, as the work can be carried on most effectively in small units.

In April, 1906, money was offered by ladies outside of Emmanuel parish for extending the work. Instead of increasing our membership, a separate class was organized. Each class has its own directing physician and a paid friendly visitor who devotes practically her entire time to the work. Nearly all of the members have been referred from the Massachusetts General Hospital. The cases taken into the class were those patients to whom other avenues of escape were closed. Either they were too poor or the disease was too far advanced for them to gain admission to the state sanatorium. Three advanced cases, rejected as unfavorable by the examining physician for Rutland, have recovered from the disease in our class and have been allowed to return to their work.

Our first member is now the friendly visitor in the Arlington Street Church Tuberculosis Class, which she has served faithfully and satisfactorily since its Organization in April, 1906. I take pleasure in reporting that she insisted on using her first savings to repay the Emmanuel Church Tuberculosis Class the money loaned in her sickness and need. Our second member, who had had a cough for five years, has completely recovered. He is a painter by trade and has not lost a day's work from illness since he graduated from the class a year ago this spring and has not lost in weight, and this in spite of the fact that he has been doing inside painting. The third member, whose case was described in detail in my first report, had been working over a year. Through the generosity of a lady of the congregation of Emmanuel Church a little tailor shop was provided for him on River street. During the spring and summer he worked with the door and window always open so that he might still get fresh air while at his trade. He has not lost an ounce of the forty pounds he gained in the class and, although he works eight or ten hours a day, he looks the picture of health.

Record Book

The record book is the invention of Dr. C. L. Minor, of Asheville, N.C., and is an essential feature of the class method. The patient records his temperature, his pulse rate, the food he eats, and every other detail of the daily life. He is required to enter in this diary the number of hours he is out of doors and the amount of milk he drinks. The book is inspected by the friendly visitor at every visit and by the physician at the weekly meeting. In my experience I have never found that keeping the records leads to introspection or depression of spirits. It is a great aid in carrying out the details of treatment. The members take pride in keeping neat records. It encourages the members to persevere.

The Weekly Meeting

This is the most important feature of the class system. It is held every Friday in a large, cheerful room at the Massachusetts General Hospital.

The class meeting is a pleasant social hour for the members. One confided to the friendly visitor that the meeting was her weekly picnic. Made up as our membership is of widely different races and different sects, they have a common bond in a common disease. A fine spirit of camaraderie has been developed. They never discuss their symptoms and are almost invariably in good spirits. Frequently our graduates drop in at the meeting to get weighed and to greet their old associates. The members are weighed each week and their pulse and temperature taken by the friendly visitor, assisted by one of the senior members. The greatest gains in weight are posted conspicuously each week on the blackboard, and the member who remains out of doors the greatest number of hours during the month has his record exhibited. One patient was out of doors 706 hours in a month, an average of nearly 23 out of the 24. Some of the sickest members gain this distinction. The favorable cases that are making rapid progress toward recovery infuse a spirit of hope in all.

After the strength of the member has been tested and increased by carefully prescribing amounts of exercise he is graduated and allowed to work. Home treatment has one advantage over the sanatorium in the fact that if health has been regained by leading the out-of-door life at home it is easy to keep up the hygienic habits after recovery. A place for sleeping out of doors and a reclining chair for resting in the recumbent posture are still available. Our graduates continue to sleep out of doors or with their heads in open windows.

In all, 52 consumptives have been admitted to the class since it was started nearly two years ago. The membership is confined to those in whom the clinical diagnosis has been confirmed either by finding tubercle bacilli in the sputum or by a positive tuberculin test. Deducting 15, the number of present members, 37 are left. Thirteen of these were in the third stage of the disease (far advanced tuberculosis). Three in this group have recovered and are now at work. Seven have died. Four of them were on the roll of the class at the time of their death. Two of the remaining three were discharged for not conforming with the rules and one is now too ill to attend the class. There were 15 moderately advanced cases. Of these one patient was sent to Rutland in an improved condition; two left the class because they considered themselves well, although the disease was not arrested and the danger of returning to work was fully explained. One of these had gained 21.25 pounds and the other 10.5 pounds in a single month. These two are the only ones that have withdrawn from the class.

Another in the group of moderately advanced cases was unable to continue treatment on account of chronic joint disease (arthritis deformans). The remaining nine patients (60 percent) of the fifteen moderately advanced cases left the class with the disease arrested. In five of these the disease was apparently cured. We had in this series nine incipient cases and in seven of the patients the disease was apparently cured and in the other two the disease was arrested. In other words, 75 percent of the patients out of the 24 incipient and moderately advanced cases recovered. No one is graduated until the disease is arrested and the member able, in the opinion of the physician in charge, to return to work. Seventeen of our members have fulfilled these requirements and have graduated. Their average gain in weight was 25.2 pounds. The greatest gain was 60 pounds. This record is held by a negro, whose weight had fallen from 200 to 146 pounds during his two years' illness. Eight have been at work 20 weeks or over and in none has the disease recurred.

******

Details of the rest treatment, including pictures of platforms and tents erected on roofs, have been omitted.

******

Other Classes

In Boston and vicinity at least five other tuberculosis classes have been organized. The Suburban and the Arlington Street Church classes have already been mentioned. In addition to these are the Cambridge and Lynn Tuberculosis Classes and one started by the Mount Sinai Dispensary of Boston intended especially for Jewish patients who can not speak English. In January, 1906, a class was formed in Providence by Dr. F. T. Fulton. Within the past six months classes have been organized by Dr. W. L. Niles in New York City, by Dr. David Riesman in Philadelphia, Dr. F. J. Ripley in Brockton, and Dr. C. Dencker in Baltimore.

The class method has proved to be economical and efficient. It is hoped that classes will be established in cities where at the present time no systematic effort is being made to cure consumption. But it must ever be borne in mind by those in charge of the classes that the necessary conditions in the treatment of pulmonary tuberculosis are, as Dr. Osler has said, "rigid regimen, a life of rules and regulations. a dominant will on the part of the doctor, willing obedience on the part of the patients and friends"—without these and without the spirit of the living creature within the wheels the system will fail.

The Basis of Group-Analysis, or the Analysis of the Reactions of Normal and Neurotic Individuals

TRIGANT BURROW, M. D., PH. D.

Trigant Burrow (1875–1950) received his medical degree at the University of Virginia, and then attended lectures in Vienna by Wagner Von Jauregg and Krafft-Ebing, two major figures in nineteenth century psychiatry. On his return he worked with Adolf Meyer at the New York State Psychiatry Institute at Ward's Island, and came into contact with Freud, Ferenczi and Jung during the 1908 Clark University lectures in Worcester, Massachusetts. This led to a year with Jung in Zurich. He was a founder member and President (1925–1926) of the American Psychoanalytic Association and considered to be a major contributor to the early analytic field. However, he became increasingly concerned about the influence of social forces on the individual, a position that led to his estrangement from the analytic establishment and to his involvement with group treatment. Burrow developed a therapeutic community called "Lyfwynn" (Joy of Life) in the Adirondacks to study his ideas about how social issues were reflected in the functioning of the small group.

Over time Burrow, working at the Henry Phipps Psychiatric Clinic in Baltimore, turned his attention to the effects of emotional tension on physiological reactions, thus combining his interest in social stress and bodily functioning. Groups offered for Burrow an opportunity both to see the effects of interpersonal isolation and to address it. It is believed that Burrow's writing influenced S.H. Foulkes's interest in the use of group methods. Burrow's ideas about the connections between social experience and brain function have a very contemporary biopsychosocial ring, now accessible to more sophisticated investigative methods. This paper was read at the Fifteenth Anniversary of the Phipps Psychiatric Clinic, Johns Hopkins Hospital, April 30, 1928. —Editor

Burrow T: The basis of group-analysis, or the analysis of the reactions of normal and neurotic individuals. *British Journal of Medical Psychology* 8:198–206, 1928.

Mental disorder is an industrial problem—a problem in how to get along. It is also an organic physiological problem—a problem in biological economy. The biological economy of an organism is the functional integrity of its parts. Mental conflict and insanity, industrial conflict and crime are disorders of economy or of adaptation that lie within us as integral parts, not outside of us as detached onlookers. They present problems not of ourselves as isolated individuals, but of ourselves as a community. They are problems in community living, in how to get along with others. These problems are physiological and economic, biological and social.

Group or social analysis is the analysis of the immediate group in the immediate moment. A social group or community consists of persons each of whom is represented under the symbol he calls 'I' or 'I, myself.' This proprietary symbol is socially accepted by the individuals of the group. It is the basis of their intercommunication. But the 'I' that is socially accepted is socially elusive of analysis. The group composed of individual 'I's is equally elusive of social analysis. The sum of impressions symbolized as 'I' would centre attention everywhere else than upon the sum of impressions thus symbolized. Group-analysis is the objective analysis of this subjective symbol as represented in the immediate group in the immediate moment.

We have long grown familiar with the dual expressions of our neurotic patients, with their manifest or apparent content in contrast with their latent or repressed content as represented in dreams, in symptoms and even in casual discourse. The group method of analysis has endeavoured to apply the same analytic principle to the manifestations of our casual social interchange and to discover in each expression of current social usage both the manifest and the latent content, the apparent and the repressed meaning. A statement is not taken upon its face value, but is subjected to the test of analysis in order to discover whatever unacknowledged content may be included in the overt expression. Where ordinarily an expression is accepted as quite *bona fide*, we now look for whatever reaction may run parallel to and beneath this manifest statement. No expression is considered complete in its surface aspect or content. But observation is directed toward whatever undisclosed proprietary motives may exist in contradistinction to our avowed statements.

The number of persons composing a group-session has come to be limited, empirically, to about ten. As now arranged, the sessions are held once weekly and continue for one hour. The object of the group-analysis is to give to the individual the opportunity to express himself in a social setting without the inhibitions of customary social images. By the social image I mean that deflection of attention which shifts the individual's focus of interest upon his awareness of himself in respect to others' awareness of him. I mean the duplicate or self-reflected image that constantly attends him in the mental and social standard he has of himself. This factor of a shift of attention has significance for us as being fundamental in the structure of the latent social content. For it would appear that by virtue of this social or duplicate image each one of us tends to enact a given role, to portray a certain character or part in the social scheme of things, and it is the object of the group-technique of analysis to enable the individual to express himself as he is—as he himself thinks and feels when utterly divorced from and unsupported by this social image of himself.[1]

In addition to the opportunity afforded each student or patient to give expression to himself apart from his social image or self-reflection, there is the opportunity for him to observe and to demonstrate in other students of the group any expression which may carry with it this latent import of the social image. In this way each student has the opportunity to bring to observation the latent social content discoverable in the manifest content of any other student. In this function he brings to evidence latent social tendencies not otherwise brought to observation. In his function toward the social analysis each student, like the psychoanalytic patient in respect to his own symptoms or dreams, discovers latent social reactions in which he must otherwise, like the patient, remain an unconscious proprietary participant.

Upon bringing to light the manifestations of the latent social content, it would seem that these manifestations consist of feelings which would tend to place each individual opposite to and in a relation of transference or moralistic dependence upon every other individual.[2] In his latent social manifestations the patient or student appears to be acutely sensitive to the impression he creates upon others. He is at all times at pains to reconcile his impression or image of himself with the image or impression which others entertain in regard to him. This marked deflection of attention toward concerns that are irrelevant to the immediate inquiry, this preoccupation with his appearance or behaviour with respect to those about him is shown to be the outstanding expression of the latent social content.

And so it would appear that a condition of self-consciousness or of preoccupation with this duplicate social image is characteristic of this latent social mood. This acutely self-conscious, moralistic attitude is plainly correlated with the moral feelings of one's early home environment. It makes connection with the earliest impressions of the family and especially of the parent–child relationship. For this fictitious social image is substituted in the childhood of each of us. Each of us is early initiated into this manifest or symbolic content of the social consciousness and under the symbol of the 'I' one's very self becomes a symbol in this manifest social expression. For each of us is made aware of his image or appearance in relation to those about him. Each is made aware of his image in the light of the image others have of him. Our place, our position among others is reckoned wholly in terms of this social image or manifest content, and in the memories of our own childhood we may trace its ancestral descent. As the student becomes more and more skilled in the technique of observation afforded by group-analysis, he is enabled to demonstrate again and again the intervention of this quite irrelevant social image and to indicate its generic place in the latent social content common to the group or community.

Let us take an instance in which a patient or student voices some complaint, offers an opinion or asks a question—instances typical of the manifest social content. The opinion, the complaint or question is not regarded in its apparently direct meaning, not any more than the symptom or dream of a patient, and it does not, therefore, receive a direct answer. Instead, one examines into its latent content, into the elements that may have prompted the question. One looks for whatever is proprietary and irrelevant. Who is the person asking the question? What is his background? Why has he asked this particular question? What will he do with the answer? Why does he direct it to this or that particular person? What is that person's especial relation to him, or what relation would the questioner like to assume toward the person addressed?—I do not mean that the student is literally confronted on every occasion with these specific demands, but they will indicate the general background against which our statements are tested. Perhaps some gesture accompanies the question, some expression of rigidity, a disclosure of uncertainty not implicit in the question itself, a fear perhaps, a suspicion; or there may be some effort of propitiation, some indirect plea for sympathy and anticipation of dependence. Perhaps the question discloses a note of competition or criticism or indicates some irritation. All these and many more such physiological accompaniments and latent intimations are material for analysis. For the repeated observation of the interreactions of individuals in groups indicates that there is never the absence of such accompaniments, and that such accompaniments are never without their conflicting symbols or images in contrast to the manifest content of the spoken word.

This over-evaluation in each individual of the self-image symbolized as 'I,' this image of oneself which one tends to carry about with him, comparing himself with the mental image he carries of others and which others carry of him, is again and again brought to open group-awareness. But always emphasis is upon the common, socially pervasive character of what the individual presumes are quite privately cherished and secretly guarded images. So that the immediate recourse of the isolated individual to elaborations of the self-image called 'I' or 'I, myself' is viewed not as specific to the individual but as generic to the group; and not to any particular group but to the community as a whole. The patient's invariable effort, therefore, to obtain attention upon himself because of what he calls his particular manifestations, clinging to them avariciously as though they were some incommodity or illness quite private to him, is consistently neutralized by distributing our group attention upon these same conditions as actually demonstrated in the group as a whole.

This feature of group-analysis I should especially like to emphasize. Under no circumstance does the procedure consist in the analysis of the individual by another individual or individuals. Whatever manifestation a student may present, in no circumstance is he made answerable for it as though it were a reaction particular to him. Whatever it may be, the manifestation is viewed as the expression of a latent content that is common to the group as a whole. Under no circumstance is the reaction of anyone regarded as isolated or separate. Nor does the group as a whole mean any particular group as differentiated from another group, but by 'group' is meant the social constellation generally with its ramifications throughout the community at large, the immediate group being but a constituent of this larger unit.

Perhaps the most interesting feature of group-analysis is its tendency to break down certain categorical demarcations in the field of mental pathology, particularly the differentiation between normal and neurotic reactions. As far as our observations have progressed, it would seem that from the basis of the group inquiry there is no difference whatever between the social images of the neurotic and social images as they occur in normal individuals. The origin and mechanism of their development would seem to be identical in both. So that from the position of the group basis of observation, the discrimination between the neurotic and the normal becomes an artificial one. Not only is the normal as completely a prey to the images comprising his latent social content, but he is quite as inaccessible to a rational attitude toward these private images occurring in himself as the neurotic is inaccessible to a rational view of these images as they occur in him. It is repeatedly observed in actual experimentation that individuals who may take a quite objective attitude toward the social images of others are utterly inaccessible to all approach when these same images are operative within themselves. In this lack of insight there is no difference between the reaction of the normal and of the neurotic. This identity between social repression existing in normality and the individual repression observable in the neurotic has naturally led to an altered evaluation of neurotic processes as to an altered technique in the effort to cope with them.

As one attempts to account for this phenomenon of the social image, one is faced with the necessity of very radical modifications of approach. These modifications are in the direction of more generic backgrounds— backgrounds that are not theoretical but actual, not historical but experimental aud immediate. Mental disorders come to be seen as the product of racial inadvertence of growth rather than as individual anomalies.[3] As elsewhere in biology, a phylogenetic basis of interpretation becomes essential in correlating ontogenetic findings, and mechanisms illustrative of the inter-social reactions of individuals as a community or race have made imperative a consideration of the origin of man's interreactions as a community or racial organism.[4]

Among the processes which mediate the functioning of the social organism must be included those physiological balances of tension and release which place the individual in conscious relationship to his environment—the process we know as attention. The chief instrument employed by man in the process of attention is the social symbol or image expressed in the spoken word. This instrument or image adopted by the race serves as sign or token of a common content of meaning. In this common meaning there is comprised the manifest content of the social consciousness.

In the evolution of man, however, and in his emergence toward higher processes of integration it would seem that this manifest content of consciousness became vitiated, and that the image or symbol represented in the spoken word too often lost its primarily common meaning. Apparently, with the introduction of the moralistic image of self, that is, the image or symbol expressed in the individual's 'good' or 'bad' appearance or behaviour and its private advantage or disadvantage to the individual, his attention became deflected from a socially common meaning or function to a private interest or wish. Instead of mediating always a common content of meaning, these social symbols were made to serve at times wholly personal, proprietary ends. So that in addition to the common content of meaning there is introduced a personal, proprietary content. While the manifest content of the spoken word remains intact as a common symbol, in so far as it has become influenced by this personal image, a wholly arbitrary and private meaning necessarily attaches to it.

In this miscarriage of the social image and in the deflection of attention it entails, the social organism has been seriously affected in its intrinsic economy. As psychopathologists, our interest has centred chiefly in those symbolic distortions and image-substitutions which Freud first traced in the manifest content of the neuroses. But in our social images or meanings there are deflections of attention which indicate a wider social impairment. It is this maladjustment among us socially which, it is felt, a group or social analysis contributes to repair.

While, then, it is the function of psychoanalysis and of psychiatry to deal with impressions and images in persons who are mentally ill or definitely ill-adapted socially, group-analysis occupies itself with social images or with images shared among people generally, regardless of whether they are designated as neurotic or normal. It places an emphasis upon the latent content of consciousness as it underlies our manifest social interchange, rather than restricting its inquiry to the reminiscent materials of consciousness as they occur in the isolated expressions of the neurotic or insane individual.

For many years it was my daily experience in personal analyses to pursue diligently the secret phantasies and symbolic irrelevancies of the individual unconscious, hunting them out from their remotest crevices with meticulous painstaking. And there is no doubt that the entertainment afforded my patients in our mutual search for various clues or associations was in many cases sufficiently diverting to constitute what is commonly called a cure. It is true that the individual patient feels that his neurosis, his sense of unworthiness and chagrin, his depression and pain, is caused by unsavoury, irrelevant preoccupations and inept tendencies that characterize him alone. He goes to his physician to receive treatment for a condition peculiar to himself—a condition in which he feels himself isolated from others. And so it was not unnatural that in its development from psychoanalytic traditions the group method of analysis tended at first also to lay stress upon the habitually repressed, reminiscent material of the individual's unconscious.

In group-analysis, however, the patient is made witness to the situation wherein these irrelevancies and secret excursions constitute a latent tendency that characterizes equally the social group about him. It becomes gradually plain to him that his adoption of a code of symbols possessing only a private latent meaning is a general social condition. He discovers that the common manifest meaning of current social usage is quite as unstable as the manifest content of his restricted personal code. Accordingly, the deflections of attention shown in the substitutions and irrelevancies, the symbolizations and conversions of the neurotic patient are interpreted as being but special manifestations of a detection of attentions existing throughout the social organism.

This interpretation has led to an increasing emphasis upon the factor of the social image as an inducement to the substitutions occurring in individuals of both the neurotic and normal reaction. With the gradual maturing of the group-method the cherished reminiscences and private ruminations of the individual have come finally to be wholly disregarded. In their stead the latent social content of consciousness, revealed beneath the manifest material represented in the habitual opinions and discussions of social interchange, have become the sole material of analysis. The only concern which occupies the group-analysis is the immediate interrelationship socially of the members composing it as expressed in the symbols of their momentary interchange. It is our group finding that in resolving these social images of common group adoption there follows the automatic restoration of group function in common social activities. For it is the interruption to this co-ordination of function within the social organism which, in our view, is the sole occasion for those states of proprietary symbolization or introversion expressed in the regressions of the neurotic individual.

The reason, therefore, for this inquiry into latent manifestations existing socially—that is, in normal as well as in neurotic persons—is the evidence that the social image of self-awareness, characteristic of the group or community, tends to obstruct the activities of individuals in their natural group inter-functioning; and, further, that those ingrowths toward secret self-satisfaction which we find to be clinically characteristic of the neurotic personality result secondarily from this wider social obstruction.

It is the daily experience of the psychopathologist that a parent brings an ill son or daughter to him for diagnosis and advice. This situation is placed in a very different light if, quite unknown to themselves, the parent of the patient and the household generally are, along with the physician himself, preserving unconsciously among them a social form of repression; and if upon analysis this social repression is shown to be the real cause of the more intense reaction expressed secondarily in the patient. As it bears upon the structure and outcome of mental disorder it makes a very great difference whether the individual patient is from infancy a constitutional neurotic, or whether the barriers to the natural inter-functioning of individuals, as these barriers exist in the social cluster comprising the family, have from childhood obstructed the patient's natural feelings of inter-communication and have forced his attention into the regressive symbols of phantasy and dream.

A programme, therefore, which would seem to me a valuable adjunct to our present endeavours in behalf of neurotic and insane patients would be one which placed upon groups of the community the responsibility of insanity as a social or community problem. Through this programme the community would endeavour to bring its own latent processes and social images to objective group-observation as a generic group condition. In such groups there would not be the situation in which certain individuals would study other individuals as presumably different in constitution from themselves, but in which all individuals would be equally responsible for the study of a constitutional condition common to all. Such a programme would, I should think, begin among groups composed of the more thoughtful element of the community. It would begin first of all, perhaps, among groups like ourselves whose interest is precisely in the field of psychopathology.

And so, if I may suggest that procedure which would seem to me of value in meeting the conflicts of the individual and the community—conflicts expressed in mental disorder and insanity, in industrial disorders and crime—it would be a programme which most closely affects the inter-reactions existing among ourselves as components in an economic social organism. This programme, in freeing us from the restrictions of latent social images and repressions, would more and more place ourselves and the community at large upon a common basis of intercommunication and function. In so doing it would render psychopathology less a psychological theory of human interrelationships and make possible the immediate expression of those interrelationships in their physiological actuality.

References

1. Social Images Versus Reality. *The Journal of Abnormal Psychology and Social Psychology*, XIX, No. 3, October–December, 1924.
2. The Problem of the Transference. *The British Journal of Medical Psychology*, VII, Part II, 1927.
3. On a Social Approach to Neurotic Conditions, by Hans C. Syz, M.D. *The Journal of Nervous and Mental Diseases*, LXVI, No. 6, December, 1927.
4. *The Social Basis of Consciousness*, Kegan Paul, Trench, Trubner and Co., London. Harcourt, Brace and Co., New York.

The Dynamics of Group Psychotherapy and Its Application

LOUIS WENDER, M.D.
Hastings-on-Hudson, NY

Louis Wender (1889–1966) was born in Lithuania and arrived in New York at the age of 11. He received his early psychiatric training with William Alanson White at St. Elizabeth's Hospital in Washington, DC and later attended Freud's seminars in Vienna where he was analyzed by an associate of Freud. In 1929 he was appointed director of the Hastings Hillside Hospital in Hastings-on-Hudson, New York. Here he found himself responsible for the care of some 40 patients suffering from what now would be termed major characterological disorders. He was eager to apply his newly obtained analytic training and the idea of psychoanalytically oriented group therapy seemed one way to address the situation. The program had many of the features of a therapeutic community, including a self-help follow-up group.

Space does not permit inclusion of a paper in this volume by Paul Schilder (1886–1940) an associate of Freud in Vienna. Schilder was a highly regarded and influential Clinical Director of Bellevue Hospital and Research Professor at New York University. He was a colleague of Wender's and they exchanged much information about their emerging methods. Schilder was interested in body image and the use of cognitive techniques. He made extensive use of structured activities such as written biographies and extensive didactic interpretations (Schilder P: The analysis of ideologies as a psychotherapeutic method, especially in group treatment. American Journal of Psychiatry 93:601–617, 1936). These two men were the pioneers in applying analytic principles in a group setting.

As outlined in this article, Wender initially used a psychoeducational approach not unlike some cognitive-behavioral techniques now in use. This gradually gave way to a less structured format. Wender described and promoted the use in group therapy of what today are called "group therapeutic factors." Aaron Stein, who is represented later in this book, was a student of Wender's and they worked and published together. This paper was read before the New York Neurological Society April 2, 1935.

—Editor

Wender L: The dynamics of group psychotherapy and its application. *Journal of Nervous and Mental Disease* 84:54–60, 1936.

Group psychotherapy has been practised at the Hastings Hillside Hospital for nearly six years. Initial experimentation with this method was prompted by the need for devising forms of therapy adapted to meeting the peculiar problems created by the segregation of mild mental patients and psychoneurotics under one roof. Carefully tested experience with this method has convinced the writer that this form of therapy is efficacious in selected situations and that it merits much wider application in hospitals where patients amenable to psychotherapy receive care.

In distinction to the method of extra-mural group analysis described by Trigant Burrows, which is psychoanalytic in technique and carries large sociological and philosophic implications, group psychotherapy is a method confined to the intra-mural treatment of certain types of mild mental disease.

In the ensuing material the writer will attempt to review some of the conditions that prompted the adoption of this approach, to define this method of therapy, to show its ideologic basis, to describe its application and scope and to evaluate its results.

In considering the treatment of patients within a hospital, one has to bear in mind that the choice between extra-mural and intra-mural care is not arbitrary. Hospitalization is the last resort, after efforts at extra-mural care have failed, and it is usually the severity of the patient's condition that precludes continued treatment on the outside. To the patient himself hospitalization is a crisis. His sporadic efforts in the direction of adjustment need no longer be maintained, since not only has his illness been acknowledged to himself, but there has been a corresponding certification to society and a meting out of "punishment." Hospitalization also deprives the patient of the attention he received from his family group and of the power he exercised over them because of his illness. He compensates for this loss by identifying the hospital with his family group (home) and proceeds to seek recognition in the new milieu. Since he no longer competes for supremacy with normal people who accede to his demands because of the illness which distinguishes him from the rest, he resorts to an intensification of his complaints, in order to focus attention on himself in the new setting, where he has to endure the competition of other sick people.

Another condition prevailing in hospitals, as in other assemblies, which requires recognition in considering approaches to therapy is the formation of friendships and cliques and the choice of "buddies." Problems are frequently analyzed and discussed among patients with greater candour than with the physician and it is a common occurrence to learn the problems and conflicts of a patient through his confidant.

McDougall's theory "that the gregarious impulse receives the highest degree of satisfaction from the presence of human beings who most closely resemble the individual, who behave in like manner and respond to the same situations with similar emotions" is amply demonstrated in hospital life. One encounters daily a group interaction, with its resultant infectiousness of symptoms and suggestibility of moods, that demands the diverting of these impulses and the utilization of group interaction into positive therapeutic channels, if we are not to promote "symptoms orgies."

In viewing intra-mural methods of therapy, one is impressed by the gap between the profound influence psychoanalytic thinking has exerted on our understanding of the individual patient and the barriers to the wide application of individual analysis to hospital patients. In this connection one must remember that as a therapeutic method psychoanalysis has a limited field of application. Hospitalization still further restricts the use of this method for the following reasons: (a) the difficulty of establishing transference where separation of patients cannot be maintained as in private practice and where patients have opportunities to compare physicians and to develop jealousies of one another while sharing a therapist; (b) the prohibitive financial cost; (c) the dearth of patients with a suitable intellectual and cultural equipment; (d) the practical barrier of extending the length of hospitalization to make possible the completion of an analysis.

The conditions enumerated, as well as many minor ones into a discussion of which we have not the time to enter, make clear the need for seeking and crystallizing methods of approach that are applicable to wider groups of patients, that are shorter in duration and that are realistically adapted to prevailing hospital conditions. To meet these requirements a proposed method of therapy would have to take cognizance not only of the individual through a psychoanalytic approach but also of the psychology of the group with its common reactions, its individual-to-individual identifications and its responses to the therapist.

Group psychotherapy is based on the assumption that the application of some of the hypotheses and methods of psychoanalysis, in combination with intellectualization, when applied to a group for the purposes of treatment under conditions of active therapeutic control, will lead to the release of certain emotional conflicts and a partial reorganization of the personality and ultimately to an increased capacity for social amalgamation. In distinction to individual psychoanalysis this method places greater emphasis on sociological factors (group interaction) and on intellectual comprehension of behaviour. The material for this form of therapy is elicited through theoretical discussions with a group of patients, affording a natural tie-up with the individual participants' experiences and problems. The base, or meeting-ground, for these patients is established through what Giddings calls "consciousness of kind." He says "that this consciousness is the basis of alliance, of rules of intercourse, of peculiarities of policy and that our conduct toward those whom we feel to be most like ourselves is instinctively and rationally different from our conduct toward others who are different from ourselves." These patients are in the same predicament; they have diminished need for concealment; in a sense, they are temporarily in a different state of society, with different mores, and their resistance to a relatively intimate sharing of problems is reduced by prevailing attitudes in the new set-up. These comments are not hypothetical. They are deductions from extended observation of patients and the progressive changes in their perspective and attitudes during hospitalization. These changes are inevitable; the only question that arises is whether one is to permit them to lie fallow or whether they are to be utilized and released through some method such as this form of therapy.

Experience has shown that group psychotherapy is applicable only to disorders in which intellectual impairment is absent and in which some degree of affect is retained. It is believed that the following groups lend themselves to this type of treatment: (a) early schizophrenics where the delusional trends are not fully systematized and in which hallucinatory phenomena are completely absent; where the splitting of the personality is not marked and there is no blocking; (b) depressions without marked retardation and those who libidinize their ideation—depression sine depression; (c) psychoneuroses, with the exception of severe compulsion neuroses of long duration.

The application of this method does not preclude the continuance of individual treatment. As a matter of fact, individual interviews are undertaken in conjunction with the patient's participating in a group and in many instances it has been found that the group stimulated the patient's desire for individual treatment and that during these interviews such patients spoke readily of experiences the discussion of which they had avoided previously.

A group consists of six to eight patients of the same sex. Attendance is entirely voluntary. The procedure is elastic. No patient is introduced into a group immediately upon his arrival in the hospital, as some degree of adaptation to the hospital is considered essential. A new patient learns soon after his arrival that this form of therapy is an established procedure and that some of his fellow patients participate in a group. Frequently requests for this form of treatment come from the patients and great tact and patience have to be exercised in explaining the exclusions. A group has two or three one-hour sessions each week and continues for a period which varies according to the needs of its members and the objectives of the therapist (usually four to five months). New patients are not admitted to a group already in session. At early meetings the group is instructed not to discuss the content of sessions with patients outside the group but they are encouraged to discuss the material freely with one another.

Sessions are begun with what is almost lecture material: a simple exposition of why we behave as we do, a description of primitive instinctual drives, conscious and unconscious elements, significance of dreams, early infantile traumata, reaction formations, repressions, rationalizations, etc. The material is presented in elementary form, with simple, every-day illustrations, the intellectual content and method of presentation being adapted to the general cultural and emotional tenor of the group, and varying accordingly. Presentations are planned with a view to arousing sincere interest in the background of everyday life without inculcating a "psychology hobby." This pitfall can be avoided by the therapist, and the response obtained from groups has always been on the level desired. The use of theoretical material in the beginning stimulates intellectual interest and serves to divert patients from their immediate problems. It also serves as an instrument of facilitating a kind of intimacy and social good will that is analogous to the reaction which we experience after spending an evening with a group in stimulating and vital conversation that gives us a feeling of closeness to people toward whom we have never felt this previously.

Even in the early period of the group's existence there are individual members who have established a transference to the therapist and there are others who have identified themselves with patients who have this transference. What occurs progressively is a common rapport, patient-to-patient transference and patient-to-therapist transference. A sense of intimacy within the group develops, greater freedom from inhibitions is observed in theoretical discussions and is followed by a spontaneous readiness on the part of some patients to discuss their own problems in relation to the theoretical material. Beginning with illustrations of individual incidents in their own lives which they regard as traumatic or significant, the patients go on to a discussion of their own and one another's symptoms and adjustments. They discuss dreams, which are interpreted on a superficial level with some of the patients participating in the interpretation. The therapist exercises no pressure and when the term "active control" is used, it is in the sense of active awareness, in distinction to any form of manipulation. Whenever resistances are observed in any particular patient, skilful guidance can divert the discussion into safe and still theoretical waters until such a time as the patients wish to resume the subject. Moreover, the use of this more generic approach minimizes resistance and trauma, since the patient is left free to accept as much as he is ready to accept as applying to him, and to the degree necessary for him is also able to project explanations painful to him on to other patients. Nevertheless, the most carefully gauged awareness as to the individual and collective reactions of the group is essential. Both the theoretical material and the guidance of the patients' own discussions have to be adapted to the changing attitudes and receptivity of the group, so that even the tempo of discussion and the duration of a group will be determined accordingly.

It is the writer's intention to make available at a later date the complete material of one group throughout its entire duration, so that the techniques may be more intensively scrutinized and evaluated. At the present time it seems expedient to summarize briefly some of the dynamics operating in group psychotherapy.

1. *Intellectualization:* In our awareness of how prominent and destructive a role the Conscious can play, we may have neglected it too completely as a factor in the healing process. While there may be no pure

intellectual acceptance and everything that may seem like logical acceptance is accompanied by emotional tone, the fact remains that a synthesis of intellect and emotion dominates every phase of our lives and is the basis of all social adjustment. Nor can we overlook entirely the fact that there are intellectual disciplines like the Yogi philosophy, the application of which results in the regulation of emotional responses through a self-determined intellectual discipline. What we term "insight" or emotional acceptance may have similar components of self-discipline. While group therapy in no way professes or strives to be an intellectual discipline, it does tend to a comprehension of emotional reactions that enables the patient to meet new situations with greater awareness and skill. The writer is convinced that intellectual awareness is a therapeutic aid as indisputable as the fact that while we may be panic-stricken at an unexpected noise coming from behind, we accept such a noise calmly when we know its origin.

   2. *Patient-to-Patient Transference:* The influence exerted by one individual on another may contain elements corresponding to the psychoanalytic transference. In group psychotherapy this patient-to-patient transference is made use of in several ways. It is used to facilitate transference to the therapist through the identification of one patient with another who has established such transference. This type of transference is encouraged, since it serves to meet the needs of the patients more permanently than the transference to the therapist which has to be abrogated for practical reasons as well as for the purpose of sustaining the patient's independence. It is also believed that the relationship which is established between patients in time takes an outward course, embracing a wider area of interests and activities (socialization).

   3. *Catharsis-in-the-Family:* In the group there is undoubtedly a transference of tendencies originally directed toward the parents and siblings. There is a possibility that the entire group set-up provides a kind of "Catharsis-in-the-Family," with an accompanying resolvement of conflicts and the displacement of parent love on to new objects. The patient finds himself sitting on terms of equality with the therapist (symbolic of the parent) and the other patients (who represent the siblings). He experiences (it may be for the first time in his life) the receiving of understanding from the just parent whom he shares with siblings who are equal in the eyes of that parent. He is not only receiving understanding but is also free to rebel openly, thus averting repression with its concomitant sense of guilt. In the writer's opinion this experience serves as a means of effecting a degree of emotional release, particularly in situations where the early traumata in child-parent relationships have remained unresolved. The fact that the actual set-up is on an adult level and that the patient is conscious of it only as a treatment process makes it acceptable to him.

4. *Group Interaction:* Group interaction is a phenomenon to which every patient was exposed prior to his hospitalization. His development, his ego ideal and his sense of values had their roots in his societal experience. In this method the patient's association with other patients, his new group experience, is made use of. Inevitably this association will influence his mode of thinking and his reactions, as manifested by the patients' competing with their respective complaints during their early sojourn. Under guidance this interaction results in the development of a changed perspective on behaviour, which in turn gives rise to new ego ideals and strivings. In the group the patient develops criteria for evaluating his own problem against the problems of others in a way that is not feasible in individual treatment. An individual who prior to his hospitalization regarded his problems as unique and peculiar to himself learns through exchange with the group that many of his fellows have similarly predicated ego conflicts and begins to view his own problems with greater detachment. The individual experiences a resultant lessening of personal tensions, his attitudes undergo modification and his whole outlook on behaviour changes. In this entire experience he is reinforced by the experience of his group.

The patient's drive to get well derives greater impetus through this method than when only individual treatment is undertaken. This drive is motivated in part by the new ego ideal which the individual has adopted and is strengthened by the apparent feasibility of attaining health, since the recovery of other members of the group presents convincing evidence.

It may be argued that suggestion is a major factor in the results gained through group interaction. If by suggestion we mean the concepts as defined by MacDougall or Freud, these types of suggestion play no greater role in this method than in any other technique. In no sense is there acceptance without logical basis or a continued infantile emotional dependence, implicit in suggestion. In the use of group psychotherapy, the patient derives an understanding of the nature and direction of his unconscious trends, experiencing simultaneously an emotional release. This is accompanied by his being exposed to observation and experience which involve himself and others, ultimately leading to a partial reorganization of his personality. In this unified process it is not an outside agent like suggestion which accomplishes the change but the saturation of the individual with the forces of his own experience.

The results yielded by this method which has been used in the treatment of about seventy-five patients over a period of six years, cannot be computed statistically. Interpretation on the basis of follow-up (in some cases for four to five years), since that is the only form of evaluation open to us in analyzing material of this nature, shows fairly conclusively that this form of therapy carries positive values for social adjustment. It has been observed repeatedly that friendships formed while groups were in session persist on the outside; that these patients retain a common bond of mutual interest, helpfulness and understanding which is a source of strength to them; and that their drive to remain well is more dynamic and characterized by a competitive quality. While the recovered patients' opinions cannot be interpreted as having scientific validity, it is significant that they attach importance to this form of therapy and attribute to the group experience their continued capacity to discuss their problems freely and their enhanced ability to deal successfully with new and difficult emotional material and experience.

Psychodrama

J. L. MORENO, M. D.

Moreno Academy, Beacon, New York

Jacob L. Moreno (1889–1974) was Rumanian born but educated in Vienna when it was still the center of the Austro-Hungarian empire and one of the leading artistic and medical centers of Europe. He received a classical nineteenth century education and had a working knowledge of five European languages as well as Latin. It is a curious paradox that this man who so valued learning should now be identified by some as one who abandoned knowledge for emotionality and display. Moreno emigrated to New York in 1925.

For Moreno, the central problem underlying psychopathology was over-control (Who Shall Survive? Foundations of Sociometry, Group Psychotherapy and Sociodrama, 2nd ed. New York: Beacon House, 1953). His theoretical approach therefore was to find ways to release a genuine personal creativity. He was drawn both by academic curiosity as well as natural predisposition to view the stage as the vehicle for accomplishing this release. He was also interested in group structure from an early point in his career and developed the techniques of sociometry to measure group forces. Moreno began his Theatre of Spontaneity in Vienna and continued it in New York with regular sessions in Carnegie Hall. This was open to the public and seems to have been particularly frequented by actors. Moreno viewed this endeavor initially as an opportunity for improvization to dramatize current events, then for educational purposes, but gradually came to concentrate on its more formal therapeutic potential. Moreno was a charismatic man who could pull people into his orbit of confidence and enthusiasm. He was highly intuitive regarding human nature and intensely concerned about the individual.

His public approach and his focus on the creative "moment" was diametrically opposed to the contemporaneous development of analytic techniques that valued privacy, patience, and the accurate cognitive interpretation. For Moreno, a creative break with the inhibitions of one's personal past was more important than a detailed understanding of historical connections. The split between the psychoanalytic and psychodramatic traditions thus has a long history. It might be noted however that these two theoretical approaches are at present considerably more integrated in most other Western countries than in America.

There is an undertone of social concern throughout Moreno's writings. He saw his ideas as having potential for social as well as individual healing (Moreno JL: The concept of sociodrama. Sociometry 6:434–449, 1943). Indeed his earliest group work was with prostitutes on the streets of Vienna. His reports on such groups as early as 1911 place him only a few years after Pratt in the intentional use of groups for therapeutic goals. His social concerns are expressed in religious language but with his customary iconoclastic twist. For Moreno, man was the Godhead and the ultimate source of creativity. Established religion was the repository of religious ideas that could be used by the individual for his own purposes.

The present selection is a condensation of material from two papers which present some of his basic ideas. The idea of "mental catharsis" through enactment of personal events is central to Moreno's approach. In addition, his extended use of the concept of "role" draws attention simultaneously to interpersonal encounters and intrapsychic meaning. While Moreno worked primarily with individuals in the group, as did many psychoanalytic group practitioners, he also formed a theory, based on Aristotle's concept of catharsis, of the value of the experience for the other group members. —Editor

Moreno JL: Mental catharsis and psychodrama. *Sociometry* 3:209–244, 1940; Psychiatry of the twentieth century: function of the universalia: time, space, reality, and cosmos. *Group Psychotherapy* 19:146–158, 1966.

Catharsis, as a concept, was introduced by Aristotle. He used this term to express the peculiar effect of the Greek drama upon its spectators. In his "Poetics" he maintains that drama tends to purify the *spectators* by artistically exciting certain emotions which act as a kind of homeopathic relief from their own selfish passions.

This concept of catharsis has undergone a revolutionary change since systematic psychodramatic work began in Vienna in 1920. This change has been exemplified by the movement away from the written (conserved) drama and toward the *spontaneous* (psycho) drama, with the emphasis shifted from the spectators to the actors.

In my treatise: "The Spontaneity Theatre" (Moreno, 1944), the new definition of catharsis was: "It (the psychodrama) produces a healing effect —not in the spectator (secondary catharsis) but in the producer-actors who produce the drama and, at the same time, liberate themselves from it."

The Historical Background

One of the most important concepts in all human thought, the concept of the moment—the moment of being, living and creating—has been the step-child of all universally known philosophical systems. The reasons for this are that the moment is difficult to define; that it has appeared to most philosophers as but a fleeting transition between past and future, without real substance; that it is intangible and unstable and therefore an unsatisfactory basis for a system of theoretical and practical philosophy. Some phenomenon on a different plan than that presented by the moment, itself, had to be found which was tangible and capable of clear definition, but to which the moment was *integrally* related. I believe that I accomplished this more than twenty years ago when, in analyzing cultural conserves, I found a concept in the light of which the dynamic meaning of the moment could be reflected and evaluated and thus become a frame of reference. Up to this time the moment had been formulated as a particle of time and space, or as a mathematical abstraction; hence it had been pragmatically useless and theoretically sterile. If the concept of the moment could be constructed against a more adequate background, the way would be open for a modern theory of the moment and a theory, perhaps, of spontaneity and creativity as well.

Spontaneity and its collaterals have reached a climax in our time, and in the course of my studies it has become clear what their meaning is and what complexes of ideas they represent. "Spontaneity" and "spontaneous" have finally come to mean a value—a human value. Spontaneity has become a biological as well as a social value. It is today a frame of reference for the scientist as well as for the politician, for the artist as well as the educator.

Here is an example: politicians, newspapermen and commentators often refer to a certain development in public opinion as a "spontaneous" movement. When they do this they really mean to say that the development in question is a genuine, sincere and truthful expression of the thoughts and wishes of the people. This term they apply to nominations, elections, political and cultural ideas, acts of revolution and acts of war. The consideration of spontaneity as a barometer of that high value, the will of the people, has become an axiom in politics. The theory behind this phenomenon is that if spontaneity is an expression of what the people think, then the man who can draw the spontaneity of the people to himself and his ideas should also have the right to exercise the greatest power over them. The desirability of even the label "spontaneous" is shown in the shrewd politician's use of propaganda to distort public opinion in his favor. Of course, after a change favorable to his plans has taken place, he will deny that propaganda or anything of the sort has been used. He will hasten to hail the new trend in public opinion as a "spontaneous" one.

Spontaneity is also used as a standard for cultural values. It is not so long ago, for instance, that an orator who came before his audience unprepared was considered arrogant and superficial, largely because the generally accepted standard of values was that a man should prepare a speech in advance in every detail and come before the public with a well-polished, finished product. During the last few years we have heard increasingly often—and with overtones of praise—that this or that address was an "impromptu" or "extemporaneous" one, with the clear implication that because it was spontaneous it must have contained the speaker's innermost and sincerest views on the subject. All this suggests that a far-reaching change in the evaluation of spontaneity is now taking place and that this change is receiving wide public recognition. This is probably one reason why my theories of spontaneity and creativity, which received little attention twenty years ago, are now more timely. A change in attitude all over the world has stimulated many other researchers to think along similar lines. A sympathetic trend towards spontaneity can be observed in cultural endeavors of all sorts—in the arts (the drama, for instance) in music and many others.

The term "spontaneous" is often used to describe subjects whose control of their actions is diminished. This is, however, a usage of the term "spontaneous" which is not in accord with the etymology of the word, which shows it to be derived from the Latin *sponte*, "of free will." Since we have shown the relationship of spontaneous states to creative functions, it is clear that the warming-up to a spontaneous state leads up to and is aimed at more or less highly organized patterns of conduct. Disorderly conduct and emotionalism resulting from impulsive action are far from being desiderata of spontaneity work. Instead, they belong more in the realm of the pathology of spontaneity.

Spontaneity is often erroneously thought of as being more closely allied to emotion and action than to thought and rest. This bias probably developed because of the assumption that a person cannot really feel something without at the same time being spontaneous and that a person who is thinking can have a genuine experience without spontaneity, but this is not the case. There seems to be a similar misconception that a person in action needs continuous spontaneity in order to keep going, but that no spontaneity is required by a person at rest. As we know now, these are fallacies. Spontaneity can be present in a person when he is thinking just as well as when he is feeling, when he is at rest just as well as when he is in action.

The Vitalizing Effect of Spontaneity Techniques on Cultural Conserves

The first significant consequence of spontaneity work is a deeper view and a vitalization of the cultural conserves. One illustration of this effect comes from religion, prayer.

A prayer consists of four components: speech, thought content, feeling and the pattern of action. The essence of prayer is true repetition; it would be sacrilegious to change the speech, thought and gestures prescribed in the prayer. But when it comes to the feeling the subject can transcend the conserve actually nullifying its repetitiousness by introducing a spontaneous factor. Feeling is the wedge by which spontaneity training can enter a religious experience. By the introjection of a spontaneous factor, the variation and intensification of feeling with which the subject accompanies a prayer may bring a depth into a stereotype—literally the same for millions of others—which may differentiate him from all other people praying at that time.

The more a cultural conserve is—in the moment of presentation—a total recapitulation of the same process, and the more a subject is conditioned to respond to it with the same feeling (in essence, the same feeling today as , let us say, ten years ago), the more the question arises as to what value the conserve has for the subject. It cannot be denied that the recall of a conserve is accompanied by great satisfaction and even joy. The periodic recapitulation seems to whisper into the subject's ear that all is the same, all is well—the world has not changed. The cultural conserve renders to the individual a service similar to that which it renders as a historical category to culture at large—continuity of heritage—securing for him the preservation and the continuity of his ego. This provision is of aid as long as the individual lives in a comparatively still world; but what is he to do when the world around him is in a revolutionary change and when the quality of change is becoming more and more a permanent characteristic of the world in which he participates?

Mental Catharsis

A change may take place at any time in the life-situation of an individual. A person may leave or a new person may enter his social atom, or he may be compelled to leave all members of his social atom behind and develop new relationships because he has migrated to a new country. A change may take place in his life-situation because of certain developments in his cultural atom. He may, for instance, aspire to a new role—that of an aviator—which brings him, among other things, face to face with the problem of mastering a new machine. Or he is taken by surprise by new roles in his son or his wife which did not seem to exist in them before. Illustrations of changes which might press upon him could easily be multiplied. Influences might threaten him from the economic, psychological and social networks around him. It can well be said that, with the magnitude of change, the magnitude of spontaneity which an individual must summon in order to meet the change must increase in proportion. If the supply (the amount of spontaneity) can meet the demand (the amount of change) the individual's own relative equilibrium within his social and cultural atoms will be maintained. As long, however, as he is unable to summon the spontaneity necessary to meet the change, a disequilibrium will manifest itself which will find its greatest expression in his inter-personal and inter-role relationships. This disequilibrium will increase in proportion to the falling-off of spontaneity and will reach a relative maximum when his spontaneity has reached its maximum point. It is a peculiarity of these disequilibria that they have their reciprocal effects. They throw out of equilibrium other persons at the same time. The wider the range of disequilibrium, the greater becomes the need for catharsis.

Catharsis in the Psychodrama

Historically there have been two avenues which led to the psychodramatic view of mental catharsis. The one avenue led from the Greek drama to the

conventional drama of today and with it went the universal acceptance of
the Aristotelian concept of catharsis. The other avenue led from the
religions of the East and the Near East. These religions held that a saint,
in order to become a savior, had to make an effort; he had, first, to save
himself. In other words, in the Greek situation the process of mental
catharsis was conceived as being localized in the spectator—a passive
catharsis. In the religious situation the process of catharsis was localized in
the individual, himself—in the actor, so to speak, his actual life becoming
his stage. This was an active catharsis. In the Greek concept the process of
realization of a role took place in the object, in a symbolic person on the
stage. In the religious concept the process of realization took place in the
subject—the living person who was seeking the catharsis. One might say
that passive catharsis is here face to face with active catharsis; aesthetic
catharsis with ethical catharsis.

These two developments which heretofore have moved along
independent paths have been brought to a synthesis by the psychodramatic concept of catharsis. From the ancient Greeks we have retained
the drama on the stage, and we have accepted the Near East's view of
catharsis; the actor has been made the locus for the catharsis. The old locus
(the spectator) has become secondary. Furthermore, as actors on our stage
we now have private persons with private tragedies, instead of the old
Greek tragedians with their masks, their make-up and their detachment
from the theme the drama.

These private tragedies may be caused by various disequilibrating
experience, one source of which may be the body. They may be caused by
the relationship of the body to the mind or by that of the mind to the body,
and result in an inadequacy of performance at the moment. They may also
be caused by an individual's thoughts and actions toward others, and by
their thoughts and actions toward him. Again, it may be caused by a
design of living which is too complicated for the amount of spontaneity
the individual is able to summon. Practically speaking, there is no sphere
of the universe imaginable, whether physical, mental, social or cultural,
from which there may not emerge, at one time or another, some cause of
disequilibrium in a person's life. It is almost a miracle that an individual
can achieve and maintain a degree of balance, and man has continually
been in search of devices which will enable to attain or increase his
equilibrium.

One of the most powerful media which can produce this effect is
mental catharsis. It can take place and bring relief from grief or fear
without change being necessary in the external situation. Large amounts of
energy are thus retained which otherwise would go into efforts to change
reality. Every disequilibrium, however, has its matrix and its locus and the
catharsis-producing agent—in order to achieve the effect intended—has to
be applied at the seat of the ailment.

Mental catharsis cannot be reproduced wholesale and on a symbolic plane to meet all the situations and relationships in which there may exist some cause for disequilibrium within a person. It has to be applied concretely and specifically. The problem has been, therefore to find a medium which can take care of the disequilibrating phenomena in the most realistic fashion, but still outside of reality; a medium which includes a realization as well as a catharsis for the body; a medium which makes catharsis as possible on the level of actions and gestures as it is on the level of speech; a medium which prepares the way for catharsis not only within an individual but also between two, three or as many individuals as are interlocked in a life-situation; a medium which opens up for catharsis the world of phantasies and unreal roles and relationships. To all these and many other problems an answer has been found in one of the oldest inventions of man's creative mind—the drama.

Spectator and Group Catharsis

We have found that persons who witness a psychodramatic performance often become greatly disturbed. Sometimes, however, they leave the theatre very much relieved, almost as if it had been their own problems which they had just seen worked out upon the stage. Experiences such as these brought us back to the Aristotelian view of catharsis—as taking place in the spectator—but from a different angle and with a different perspective.

The audience in a therapeutic theatre was originally limited to persons necessary to accomplish the treatment. This is still considered the classic approach. At first we concerned ourselves with what this group meant to the actor-patients on the stage. It was soon discovered that they represented the world—public opinion. The amount and the kind of influence which the group exerted upon the conduct of a patient on the stage became an object of research, but in the course of time we made another discovery—the effect of psychodramatic work upon a spectator. This effect is bound to have important consequences for the psychodramatic treatment of groups.

Mental patients show a remarkable sensitivity for one another in daily life, a tele-relation for one another's actions and words which is often surprising to the staff, and which amounts to a high appreciation of their various ideological and emotional patterns. This heightened sensitivity was brought to a true test when we began to permit mental patients to witness a delusionary or a hallucinatory, a depressive or a paranoid experience of another patient, reproduced on the psychodramatic stage.

The discovery of a spectator-catharsis in mental patients opened up a prospect of treating them at the same time as the patient on the stage. The latter became more and more a prototype of pathological mental processes for the entire group of patients in the audience. Patients who suffered from similar complaints or who had similar patterns of delusion and hallucination were selected to sit together in the audience. They then had similar cathartic experiences when a patient with a problem resembling their own was being treated on the stage.

The importance of this approach as a method of group psychotherapy is evident. At times, instead of using the mental patient as a prototype, specially-trained psychodramatic assistants—so-called "auxiliary egos"—have been used with equally beneficial results. Methodically, the use of the auxiliary ego was an advantage because of the frequent difficulty of influencing more or less non-cooperative mental patients to choose situations or plots which were fruitful for the whole group and not merely for themselves. The employment of auxiliary egos who were under our own control and sufficiently sensitive to the experiences of the psychotic, marked an important step forward in the technique of "group catharsis."

In contradistinction to the conventional theatre, the spectators of this psychodrama are then witnessing a performance which is expressly intended to relate (and which, in fact, does relate) to their specific individual problems. The reactions of the spectators during and immediately following the performance can be made the basis for individual psychodramatic treatments. Thus is Aristotle's concept of catharsis brought to its rightful, logical culmination.

The therapeutic aspect of the psychodrama cannot be divorced from its aesthetic aspect nor, ultimately from its ethical character. In the therapeutic theatre an anonymous, average man becomes something approaching a work of art—not only for others but for himself. A tiny, insignificant existence is here elevated to a level of dignity and respect. Its private problems are projected on a high plane of action before a special public—a small world, perhaps, but *the* world of the therapeutic theatre. The world in which we all live is imperfect, unjust and amoral, but in the therapeutic theatre a little person can rise above our everyday world. Here his ego becomes an aesthetic prototype—he becomes representative of mankind. On the psychodramatic stage he is put into a state of inspiration—he is the dramatist of himself.

Comments and Conclusions

At this juncture it is logical to consider what processes in other types of psychotherapy are used to attain mental catharsis. Throughout this paper it has been my purpose to demonstrate the close relationship between spontaneity and mental catharsis, the material being largely drawn from actual psychodramatic experiences and studies. It can readily be assumed that any other genuine psychotherapeutic approach to the same problems must disclose similar basic conditions and that catharsis will be attained by similar devices.

An interested investigator can observe a plain relationship between other types of psychotherapy (such as hypnosis, suggestion or psychoanalysis) and the psychodrama. The spontaneous factor operates in all psychotherapies up to certain limits. It operates in the "free association" technique used in psychoanalysis, in suggestion therapy or during a hypnotic session. On the basis of the conclusions reached in this paper, there must be a relationship between the spontaneity quotient of any type of psychotherapy and the extent of mental catharsis it achieves. Similarly, the other principles discussed, such as the patterns of roles and *role-relationships* which are given so much prominence in psychodramatic work, can be discerned as operating—even if only in a fragmentary fashion—in every psychotherapeutic technique.

Psychotherapy and Psychopathology of Time

From the point of view of therapeutic procedures, to what extent does the time dimension enter into and function in psychotherapeutic settings? Man lives in time—past, present and future. He may suffer from a pathology related to each. The problem is how to integrate all three dimensions into significant therapeutic operations. It is not sufficient that they figure as "abstract" references: they must be made alive within treatment modalities. The psychological aspects of time must reappear in toto.

Let us look first at psychoanalysis. When I speak of psychoanalysis, I refer to the orthodox Freudian tradition. Time, in the psychoanalytic doctrine, is emphasized in terms of the *past*. Freud, an exponent of genetic psychology and psychobiology, found going back and trying to find the causes of things of particular interest. Often, the farther back he went, the more he thought he would find something which is worthwhile as a causation. And soon, psychoanalysts began to go farther and farther back, into the womb, and, if possible, even beyond that, until they got tired of this futile "recherche du temps perdu," and began to come back.

However important that past is as a dimension of time, it is a one-sided position, a "reduced time" which neglects and distorts the total influence which time has upon the psyche. Here we come to my first conflict with the Freudian view. I have pointed out that time has other phases which are important, one of which is the *present*, the dynamics of the present, of the Here and Now, *hic et nunc*. The experiences which take place continuously in the context of the Here and Now have been overlooked, distorted, or entirely forgotten. Therefore, early in my writings (1914–1924), in fact already in my first book in 1914, I began to emphasize the moment, the dynamics of the moment, the warming up to the moment, the dynamics of the present, the Here and Now, and all its immediate personal, social and cultural implications. But again, I considered these not only from the point of view of philosophy and phenomenology, but from the viewpoint of the therapeutic process as it takes place in connection with patients, in patient groups, the *Encounter*. The Encounter is a telic phenomenon. The fundamental process of tele is reciprocity—reciprocity of attraction, reciprocity of rejection, reciprocity of excitation, reciprocity of inhibition, reciprocity of indifference, reciprocity of distortion.

> A meeting of two: eye to eye, face to face.
> And when you are near I will tear your eyes out
> and place them instead of mine,
> and you will tear my eyes out
> and will place them instead of yours,
> then I will look at you with your eyes . . .
> and you will look at me with mine.
>
> (Moreno, 1914)

There is another dimension of therapeutic time which has been neglected until recently—the *future*. Yet it is an important aspect of living, for we certainly live in the future, rather than in the past. Since early this morning, I have been concerned with being on time to meet you. But it is one thing to consider the expectancies of future happenings in our own mind and another thing to "simulate" them, to construct techniques which enable us to live in the future, to act as if the future is on hand, right here, "à la recherche du temps de l'avenir." For instance, via our therapeutic future techniques, I can act out a situation which I expect to happen tomorrow, with a new friend, or an appointment with a prospective employer, to simulate the morrow as concretely as possible, so as to predict it or perhaps to be better prepared for it.

I have often had clients who suffered from an employment neurosis or an unemployment neurosis, who are anxious about getting a job, or having an interview with a boss asking for higher wages. Often we rehearse such a client a week in advance for what may happen; it is a sort of "rehearsal for life." This rehearsal for life technique is also effective with clients concerned over affairs of the heart—whether it be a prospective marriage, divorce, new baby, or whatever. The problem is how to integrate these expectancies and concerns of the client into the therapeutic operation as actualities, so as to be of value for both client and therapist.

The importance of the future as a perception and as a dynamic meaning has been emphasized by others in the course of years, for instance, Adler, Horney, and Sullivan. But the special configuration around and inside the future situation remained unstructured and impersonal.

Thus *all three dimensions of time*—past, present and future are brought together in psychodrama, as they are in life, from the point of view of functional therapy.

Psychopathology and Psychotherapy of Space

If you go into an office in which any of the current varieties of psychotherapy are practised, you may find only a chair. The space in which the protagonist experiences his traumas has no place in that setting. The idea of a psychotherapy of space has been pioneered by psychodrama, which is *action-centered* and comprehensively tries to integrate all the dimensions of living into itself. It is a sort of "recherche de l'espace concret, vécu." If a client steps into the therapeutic space, we insist on a description, delineation, and actualization of the space in which the ensuing scene is to be portrayed, its horizontal and vertical dimensions, objects in it, and their distance and relationship to one another.

I cannot emphasize sufficiently that in our research the configuration of space as a part of the therapeutic process is of utmost importance. It warms up the protagonist to be and to act himself in an environment which is modeled after that in which he lives.

Psychopathology and Psychotherapy of Reality

Surplus Reality

We come to yet another level of structuring which represents the intangible, invisible dimensions of intra- and extra-psychic life, which I have called "surplus reality." Surplus reality is only an analogous term; in our case it means that there are certain invisible dimensions in the reality of living, not fully experienced or expressed, and that is why we have to use surplus operations and surplus instruments to bring them out in our therapeutic settings.

One of the most popular surplus reality technique in psychodrama is that of *role reversal*. If, for instance, a husband and wife fight in the reality of daily life, each remains in his own role, in his own life situation. The perceptions, the expectations, fears, disappointments, or whatever, of each, remain unchanged. And even if both parties come to some point of agreement or disagreement, they still maintain the same relative status which they have in life. The husband remains the husband, the wife remains the wife. But in role reversal we request the wife to take the part of the husband, and the husband to take the part of the wife. We expect them to do this not only nominally, but to make an effort to go through the actual process of reversing roles, each one to try and feel his way into the thinking, feeling, and behavior patterns of the other.

One of the basic instruments in constructing a patient's psychodramatic world is that of the *auxiliary ego*, which is well known as the representation of absentees, individuals, delusions, hallucinations, symbols, ideals, animals, and objects. They make the protagonist's world real, concrete, and tangible. However, in the course of making this world real and dynamic, numerous problems emerge, as for instance the use of *bodily contact*. Now, bodily contact has been, to some extent, a taboo in all psychotherapies. Yet, when a nurse sees a patient suffering, she cannot help but touch him and say, "Now Jack, don't worry, it will be all right." Her touch may mean more to the boy than the words she speaks, not in an overtly sexual way, but as a sort of maternal, protective approach to him. But a psychoanalyst who would become in any way physically personal with his patient, would be ostracized.

However, in the psychodramatic approach to human relations we are interested in following the model of life, itself, and within limits, in making therapeutic use of the bodily contact technique. This technique is obviously contra-indicated if it is used to gratify the need of the therapist, but most indicated if it gives the patient the warmth and immediacy of pulsating life in an area in which he is in need, not only in words, but in action.

Role playing is another important surplus reality technique. Here a person may be trained to function more effectively in his reality roles, e.g. employer, employee, student, instructor, parent, child, mate, lover, friend, etc. In the therapeutic setting of psychodrama, the protagonist is free to try and fail in his role, for he knows he will be given the opportunity to try again, another alternative, and another, until he finally learns new approaches to the situations which he fears, approaches which he can then apply in situ, in life itself.

Psychopathology and Psychotherapy of the Cosmos

Now we come to the fourth universal—the *cosmos*. Early in the twentieth century, during my youth, two philosophies of human relations were particularly popular. One was the philosophy that everything in the universe is all packed in the single individual, in the individual psyche. This was particularly emphasized by Sigmund Freud, who thought that the group was an epi-phenomenon. For Freud, everything was epi, only the individual counted. The other philosophy was that of Karl Marx. For Marx everything ended with the social man, or more specifically, the socio-economic. It was as if that were all there were in the world. Very early in my career I came to the position that there is another area, a larger world

beyond the psychodynamics and sociodynamics of human society—
"*cosmodynamics.*"

Since time immemorial, man has tried to understand his position in
the universe at large, and, if possible, to control the phenomena that
determine this position—evolution, birth, death, sex, and the function of
the Creator of the world, himself. To do this, man has, in the past, invented
religions, myths, fables. He has submitted himself to stark regimentation
in order to comply with the laws of the universe as he conceived them.
Budda's Rules, the Ten Commandments of Moses, the numerous rituals of
the various illiterate cultures, are all testimony for the profound anxiety of
man to comply with an invisible value system.

Just like the functions of time, space, and reality, the function of the
cosmos must be so integrated into the therapeutic setting that it has
experiential and existential value for the protagonist. Within the
framework of psychodrama, by means of its numerous methods, cosmic
phenomena can be integrated into the therapeutic process. A therapeutic
method which does not concern itself with these enormous cosmic
implications, with man's very destiny, is incomplete and inadequate. Just
as our forefathers encountered these changes by means of fables and myths,
we have tried to encounter them in our own time with new devices. It is
at this point that surplus reality techniques in cosmodynamics come to the
fore. In the psychodramatic world the differentiation between the sexes is
overlooked and surpassed. There is no sex in psychodrama. The differences
in age are overlooked. There is no age in psychodrama. The factualities of
birth and death are overlooked. There is no death in psychodrama. The
unborn and the dead are brought to life or live again on the psychodrama
stage. It is a form of surplus art applied to cosmodynamics!

This is not a plea for "illusionism" or an escape from reality, but, just
the opposite, a plea for creativity of man and the creativity of the universe.
It is, therefore, through man's faith in the infinite creativity of the cosmos,
that what he embodies in a psychodramatic world may one day actually
become true. And so, as Goethe's Faust, at the end of his life, looked into
the future in a visionary way and said, "What will be, then, someday in the
distant future, I am already experiencing now," psychodrama makes it
possible for man to anticipate life in a very distant future without having
to wait until it becomes reality.

In the psychodramatic world the fact of embodiment is central,
axiomatic, and universal. Everyone can portray his version of God through
his own actions and so communicate his own version to others. That was
the simple meaning of my first book, in which I proclaimed the "*I-God.*"
None of my inspirations and pronouncements however, have been more
severely criticized, misunderstood, and ridiculed, than the idea that I
proclaimed myself as God, as the Father of my mother and father, of my
ancestors, and of everything which lives. Had I presented God as a "He"
or at least as a "Thou," like Christ, my book may have been praised, as the

English poet Christopher Isherwood said after reading it, "the greatest prophetic poem of our time." But it is the *I* which matters; it is the *I* which was provocative and new. And it is the I-God with whom we are all connected. It is the *I* which becomes the *We*.

It is amusing to think retroactively that my proclamation of the *I* was considered as the most outstanding manifestation of megalomania from my side. Actually, when the I-God is universalized, as it is in my book, the whole God concept becomes one of humbleness, weakness, and inferiority, a micromania rather than a megalomania. God has never been so lowly described and so universal in his dependence as he is in my book. It was a significant transformation from the cosmic God of the Hebrews, the He-God, to the living God of Christ, the Thou-god. But it was an even more challenging transformation from the Thou-God to the I-God, which puts all responsibility upon me and us, the I and the group.

We live within the framework of time, space and reality, but time learning, space learning, and reality learning cannot take place and be improved unless they are tested in an experimental setting, where they are experienced, expressed, practised, and reintegrated within the framework of a psychotherapy which is modeled after life, itself. Otherwise, the split between the experiences of time, space, and reality in life, itself and their representations within the therapeutic process may remain unrelated. Thus it is imperative that we transfer these phenomena from life itself into the therapeutic setting and back from the therapeutic setting into life itself.

References

Moreno J. L. (1914). *Einladung zu einer Begegnung.*
Moreno J. L. (1944). *The theater for spontaneity* (Trans. from *Das Stegreiftheater*. Berlin: Verlag Gustav Kiepenheuer, 1923). Psychodrama Monographs: No. 4. Beacon, NY: Beacon House.

Intra-Group Tensions in Therapy: Their Study as the Task of the Group

W. R. BION, D.S.O., B.A. OXFORD, M.R.C.S., MAJOR RAMC
JOHN RICKMAN, M.D. CAMBRIDGE, MAJOR RAMC

Wilfred Bion (1897–1979) was a British Kleinian analyst who became interested in group phenomena when he was stationed at the Northfield Military Neurosis Centre in Birmingham during the Second World War. This facility was created for the management of men experiencing neurotic reactions to the war, generally accompanied by low morale. The Northfield experiment consisted of treating the entire unit as a large group with the use of an ambiguous and nondirective leadership style that shifted the responsibility for the program onto the participants. Not surprisingly, this approach was less than enthusiastically received by the military.

Following Bion, the Northfield program was continued by a group of analytically trained psychiatrists who built upon his ideas. These included Joshua Bierer, who began one of the first Day Hospital programs; Henry Ezriel, who developed the early ideas about group focal conflict theory; Henry Foulkes, the founder of the British Group Analytic Society; Tom Main, who coined the term "therapeutic community"; and Jock Sutherland, later to become Director of the Tavistock Clinic.

This group produced a body of theory that eventually crossed the Atlantic in the 1960s, particularly following the publication of D. S. Whitaker and M. A. Lieberman's text "Psychotherapy through the Group Process" (New York: Atherton, 1964). This British tradition has been particularly associated in America with Group Relations training experiences as developed by the A. K. Rice Institute.

Bion's central contribution to the group literature lies in his description of how a group fluctuates between working and resistant attitudes. In the group resistant states, the individual becomes caught up in group emotion and loses a sense of personal autonomy. This core idea of a collective unconscious process that unites the members and to which each individual contributes has had a continuing impact on the field, even though defined in slightly different ways by others. Unfortunately Bion's therapeutic approach has not proved useful, at least not in the rather stark manner he espoused. It runs counter to a substantial literature concerning the importance of group supportive functions. Bion himself soon moved away from group involvement to pursue his interests in psychotic thought disorder. He moved to California in 1968, at the age of 70, for the "adventure" of spreading the concepts of Melanie Klein.

This is Bion's first published article describing the setting that stimulated his ideas about group phenomena. John Rickman was Bion's first personal analyst as well as a colleague in Northfield. Close reading will reveal the roots of numerous group concepts that have become more specifically articulated in later years. —Editor

61

Bion WR, Rickman J: Intra-group tensions in therapy: their study as the task of the group. *Lancet* 245:678–681, 1943.

The term "group therapy" can have two meanings. It can refer to the treatment of a number of individuals assembled for special therapeutic sessions, or it can refer to a planned endeavour to develop in a group the forces that lead to smoothly running cooperative activity.

The therapy of individuals assembled in groups is usually in the nature of explanation of neurotic trouble, with reassurance; and sometimes it turns mainly on the catharsis of public confession. The therapy of groups is likely to turn on the acquisition of knowledge and experience of the factors which make for a good group spirit.

A Scheme for Rehabilitation (W. R. B.)

In the treatment of the individual, neurosis is displayed as a problem of the individual. In the treatment of a group it must be displayed as a problem of the group. This was the aim I set myself when I was put in charge of the training wing of a military psychiatric hospital. My first task therefore was to find out what the pursuit of this aim would mean in terms of time-table and organisation.

I was not able to work at this task in an atmosphere of cloistered calm. No sooner was I seated before desk and papers than I was beset with urgent problems posed by importunate patients and others. Would I see the NCOs in charge of the training wing and explain to them what their duties were? Would I see Private A who had an urgent need for 48 hours' leave to see an old friend just back from the Middle East? Private B, on the other hand, would seek advice because an unfortunate delay on the railway had laid him open to misunderstanding as one who had overstayed his leave. And so on.

An hour or so of this kind of thing convinced me that what was required was discipline. Exasperated at what I felt to be a postponement of my work I turned to consider this problem.

Discipline for the Neurotic

Under one roof were gathered 300–400 men who in their units already had the benefit of such therapeutic value as lies in military discipline, good food and regular care; clearly this had not been enough to stop them from finding their way into a psychiatric hospital. In a psychiatric hospital such types provide the total population and by the time they reach the training wing they are not even subject to such slight restraint as is provided by being confined to bed.

I became convinced that what was required was the sort of discipline achieved in a theatre of war by an experienced officer in command of a rather scallywag battalion. But what sort of discipline is that? In face of the urgent need for action I sought, and found, a working hypothesis. It was, that the discipline required depends on two main factors: (1) the presence of the enemy, who provides a common danger and a common aim; and (2) the presence of an officer who, being experienced, knows some of his own failings, respects the integrity of his men, and is not afraid of either their goodwill or their hostility.

An officer who aspires to be the psychiatrist in charge of a rehabilitation wing must know what it is to be in a responsible position at a time when responsibility means having to face issues of life and death. He must know what it is to exercise authority in circumstances that make his fellows unable to accept his authority except in so far as he appears to be able to sustain it. He must know what it is to live in close emotional relationship with his fellow men. In short, he must know the sort of life that is led by a combatant officer. A psychiatrist who knows this will at least be spared the hideous blunder of thinking that patients are potential cannon-fodder, to be returned as such to their units. He will realise that it is his task to produce self-respecting men socially adjusted to the community and therefore willing to accept its responsibilities whether in peace or war. Only thus will he be free from deep feelings of guilt which effectually stultify any efforts he may otherwise make towards treatment.

What common danger is shared by the men in the rehabilitation wing? What aim could unite them?

There was no difficulty about detecting a common danger; neurotic extravagances of one sort and another perpetually endanger the work of the psychiatrist or of any institution set up to further treatment of neurotic disorders. The common danger in the training wing was the existence of neurosis as a disability of the community. I was now back at my starting-point—the need, in the treatment of a group, for displaying neurosis as a problem of the group. But, thanks to my excursion into the problem of discipline, I had come back with two additions. Neurosis needs to be displayed as a danger to the group; and its display must somehow be made the common aim of the group.

But how was the group to be persuaded to tackle neurotic disability as a communal problem?

The neurotic patient does not always want treatment, and when at last his distress drives him to it he does not want it wholeheartedly. This reluctance has been recognised in the discussion of resistance and allied phenomena; but the existence of comparable phenomena in societies has not been recognised.

Society has not yet been driven to seek treatment of its psychological disorders by psychological means because it has not achieved sufficient insight to appreciate the nature of its distress. The organisation of the training wing had to be such that the growth of insight should at least not be hindered. Better still if it could be designed to throw into prominence the way in which neurotic behaviour adds to the difficulties of the community, destroying happiness and efficiency. If communal distress were to become demonstrable as a neurotic by-product, then neurosis itself would be seen to be worthy of communal study and attack. And a step would have been taken on the way to overcome resistance in the society.

Two minor, but severely practical, military requirements had to be satisfied by the training wing. The organization should if possible provide a means by which the progress of the patients could be indicated, so that the psychiatrist could tell if a man were fit for discharge. It would also be useful to have an indication of the patient's direction, of his effective motivation, so that an opinion could be formed about the sort of work to which he should be discharged.

I found it helpful to visualize the projected organization of the training wing as if it were a framework enclosed within transparent walls. Into this space the patient would be admitted at one point, and the activities within that space would be so organised that he could move freely in any direction according to the resultant of his conflicting impulses. His movements as far as possible were not to be distorted by outside interference. As a result his behaviour could be trusted to give a fair indication of his effective will and aims, as opposed to the aims he himself proclaimed or the psychiatrists wished him to have.

It was expected that some of the activities organized within the "space" would be clearly war-like, others equally clearly civilian, others again merely expressions of neurotic powerlessness. As the patient's progress was seen to run along one or other of these paths so his "assets and liabilities" to use a phrase employed in the sphere of officer selection by Major Eric Wittkower, could be assessed with reasonable objectivity. As his progress appeared to be towards one or other of the possible exits from this imaginary space, so his true aim could be judged.

At the same time the organisation could be used to further the main aim of the training wing—the education and training of the community in the problems of interpersonal relationships. If it could approximate to this theoretical construct it would enable the members of the training wing to stand (as it were) outside the framework and look with detachment and growing understanding upon the problems of its working.

The Experiment

The training wing, consisting of some hundred men, was paraded and was told that in future the following regulations would apply:

1. Every man must do one hour's physical training daily unless a medical certificate excused him.
2. Every man must be a member of one or more groups—the groups designed to study handicrafts, Army correspondence courses, carpentry, map reading, sand-tabling, etc.
3. Any man could form a fresh group if he wanted to do so either because no group existed for his particular activity or because, for some reason or other, he was not able to join an existing similar group.
4. A man feeling unable to attend his group would have to go to the rest-room.
5. The rest-room would be in charge of a nursing orderly, and must be kept quiet for reading, writing or games such as draughts. Talking in an undertone was permitted with the permission of the nursing orderly but other patients must not be disturbed; couches were provided so that any men who felt unfit for any activity whatever could lie down. The nursing orderly would take the names of all those in the rest-room as a matter of routine.

It was also announced that a parade would be held every day at 12:10 for making announcements and conducting other business of the training wing. Unknown to the patients, it was intended that this meeting, strictly limited to 30 minutes, should provide an occasion for the men to step outside their framework and look upon its working with the detachment of spectators. In short, it was intended to be the first step towards the elaboration of therapeutic seminars.

For the first few days little happened; but it was evident that among the patients a great deal of discussion, and thinking, was taking place. The first few 12:10 meetings were little more than attempts to gauge the sincerity of the proposals; then the groups began to form in earnest. Among other more obvious activities there was a programme group to chart out working hours of groups and their location, to make announcements and to allocate tickets for free concerts and such-like. In a very short time the programme room, which showed by means of flags on a work-chart the activities of every man in the training wing, now growing rapidly in size, became almost vernal in its display of multi-coloured flags of patterns suggested by the ingenuity of the patients. By a happy thought a supply of flags bearing the skull and crossbones was prepared, ready for the use of such gentlemen as felt compelled to be absent without leave.

The existence of this brave display gave occasion for what was probably the first important attempt at therapeutic cooperation at a 12:10. meeting. It had been my habit, on going the rounds of the groups, to detach one or two men from their immediate work and take them with me "Just to see how the rest of the world lived." I was therefore able to communicate to this meeting an interesting fact observed by myself and others who had gone round with me. Namely, that, although there were many groups and almost entire freedom to each man to follow the bent of his own inclinations, provided he could make a practical proposal, yet very little was happening. The carpenter's shop might have one or two men at most; car maintenance the same; in short, I suggested it almost looked as if the training wing was a facade with nothing behind it. This, I said, seemed odd because I remembered how bitterly the patients in the training wing had previously complained to me that one of their objections to the Army was the "eyewash." Its presence in the training wing, therefore, really did seem to be a point worth study and discussion.

This announcement left the audience looking as if they felt they were being "got at." I turned the discussion over at that point as a matter of communal responsibility and not something that concerned myself, as an officer, alone.

With surprising rapidity the training wing became self-critical. The freedom of movement permitted by the original set-up allowed the characteristics of a neurotic community to show with painful clarity; within a few days men complained that the wards (hitherto always claimed to be spotless) were dirty and could not be kept clean under the present system of a routine hour for ward fatigues. They asked and were allowed to organise under the programme group an "orderly group," whose duties it would be to keep the wards clean throughout the day. The result of this was that on a subsequent weekly inspection the Commanding Officer of the hospital remarked on the big change in cleanliness that had taken place.

Some Results

It is impossible to go into details about the working of all the therapeutic aspects of the organisation; but two examples of method and result may be given.

Shortly after the new arrangement started, men began to complain to me that patients were taking advantage of the laxity of the organization. "Only 20%," they said, "of the men are taking part and really working hard. The other 80% are just a lot of shirkers". They complained that not only was the rest-room often filled with people simply loafing, but that some men even cut that. I was already aware of this, but refused, at least outwardly, to have its cure made my responsibility. Instead, I pointed out that, at an ABCA meeting some weeks before, the discussion had at one point centred on just that question—namely, the existence in communities (and the community then under discussion was Soviet Russia) of just such uncooperative individuals as these and the problem presented to society by their existence. Why, then, did they sound so surprised and affronted at discovering that just the same problem afflicted the training wing?

This cool reply did not satisfy the complainants—they wanted such men to be punished, or otherwise dealt with. To this I replied that no doubt the complainants, themselves, had neurotic symptoms, or they would not be in hospital; why should their disabilities be treated in one way and the disabilities of the 80% treated in another? After all, the problem of the "80%" was not new; in civil life magistrates, probation officers, social workers, the Church and statesmen had all attempted to deal with it, some of them by discipline and punishment. The "80%," however, were still with us; was it not possible that the nature of the problem had not yet been fully elucidated and that they (the complainants) were attempting to rush in with a cure before the disease had been diagnosed? The problem, I said, appeared to be one that concerned not only the training wing, or even the Army alone, but to have the widest possible implications for society at large. I suggested that they should study it and come forward with fresh proposals when they felt they were beginning to see daylight.

It is worth remarking at this point that my determination not to attempt solution of any problem until its borders had become clearly defined helped to produce, after a vivid and healthy impatience, a real belief that the unit was meant to tackle its job with scientific seriousness. One critic expostulated that surely such a system of patient observation would be exceedingly slow in producing results, if indeed it produced results at all. He was answered by reminding him that only a few days previously the critic himself had spontaneously remarked that the military discipline and bearing of the training wing had improved out of all recognition within the short period of a month.

The second example illustrates the development of an idea from the stage of a rather wild, neurotic impulse to practical common-sense activity.

By far the largest group of men proposed the formation of a dancing class. Despite the veneer of a desire to test my sincerity in promising facilities for group activity, the pathetic sense of inferiority toward women that underlay this proposal, by men taking no part in fighting, was only too obvious. They were told to produce concrete proposals. The steps by which this was done need not detain us; in the end the class was held during hours usually taken up by an evening entertainment; it was confined, by the volition of the men themselves, only to those who had no knowledge of dancing and the instruction was done by ATS staff. In short, a proposal, which had started as a quite unpractical idea, quite contrary to any apparently serious military aim, or sense of social responsibility to the nation at war, ended by being an inoffensive and serious study carried out at the end of a day's work. Furthermore, the men concerned had had to approach the Commanding Officer, the ATS officers and the ATS, as a matter of discipline in the first place and social courtesy in the second.

In the meantime, the 12:10 parades had developed very fast into business-like, lively and constructive meetings and that in spite of the fact that the wing was now receiving heavy reinforcements of patients new to the organisation, as well as losing others who had been discharged from hospital, often when they had become very useful.

Within a month of the inception of the scheme big changes had taken place. Whereas at first it almost seemed difficult to find ways of employing the men, at the end of the month it was difficult to find time for the work they wanted to do. Groups had already begun to operate well outside what were ordinarily considered parade hours; absence without leave was for a considerable period non-existent, and over the whole period there was only one case; patients not in the training wing became anxious to come over to it; and despite the changing population, the wing had an unmistakable esprit-de-corps, which showed itself in details such as the smartness with which men came to attention when officers entered the room at the 12:10 meetings. The relationship of the men to the officers was friendly and cooperative; they were eager to enlist the officers' sympathy in concerts and other activities which they were arranging. There was a subtle but unmistakable sense that the officers and men alike were engaged on a worth-while and important task even though the men had not yet grasped quite fully the nature of the task on which they were engaged. The atmosphere was not unlike that seen in a unit of an army under the command of a general in whom they have confidence, even though they cannot know his plans.

Comment

It is not possible to draw many conclusions from an experiment lasting, in all, six weeks. Some problems that arose could not be fully explored in the time; others may not be openly discussed while the war is still in progress.

It was evident that the 12:10 meetings were increasingly concerned with the expression, on the part of the men of their ability to make contact with reality and to regulate their relationships with others, and with their tasks, efficiently. The need for organisation of seminars for group therapy had become clear, and the foundation of their commencement appeared to be firmly laid.

The whole concept of the "occupation" of the training wing as a study of, and a training in, the management of interpersonal relationships within a group seemed to be amply justified as a therapeutic approach. Anyone with a knowledge of good fighting regiments in a theatre of war would have been struck by certain similarities in outlook in the men of such a unit and the men of the training wing. In these respects the attempt could be regarded as helpful; but there were also lessons to be learnt.

Some of these raised serious doubts about the suitability of a hospital milieu for psychotherapy. It was possible to envisage an organisation that would be more fitly described as a psychiatric training unit, and, indeed, some work had been done in the elaboration of an establishment and a modus operandi of such a unit. With regard to the psychiatrist, also, there was room for some readjustment of outlook. If group therapy is to succeed it appears necessary that he should have the outlook, and the sort of intuitive sympathetic flair, of the good unit commander. Otherwise there will always be a lingering suspicion that some combatant officers are better psychiatrists, and achieve better results, than those who have devoted themselves to the narrow paths of individual interview.

Finally, attention may be drawn again to the fact that society, like the individual, may not want to deal with its distresses by psychological means until driven to do so by a realisation that some at least of these distresses are psychological in origin. The community represented by the training wing had to learn this fact before the full force of its energy could be released in self-cure. What applied to the small community of the training wing may well apply to the community at large; and further insight may be needed before wholehearted backing can be obtained for those who attempt in this way to deal with deep seated springs of national morale.

Applications of Group Therapy on a Small Ward (J. R.)

An experiment in the application of group therapy, in the newer sense, to patients in a ward of 14–16 beds was made in the hospital division of the same institution. Each patient had an initial interview with the psychiatrist in which a personal history was taken in the usual way; thereafter there were group discussions every morning before the hour's "route march"; and after it, as the patients returned to the ward, they could call in at the psychiatrist's room to discuss privately the topic of the group discussion, which had usually been the subject of conversation on the "route march" and their personal feelings about it.

The therapeutic talks centred on their personal difficulties in putting the welfare of the group in the first place during their membership of the group. The topics of the group discussion included the following:

(a) Since residence in this ward is temporary, some going into the training wing and others coming from the admission ward to take their place, how is this changing situation to be met? We—the distinction between physician and patient, officer and other ranks was another special topic—should have to accommodate ourselves to people entering our group to whom our attitude to our ward (it was always referred to as "our ward") meant nothing at all; either we could regard them as outsiders or as imperfectly accommodated insiders. So too with those who "went out"

into the training wing; they could not expect to retain the ward-group
attitudes indefinitely, nor could they expect to include the much larger
training wing in their ward group; they would have to find their place in
the new groupings and allow their ward experience to be but a memory,
but it was to be hoped helpful memory. Then there was the further point,
whether those in the training wing should come back to the daily group
discussions, the question being not what they would get out of them (there
seemed little doubt they were among the most interesting experiences we
had ever had) but whether, coming from another group-formation, or
while losing their ward contact, they might not prove a distraction to those
who were finding their feet in the ward group.

(b) How far were the differences of rank acquired "outside" to
determine the behaviour of the members of the group to one another while
in the ward? Would an attempt at equality work, or would it be better,
while not forgetting the rank acquired outside, to consider what
equivalents of rank emerge when in the ward, and if so the basis of these
equivalents?

(c) What makes for discontent in the ward? Is it something peculiar
to this ward, or any ward, or to any association of people?

(d) What makes for content and happiness in the ward? Is it the
exercise of individual initiative having for its soul criterion the free
expression of the person's own private enterprises, or does that come only
after recognition of what the ward needs from the individual? Is there a
fundamental incompatibility between these two points of view, and if so
does it apply to all or only some members? If to only some, what causes it
to appear in these and is it a characteristic they carry through in their lives
all the time or is it sometimes more strong than at others? If it varies, can
the ward diminish it without being oppressive to those individuals so
endowed?

The effect of this approach to the problem of neurosis was
considerable. There was a readiness, and at times an eagerness, to discuss
both in public and in private the social implications of personality
problems. The neurotic is commonly regarded as being self-centred and
averse from cooperative endeavour; but perhaps this is because he is seldom
put in an environment in which *every* member is on the same footing as
regards interpersonal relationships.

The experiment was interrupted by posting of personnel, so I cannot
give clinical or statistical results; but it seemed to show that it is possible
for a clinician to turn attention to the structure of a group and to the forces
operating in that structure without losing touch with his patients, and
further that anxiety may be raised either inside or outside the group if this
approach is made.

Conclusions

We are now in a better position to define the "good group spirit" which has been our aim.

It is as hard to define as is the concept of good health in an individual; but some of its qualities appear to be associated with:

(a) A common purpose, whether that be overcoming an enemy or the defending and fostering an ideal or a creative construction in the field of social relationships or in physical amenities.

(b) Common recognition by members of the group of the "boundaries" of the group and their position and function in relation to that of larger units or groups.

(c) The capacity to absorb new members and to lose members without fear of losing group individuality—i.e., "group character" must be flexible.

(d) Freedom from internal subgroups having rigid (ie., exclusive) boundaries. If a subgroup is present it must not be centred on its members nor on itself—treating other members of the main group as if they did not belong within the main group barrier—and the value of the subgroup to the function of the main group must be generally recognized.

(e) Each individual member is valued for his contribution to the group and has free movement within it, his freedom of locomotion being limited only by the generally accepted conditions devised and imposed by the group.

(f) The group must have the capacity to face discontent within the group and must have means to cope with discontent.

(g) The minimum size of a group is three. Two members have personal relationships; with three or more there is a change of quality (interpersonal relationship).

These experiments in a rehabilitation wing of a military psychiatric neurosis hospital suggest the need for further examination of the structure of groups and the interplay of forces within the groups. Psychology and psychopathology have focused attention on the individual often to the exclusion of the social field of which he is a part. There is a useful future in the study of the interplay of individual and social psychology (viewed as equally important interacting elements), and war-time makes this study an urgent issue.

Frontiers in Group Dynamics: Concept, Method and Reality in Social Science; Social Equilibria and Social Change

KURT LEWIN, PH. D.

Kurt Lewin (1890–1947), a German psychologist, moved to America in the early 1930s and eventually settled at the University of Michigan where he formed the Research Center for Group Dynamics. His profound impact on the field of social psychology was continued by a generation of students including Kenneth Benne, Leland Bradford, Dorwin Cartright, Ronald Lippitt, Herbert A. Thelen, and Ralph K. White. Lewin also influenced Jerome Frank, represented in this volume, and George R. Bach, who wrote one of the early texts in clinical group psychotherapy (Intensive Group Psychotherapy. New York: Ronald Press, 1954).

Lewin developed the National Training Laboratories in Bethel, Maine, where the T-group originated. The idea behind these training experiences was to provide a social field where individuals could explore their definition of self, not by a restatement of old roles, but in the reality of their current interaction. The parallels with Moreno's idea of the importance of the "moment" are obvious; Lewin drew upon Moreno's techniques of sociometry. Carl Rogers was also strongly influenced by this tradition and became a major figure in the subsequent encounter group movement which swept through America in the 1960s.

This is Lewin's last major paper, published shortly before his death. It was the lead article in the first issue of the journal Human Relations , which was created by the joint efforts of Lewin and the Tavistock Institute of Human Relations. Lewin introduces some of his ideas about the importance of immediate social influences on determining how the individual views himself and his interpersonal world, as well as his core concept of the "field theory" of small group functioning, a precursor of general systems theory. The paper also summarizes some of the work concerning the impact of leadership style on group behavior, material that is echoed in Yalom's paper on encounter group casualties in this volume . Lewin provides an interesting look at the social culture of scientific enquiry at the beginning of the postwar explosion of knowledge. The original paper is much longer; technical details and background material have been deleted.

—Editor

Lewin K: Frontiers in group dynamics: Concept, method, and reality in social science: Social equilibria and social change. *Human Relations 1*:5–41, 1947.

One of the byproducts of World War II of which society is hardly aware is the new stage of development which the social sciences have reached. This development indeed may prove to be as revolutionary as the atom bomb. Applying cultural anthropology to modern rather than "primitive" cultures, experimentation with groups inside and outside the laboratory, the measurement of sociopsychological aspects of large social bodies, the combination of economic, cultural, and psychological fact-finding, all of these developments started before the war. But, by providing unprecedented facilities and by demanding realistic and workable solutions to scientific problems, the war has accelerated greatly the change of social sciences to a new development level.

The scientific aspects of this development center around three objectives:

1. Integrating social sciences.
2. Moving from the description of social bodies to dynamic problems of changing group life.
3. Developing new instruments and techniques of social research.

Theoretical progress has hardly kept pace with the development of techniques. It is, however, as true for the social as for the physical and biological sciences that without adequate conceptual development, science cannot proceed beyond a certain stage. It is an important step forward that the hostility to theorizing which dominated a number of social sciences ten years ago has all but vanished. It has been replaced by a relatively wide-spread recognition of the necessity for developing better concepts and higher levels of theory. The theoretical development will have to proceed rather rapidly if social science is to reach that level of practical usefulness which society needs for winning the race against the destructive capacities set free by man's use of the natural sciences.

I should like to survey certain concepts and theories which have emerged mainly from experimental research. They concern:

(a) Quasi-stationary social equilibria and social changes.
(b) Locomotion through social channels.
(c) Social feedback processes and social management.

The last two of these will be dealt with in a later article. A cursory introductory discussion of certain aspects of the present state of affairs in social science is included here for those readers who are interested in the general background of these concepts and in the problems from which they have sprung.

Concept, Method, and Reality in
Social Science

Developmental Stages of Science

For planning and executing research a clear insight into the present stage of scientific development is needed. Research means taking the next step from the known into the jungle of the unknown. To choose scientifically significant objectives and procedures it does not suffice to be acquainted with the factual knowledge available at a given stage. It is also necessary to free oneself from the scientific prejudices typical of a given developmental stage.

The type of obstacles which have to be overcome when proceeding to a next scientific step are frequently quite different from what one may expect. Looking backwards it is often hard to understand how anyone could have been influenced by those arguments which have delayed scientific progress for considerable time.

The Problem of Existence in an Empirical Science

Arguments about "existence" may seem metaphysical in nature and may therefore not be expected to be brought up in empirical sciences. Actually the opinions about existence or non-existence are quite common in the empirical sciences and have greatly influenced scientific development in a positive and a negative way. Labeling something as "non-existing" is equivalent to declaring it "out of bounds" for the scientist. Attributing "existence" to an item automatically makes it a duty of the scientist to consider this item as an object of research; it includes the necessity of considering its properties as "facts" which cannot be neglected in the total system of theories; finally, it implies that the terms with which one refers to the item are accepted as scientific "concepts" (rather than as "mere words").

Beliefs regarding "existence" in social science have changed in regard to the degree to which "full reality" is attributed to psychological and social phenomena, and in regard to the reality of their "deeper," dynamic properties.

In the beginning of this century, for instance, the experimental psychology of "will and emotion" had to fight for recognition against a prevalent attitude which placed volition, emotion, and sentiments in the "poetic realm" of beautiful words, a realm to which nothing corresponds which could be regarded as "existing" in the sense of the scientist. Although every psychologist had to deal with these facts realistically in his private life they were banned from the realm of "facts" in the scientific sense. Emotions were declared to be something too "fluid" and "intangible" to be pinned down by scientific analysis or by experimental procedures. Such a methodological argument does not deny existence to the phenomenon but it has the same effect of keeping the topic outside the realm of empirical science.

Like social taboos, a scientific taboo is kept up not so much by a rational argument as by a common attitude among scientists; any member of the scientific guild who does not strictly adhere to the taboo is looked upon as queer; he is suspected of not adhering to the scientific standards of critical thinking.

The Reality of Social Phenomena

Before the invention of the atom bomb the average physical scientist was hardly ready to concede to social phenomena the same degree of "reality" as to a physical object. Hiroshima and Nagasaki seem to have made many physical scientists ready to consider social facts as being perhaps of equal reality. This change of mind was hardly based on philosophical considerations. The bomb has driven home with dramatic intensity the degree to which social happenings are both the result of, and the conditions for the occurrence of, physical events. Gradually, the period is coming to an end when the natural scientist thinks of the social scientist as someone interested in dreams and words, rather than as an investigator of facts, which are not less real than physical facts, and which can be studied no less objectively.

The social scientists themselves, of course, have had a stronger belief in the "reality" of the entities they were studying. Still, this belief was frequently limited to the specific narrow section with which they happened to be familiar. The economist, for instance, finds it a bit difficult to concede to psychological to anthropological or to legal data that degree of reality which he gives to prices and other economic data. Some psychologists still view with suspicion the reality of those cultural facts with which the anthropologist is concerned. They tend to regard only individuals as real and they are not inclined to consider a "group atmosphere" as something which is as real and measurable as, let us say, a physical field of gravity. Concepts like that of "leadership" retained a halo of mysticism even after it had been demonstrated that it is quite possible to measure, and not only to "judge," leadership performance.

The denial of existence of a group, or of certain aspects of group life, is based on arguments which grant existence only to units of certain size, or which concern methodologic–technical problems, or conceptual problems.

Reality and Dynamic Wholes

Cassirer (7) discusses how, periodically throughout the history of physics, vivid discussions have occurred about the reality of the atom, the electron, or whatever else was considered at that time to be the smallest part of physical material. In the social sciences it has usually been not the part but the whole, whose existence has been doubted.

Logically, there is no reason to distinguish between the reality of a molecule, an atom, or an ion, or more generally between the reality of a whole or its parts. There is no more magic behind the fact that groups have properties of their own, which are different from the properties of their subgroups or their individual members than behind the fact that molecules have properties, which are different from the properties of the atoms or ions of which they are composed.

Structural properties are characterized by *relations* between parts rather than by the parts or elements themselves. Cassirer emphasizes that throughout the history of mathematics and physics problems of constancy of relations rather than of constancy of elements have gained importance and have gradually changed the picture of what is essential. The social sciences seem to show a very similar development.

Reality and Methods. Recording and Experimentation

If recognition of the existence of an entity depends upon this entity's showing properties or constancies of its own, the judgment about what is real or unreal should be affected by changes in the possibility of demonstrating social properties.

The social sciences have considerably improved techniques for reliably recording the structure of small or large groups and of registering the various aspects of group life. Sociometric techniques, group observation, interview techniques, and others are enabling us more and more to gather reliable data on the structural properties of groups, on the relations between groups or sub-groups, and on the relation between group and the life of its individual members.

The taboo against believing in the existence of a social entity is probably most effectively broken by handling this entity experimentally. As long as the scientist merely describes a leadership form he is open to the criticism that the categories used reflect merely his "subjective views" and do not correspond to the "real" properties of the phenomena under consideration. If the scientist experiments with leadership and varies its form, he relies on an "operational definition" which links the concept of a leadership form to concrete procedures of creating such a leadership form or to the procedures for testing its existence. The "reality" of that to which the concept refers is established by "doing something with" rather than "looking at," and this reality is independent of certain "subjective" elements of classification. The progress of physics from Archimedes to Einstein shows consecutive steps by which this "practical" aspect of the experimental procedure has modified and sometimes revolutionized the scientific concepts regarding the physical world by changing the beliefs of the scientists about what is and is not real (7).

To vary a social phenomenon experimentally the experimenter has to take hold of all essential factors even if he is not yet able to analyze them satisfactorily. A major omission or misjudgment on this point makes the experiment fail. In social research the experimenter has to take into consideration such factors as the personality of individual members, the group structure, ideology and cultural values, and economic factors. Group experimentation is a form of social management. To be successful it, like social management, has to take into account all of the various factors that happen to be important for the case in hand. Experimentation with groups will therefore lead to a natural integration of the social sciences, and it will force the social scientist to recognize as reality the totality of factors which determine group life.

Social Reality and Concepts

It seems that the social scientist has a better chance of accomplishing such a realistic integration than the social practitioner. For thousands of years kings, priests, politicians, educators, producers, fathers and mothers—in fact, all individuals, have been trying day by day to influence smaller or larger groups. One might assume that this would have led to accumulated wisdom of a well integrated nature. Unfortunately nothing is farther from the truth. We know that our average diplomat thinks in very one-sided terms, perhaps those of law, or economics, or military strategy. We know that the average manufacturer holds highly distorted views about what makes a work-team "tick." We know that no one can answer today even such relatively simple questions as what determines the productivity of a committee meeting.

If one tries to transform these sentiments into scientific language, they amount to the following statements: (a) Social events depend on the social field as a whole, rather than on a few selected items. This is the basic insight behind the field theoretical method which has been successful in physics, which has steadily grown in psychology and, in my opinion, is bound to be equally fundamental for the study of social fields, simply because it expresses certain basic general characteristics of interdependence. (b) The denial of "simple rules" is partly identical with the following important principle of scientific analysis. Science tries to link certain observable (phenotypical) data with other observable data. It is crucial for all problems of interdependence, however, that—for reasons which we do not need to discuss here—it is, as a rule, impracticable to link one set of phenotypical data *directly* to other phenotypical data. Instead it is necessary to insert "intervening variables" (29). To use a more common language: the practitioner as well as the scientist views the observable data as mere "symptoms." They are "surface" indications of some "deeper-lying" facts. He has learned to "read" the symptoms, like a physicist reads his instruments. The equations which express physical laws refer to such deeper-lying dynamic entities as pressure, energy, or temperature rather than to the directly observable symptoms such as the movements of the pointer of an instrument (7).

The dynamics of social events provides no exception to this general characteristic of dynamics. If it were possible to link a directly observable group behavior with another behavior then simple rules of procedure for the social practitioner would be possible. When the practitioner denies that such rules can be more than poor approximations he seems to imply that the function is complicated. I am inclined to interpret his statement actually to mean that in group life, too, "appearance" should be distinguished from the "underlying facts," that similarity of appearance may go together with dissimilarity of the essential properties, and vice-versa, and that laws can be formulated only in regard to these underlying dynamic entities: where the units refer not to behavioral symptoms but to intervening variables (13).

For the social scientist this means that he should give up thinking about such items as group structure, group tension, or social forces as nothing more than a popular metaphor or analogy which should be eliminated from science as much as possible. While there is no need for social science to copy the specific concepts of the sciences, the social scientist should be clear that he, too, needs intervening variables, and that these dynamic facts rather than the symptoms and appearances, are the important points of reference alike for him and for the social practitioner.

"Subjective" and "Objective" Elements in the Social Field: The Three Step Procedure

One last point concerning conceptualization and general methodology may be mentioned. For instance, the analysis of the history of a marriage might proceed in a series of three steps: first, a separate analysis of the psychological situation of the husband and that of the wife, at time 1 with the purpose of deriving the next behavior of each. Second, representing the resultant sociological ("objective") situation at time 2. Third, deriving with the help of the laws of perception the resultant psychological situation for husband and wife at time 2. This would give the basis for the next sequence of three steps, starting with the analysis of the psychological situation of the persons involved predict their actual next step.

Such a procedure looks involved, particularly if we consider groups composed of many members. Is it possible to eliminate the "objective", or the "subjective," aspect of this analysis? Actually, social science faces here two types of question; one concerning the size of units, the other concerning the role of perception in group life. It would be prohibitive if the analysis of group life always had to include analysis of the life space of each individual member.

Analysis of group life, can proceed rather far on the basis of relatively larger units. In the end, of course, the theory of small and large units has to be viewed in social science as well as in physical science, as one theoretical system. But this stage can be reached only after an attack on both the larger and the smaller units.

Unfortunately, treating groups as units does not eliminate the dilemma between "subjective" and "objective" aspects of social fields. It seems to be impossible to predict group behavior without taking into account group goals, group standards, group values and the way a group "sees" its own situation and that of other groups. Group conflicts would have quite different solutions if the various groups concerned did not perceive differently the situation existing at a given time. To predict or to understand the steps leading to war between two nations A and B it seems to be essential to refer to the group life space of A and to the different group life space of B. This means that the analysis of group interaction has again to follow a three step procedure, moving from the separate analysis of the life space of each group to the group conduct in the total social field and from there back again to the effect on the group life space.

This procedure of analysis which swings from an analysis of "perception" to that of "action," from the "subjective" to the "objective," and back again is not an arbitrary demand of scientific methodology, nor is it limited to the interaction between groups or between individuals. The procedure mirrors one of the basic properties of group life. Any kind of group action or individual action, even including that of the insane, is regulated by circular causal processes of the following type: individual perception or "fact-finding"—for instance, an act of accounting—is linked with individual action or group action in such a way that the content of the perception or fact-finding depends upon the way in which the situation is changed by action. The result of the fact-finding in turn influences or steers action.

Quasi-Stationary Equilibria in Group Life and the Problem of Social Change

Periods of social change may differ quite markedly from periods of relative social stability. Still, the conditions of these two states of affairs should be analyzed together for two reasons: (a) Change and constancy are relative concepts; group life is never without change, merely differences in the amount and type of change exist. (b) Any formula which states the conditions for change implies the conditions for no-change as limit, and the conditions of constancy can be analyzed only against a background of "potential" change.

Constancy and Resistance to Change

It is important to distinguish two questions which are generally not sufficiently separated; the one concerns actual change or lack of change, the other concerns resistance to change. A given group may show little change during a period of, let us say, two weeks. The group may be composed of friends on an island in the middle of their vacation, or a work-team in a factory. Let us assume that the conditions under which this group lives happen to stay constant during this period: no individual leaves or joins the group, no major friction occurs, the facilities for activities or work remain the same, etc. Under these circumstances the constancy of group life, for instance, the unchanged level of production does not require any other "explanation" than the reference to the principle: the same conditions lead to the same effect. This principle is identical with the general idea of lawfulness of group life.

The case would be different if the production level of the work-team were maintained in spite of the fact that a member of the work-team took sick or that inferior or superior material was provided. If, in spite of such changes in the group life setting, production is kept at the same level then can one speak of "resistance" to change of the rate of production. The mere constancy of group conduct does not prove stability in the sense of resistance to change, nor does much change prove little resistance. Only by relating the actual degree of constancy to the strength of forces toward or away from the present state of affairs can one speak of degrees of resistance or "stability" of group life in a given respect.

The practical task of social management, as well as the scientific task of understanding the dynamics of group life, require insight into the desire for and resistance to, specific change. To solve or even to formulate these questions adequately we need a system of analysis which permits the representation of social forces in a group setting. The following considerations are directed more toward the improvement of these analytical tools than toward the analysis of a particular case.

Social Fields and Phase Spaces

A basic tool for the analysis of group life is the representation of the group and its setting as a "social field." This means that the social happening is viewed as occurring in, and being the result of, a totality of coexisting social entities, such as groups, subgroups, members, barriers, channels of communication, etc. One of the fundamental characteristics of this field is the relative position of the entities, which are parts of the field. This relative position represents the structure of the group and its ecological setting. It expresses also the basic possibilities of locomotion within the field.

What happens within such a field depends upon the distribution of forces throughout the field. A prediction presupposes the ability to determine for the various points of the field the strength and directions of the resultant forces.

According to general field theory the solution of a problem of group life has always to be finally based on an analytical procedure of this type. Only by considering the groups in question in their actual setting, can we be sure that none of the essential possible conduct has been overlooked.

Certain aspects of social problems, however, can be answered through a different analytical device called *"phase space."* The phase space is a system of coordinates, each corresponding to different amounts of intensities of the "property." The phase space does not intend to represent the layout of a field composed of groups, individuals and their ecological setting, but concentrates on one or a few factors. It represents by way of graphs or equations, the quantitative relation between these few properties, variables or aspects of the field, or of an event in it. For the discussion of the conditions of change we make use of such a phase space, realizing that one has finally to refer back to the actual social field.

Example of Quasi-Stationary Equilibrium in Different Areas of Group Life

The following examples are not intended to prove the correctness of a theory for the given case. They are intended mainly to illustrate principles and to prepare the way for the quantitative measurement of social forces. In regard to the specific case they represent hypotheses which have to be tested experimentally.

Level of Aggressiveness in Democratic and Autocratic Atmospheres

Lippitt (21) and Lippitt and White (23) have compared the amount of intermember aggression of the same groups of boys in democratic and autocratic atmospheres. Since the personalities and types of activities were kept constant, the change can be attributed to the different social climate or form of leadership. They found that the group average of intermember aggressiveness in autocracy is either very high or very low; in democracy it is on a more medium level.

Let us assume that each of these levels of aggressiveness is a quasi-stationary equilibrium, and ask which forces tend to raise and which to lower the level. One factor is the type of activity: a wild game gives more chance for clashes than quiet work; a certain amount of fighting might be fun for boys. Forces against intergroup aggression might be: friendship between members; the presence of an adult leader; the dignified character of the setting. The actual conduct indicates that in the democratic atmosphere these conflicting forces lead to an equilibrium.

If we use the force field in the democratic atmosphere as our base for comparison, the higher level of aggressiveness in aggressive autocratic could be explained by an increase in the strength of forces toward more aggression or by a diminishing of the forces toward less aggression. Actually both forces seem to have been altered in autocracy: the style of leadership and the irritation due to the restriction of the space of free movement increases the force toward aggressiveness. Lippitt found that the we-feeling which tends to decrease intermember aggression is diminished in autocracy. This would suffice to explain why the level of aggression increases in autocracy. If there were no other changes involved, we could even derive a statement concerning the gradient of the force field in the democratic situation.

How then can aggressiveness in apathetic autocracy be low? Lippitt and White (23) found the we-feeling to be low in both types of autocracy; it is unlikely that the irritating effect of the frustrating autocratic leadership should not exist. We are inclined rather to assume that the autocratic leadership form implies an additional force which corresponds to the higher degree of authoritarian control and which in these situations has the direction against open aggression.

As a rule we can assume that the force is rather strong. This autocratic control would keep open aggression very low in spite of the greater force toward aggressions. Only if this control were for one reason or other, sufficiently weakened would the increased tendency toward aggression come into the open.

From this theory one could conclude that the opposing components which make up the resultant forces are greater than in the case of democracy. The strength of this additional component is—compared with that in the democratic situation—*ceteris paribus* equal to the pressure of the autocratic control plus the force due to the difference in we-feeling. In other words we would expect *a high degree of inner tension existing in apathetic autocracy in spite of its appearance of quietness and order.*

Since an autocratic atmosphere is less permissive than the democratic atmosphere one may wonder how a high level of in-group aggression can occur in autocracy. The answer lies in the fact that the restrictive character of autocracy has two contradictory effects: (a) It leads to frustration of the group members and therefore to an increase in the direction of more aggression. (b) The control aspect of restriction is equivalent to a restraining force against in-group aggression. This inner contradiction is inherent in every autocratic situation and is the basis of the higher tension level.

An Atmosphere Affecting Individual Levels of Conduct

One can represent the amount of dominating behavior of a member of an aggressive autocratic group and a member of a democratic group. After an equality at the first meeting the conduct of the individuals changed in line with the social atmosphere. The two members were changed from one group to the other after the ninth meeting. The fact that after transfer each member rapidly displayed the level of conduct shown by the other member before change, indicates that the strength and the gradient of the resultant force field corresponding to the two atmospheres was approximately the same for both individuals.

Scapegoating and the Interdependence of Levels of Conduct

Data regarding the amount of dominance given and received by individual members of an aggressive autocratic group can serve as an illustration for several general points concerning quasi-stationary processes.

Levels of Received Hostility as Equilibria: It is appropriate to consider such a *passive* property as "being attacked" as a quasi-stationary equilibrium. The amount of aggression received depends partly on the degree to which the individual provokes or invites aggression and the way he fights or does not fight back. Other factors are the aggressiveness of the other members, the social atmosphere, etc. On the whole then, the constellation is the same as in the forces in other cases of equilibrium: the forces always depend on the characteristics of the group or the individual in question and on his relation to the surroundings.

Quitting and the Range of the Central Force Field: Scapegoat B quits membership in the club on the sixth day, scapegoat C on the ninth day. These happenings are examples of the general fact that a sufficiently large change of the level of equilibrium leads to a basic change in the character of the total situation: too much received dominance makes the member leave.

One may be tempted to represent the tendency of the individual to leave the club after too much received hostility by means of a central force field with a definite range beyond which the resultant forces are directed away from the level of equilibrium. Such a representation could not indicate, however, that the individual leaves the club since the co-ordinates of the phase space refer only to time and to the amount of received dominance. To represent this fact one has either to refer to the force constellation in the actual social field or to introduce the degree of "eagerness to belong to the club" as a third dimension of the phase space.

Interaction and Circular Causal Processes: The scapegoats A and B who received much dominating behavior themselves showed much dominating behavior. This indicates a close relation between being attacked and attacking. This relation has the character of a circular causal process: the attack of A against B increases B's readiness to attack; the resultant attacks of B raise A's readiness, etc. This would lead to a continuous heightening of the level of equilibrium for A, for B, and for the group as a whole. This holds, however, only within certain limits: if the attack of A is successful B might give in (3). This is another example of the fact that the change of a social process which results from the change of the force field determining the level of equilibrium may in itself effect the total situation in the direction of a further change of the force field. This example can, of course, be regarded as a case of non-equilibrium which corresponds to a constellation of forces away from the present level.

The Creation of Permanent Changes

In discussing the means of bringing about a desired state of affairs one should not think in terms of the "goal to be reached" but rather in terms of a change "from the present level to the desired one." The discussion thus far implies that a planned change consists of transplanting the force field corresponding to an equilibrium at the beginning level by a force field having its equilibrium at the desired level. It should be emphasized that the total force field has to be changed at least in the area between them.

The techniques of changing a force field cannot be fully deduced from the representation in the phase space. To change the level of velocity of a river its bed has to be narrowed down or widened, rectified, cleared from rocks, etc. To decide how best to bring about such an actual change, it does not suffice to consider one property. The total circumstances have to be examined. For changing a social equilibrium, too, one has to consider the total social field: the groups and subgroups involved, their relations, their value systems, etc. The constellation of the social field as a whole has to be studied and so reorganized that social events flow differently. The analysis by way of phase space indicates more what type of effect has to be accomplished than how this can be achieved.

The use of a phase space for treating a social equilibrium makes it necessary to clarify certain technical questions of analysis, such as the relation between the strength of the opposing forces at a given level of the process, the structure of the force field inside and outside of the neighbouring range, the formal conditions of fluctuation and of individual differences, the relation between forces and capacities, and the relation between forces and tension.

This technical analysis makes it possible to formulate in a more exact way problems of planned social changes and of resistance to change. It permits general statements concerning some aspects of the problem of selecting specific objectives in bringing about change, concerning different methods of bringing about the same amount of change, and concerning differences in the secondary effects of these methods. A theory emerges that one of the causes of resistance to change lies in the relation between the individual and the value of group standards. This theory permits conclusions concerning the resistance of certain types of social equilibria to change, the unfreezing, moving, and freezing of a level, and the effectiveness of group procedures for changing attitudes or conduct.

The analytic tools used are equally applicable to cultural, economic, sociological and psychological aspects of group life. They fit a great variety of processes such as production levels of a factory, a work-team and an individual worker; changes of abilities of an individual and of capacities of a country; group standards with and without cultural value; activities of one group and the interaction between groups, between individuals, and between individuals and groups. The analysis concedes equal reality to all aspects of group life and to social units of all sizes. The application depends upon the structural properties of the process and of the total situation in which it takes place.

Our consideration of quasi-stationary equilibrium has been based on analytic concepts which, within the realm of social sciences, have emerged first in psychology. The concepts of a psychological force, of tension, of conflicts as equilibria of forces, of force fields and of inducing fields, have slowly widened their range of application from the realm of individual psychology into the realm of processes and events which had been the domain of sociology and cultural anthropology. From what I have been able to learn recently about the treatment of equilibria by mathematical economics, I am convinced that this treatment, although having a different origin and being based perhaps on a different philosophy, is also fully compatible with our considerations.

The ease of quantitatively measuring economic data on the one hand, and the disturbing qualitative richness of psychological and cultural events on the other has tended to keep the methods of investigating these areas separated. Perhaps, this situation has driven some mathematical economists into an attempt to develop an economics without people and without culture, much in the way that some mathematically inclined psychologists have tried to develop a theory of learning without organisms (12). It is possible, however, to leave the philosophical interpretation in abeyance and to regard the equations of mathematical economics as a treatment of certain aspects, of events which are methodologically similar to our treatment of certain aspects of social processes by way of phase spaces; in both cases one has to realize that for prediction it is necessary to refer finally to the total social field with all its essential properties. If one is conscious of the limitation of the separate analytic treatment of certain aspects of the social field, this treatment is a useful and indeed necessary step.

The analytic tools of mathematical economics should be of great help for carrying through the task of measuring social forces, a task which thus far has been accomplished only in a limited area of individual psychology (6). This task implies three steps; a sufficient development of analytical concepts and theories concerning social forces, their quantification in principle through equations, and measuring concrete cases. It seems that the first step in the treatment of group life has sufficiently progressed to permit a collaboration with the various branches of the social sciences for the second and third task.

For economics the fusion implies the possibility of taking into account the cultural and psychological properties of the population involved and, therefore, of improving greatly the ability of analyzing concrete cases and making correct predictions. Economics may have to be ready to complicate the analytic procedures at certain points; particularly, it will have to recognize the cognitive problems mentioned above in the discussion of the three step procedure.

The fusion of the social sciences will make accessible to economics the main advantages which the experimental procedure offers for testing theories and for developing new insight. The combination of experimental and mathematical procedures has been the main vehicle for the integration of the study of light, of electricity, and of the other branches of physical science. The same combination seems to be destined to make the integration of the social sciences a reality.

References

1. Allport, G. W. Catharsis and the reduction of prejudice. In Problems of re-education. *J. of Soc. Issues*, August 1945, 3–10.
2. Barker, R., Dembo, T., and Lewin, K. Frustration and regression: an experiment with young children. *Studies in topological and vector psychology II.* Univ. of Iowa Press, 1941.
3. Bateson, G. *Naven.* Cambridge Univ. Press, 1936.
4. Bavelas, A. Morale and the training of leaders. In *Civilian morale* (Watson, Ed.) Houghton Mifflin, 1942.
5. Bavelas, A. Unpublished manuscript.
6. Cartwright, D., and Festinger, L. A quantitative theory of decision. *Psychol. Rev.,,* 1943, 50, 595/n-/621.
7. Cassirer, E. *Substance and function.* (Tr. by W. C. and M. C. Swab) Chicago and London: Open Court, 1923.
8. Hicks, J. R. *Value and capital.* Oxford: Clarendon Press, 1939.
9. Klisurich, D. Concepts and sanctions related to milk. Unpublished Master's Thesis deposited in the Library of the State Univ. of Iowa, 1944.
10. Kohler, W. *The place of value in a world of fact.* New York: Liveright, 1938.
11. Lange, O. *Price flexibility and employment.* Univ. of Chicago Press, 1945.
12. Leeper, R. W. *Lewin's topological and vector psychology.* Eugene, Oregon: Univ. of Oregon Press, 1943.
13. Lewin, K. *A dynamic theory of personality.* (Tr. by D. Adams and K. Zener). New York: McGraw-Hill, 1935.

14. Lewin, K. The conceptual representation and the measurement of psychological forces. *Contributions to psychological theory*, Vol. I, No. 4. Duke Univ. Press, 1938.
15. Lewin, K. Field theory of learning. In *The psychology of learning* (H. B. Nelson, Ed.). Forty-first yearbook of the Nat. Society for the Study of Education, Part II. Bloomington, Ill: Public School Publishing Co., 1942.
16. Lewin, K. Forces behind food habits and methods of change. *Bulletin of the National Research Council*, 1943, *108*, 35–65.
17. Lewin, K. Action research and minority problems. *J. of Soc. Issues*, 1946, *2*.
18. Lewin, K., Dembo, T., Festinger, L., and Sears, P. Level of aspiration. In *Personality and the behavior disorders*, Vol I. (J. M. Hunt, Ed.). New York: Ronald Press, 1944.
19. Lewin, K., and Grabbe, P. (Eds.). Problems of re-education. *J. of Soc. Issues*, August, 1945.
20. Lewin, K., Lippitt, R., and White, R. Patterns of aggressive behavior in experimentally created "social climates." *J. of Soc. Psychol.,*, 1939, *10*, 271–299.
21. Lippitt, R. An experimental study of authoritarian and democratic group atmospheres. *Studies in topological and vector psychology* I, Univ. of Iowa Press, 1940.
22. Lippitt, R, and White, R. Unpublished manuscript reported by White at 1938 meetings of the American Psychological Association.
23. Lippitt, R., and White, R. The "social climate" of children's groups. In *Child behavior and development* (R. Barker, J. Kounin, and B. Wright, Eds.). New York: McGraw-Hill, 1943.
24. Maier, N. *Psychology in industry*. Houghton Mifflin, 1946.
25. Radke, M., and Klisurich, D. Experiments in changing food habits. Unpublished manuscript.
26. Redl, F. Clinical group work with children. In *Group work and the social scene today*. New York: Association Press, 1943.
27. Roethlisberger, F. J., and Dickson, W. J. *Management and the worker*. Cambridge: Harvard Univ. Press, 1939.
28. Samuelson, P. A. The stability of equilibrium: linear and non-linear systems. *Econometrica*, 1942, *10*, 1-25.
29. Tolman, E. C. The determiners of behavior at a choice point. *Psychol. Rev.,*, 1938, *45*, 1–41.
30. Von Neumann, J., and Morgenstern, O. *Theory of games and economic behavior*. Princeton Univ. Press, 1944.

Emotional Catharsis and Re-Education in the Neuroses with the Help of Group Methods

MAXWELL JONES, M. D.

Maxwell Jones is not customarily included in the group literature. This seems inappropriate since his work on developing "therapeutic communities" based on social system ideas had a major influence on the development of group-based intensive programming patterns throughout the 1960s and 1970s. Jones began his interest in therapeutic communities in the United Kingdom (The Therapeutic Community: A New Treatment Method in Psychiatry. New York: Basic Books, 1953). He then became Consultant to the Fort Logan Mental Health Center in Denver during the 1970s when it was in the forefront of such developments in America. This format has been ambivalently received by the larger mental health professional community, the principal concern being an excessive diffusion of clinical responsibility. The direct confrontation of here-and-now behavior with attendant high affect did not sit well with a more conservative and cognitive tradition. Jones addressed the issue squarely: "The traditional attitudes which may be relevant in a surgical ward or operating theatre are harmful rather than helpful when we consider the psychological and social factors which represent such a large part of psychiatry"(p.ii) (Margolis PM: Patient Power. Springfield, IL: Charles C Thomas, 1973).

This is an early paper that appeared shortly after World War II at the same time that Day Hospital programs were being developed by Ewen Cameron in Montreal and Joshua Bierer in London. While not directly quoting Moreno, Jones applies many of the principles of psychodrama, including a secretary with acting experience. In this paper, one can sense the directness of Jones's approach and his integration of cognitive, affective, and action components. The paper was read at the Psychiatric Section of the Royal Society of Medicine on February 11, 1947. Note Jone's avoidance of the formality that was at the time the norm for this type of presentation. The basic ingredients of a therapeutic community are evident but not specifically labelled as such.
—Editor

Jones M: Emotional catharsis and re-education in the neuroses with the help of group methods. *British Journal of Medical Psychology* 21:104–110, 1948.

Group methods of treatment are still too undeveloped to have evolved any specific treatment techniques. Experimentation must proceed for years before the various schools of thought have produced serious arguments to support their claims. It seems to me that no good purpose would be served by reviewing the present trends in group treatment when they are in such a state of flux—I would prefer to describe to you the story of a group of six men at present under treatment at Sutton Emergency Hospital and let you form your own judgements regarding the value, disadvantages, and possible dangers of this form of treatment. For these reasons I shall not here refer to the large volume of publications on Group Treatment.

First let us consider the setting. The group meets daily for an hour, 10–11 a.m., in my consulting room, which is a large room with an alcove leading to a communicating door and to the secretary's office. This arrangement is convenient for our impromptu acting as will be described later. The group includes the six male patients, myself, usually another psychiatrist in training, and two girls with experience in acting—one is a nurse, and the other a secretary. We sit around in a rough circle in an entirely informal way.

Now as to procedure—this follows no fixed pattern and we are always experimenting with new methods. Generally, however, we start the hour by free discussion of any material raised by the patients; the men are encouraged to talk about their emotional problems, and it is certainly advantageous to the group, if the main aspects of the clinical histories of each patient becomes known at an early date. When the group has achieved a certain degree of integrity, after say 10 hours (2 weeks), we like to start impromptu acting. At the moment we use the acting with two main objects in view: Re-education and Catharsis.

Re-education: To re-create social situations which have caused minor emotional difficulties to patients, and act them out; then to discuss subjective and objective reactions by the members of the group, and attempt to modify the patient's attitude, or at least indicate a more desirable pattern of behaviour, when faced by the social situation in question. The same difficulty is then acted out again, discussed further, and so on until the situation can be faced more adequately by the individual.

Catharsis: To re-enact a strong emotional experience by placing the patient in a situation which resembles the original one, and asking him to re-live the experience if possible. This cathartic technique is obviously more difficult to apply than the previous one; again the group discusses the scene enacted, and by explanation and emotional support, aims at strengthening the patient's ego, so that the situation can no longer overwhelm him.

The present group of male patients started eight weeks ago. The group was chosen at random, in that I simply formed a group comprising all of the patients I had under my care in the wards at that time. There were originally ten men but the number is now reduced to six—one schizophrenic was put on insulin coma treatment, and another schizophrenic attended the group meetings so irregularly that he was taken out of the group. Two other patients who had been members of my previous group were well enough to leave hospital shortly after the present group was formed. The remaining six patients I shall describe briefly, and try at the same time to indicate how their problems are handled and influenced by the group.

******

Only two of the six patient stories are included.

******

Parsons, a red-faced startled looking man aged 26 has an I.Q. of 100. He has never had much confidence in himself, and always blushed fairly readily. He was an errand boy before conscription, and was used to a good deal of ragging at his place of work. He was none too happy in the Army, but managed fairly well until 1941 when, during the siege of Malta, he began to get excessively self-conscious. He blushed far more than ever before, and was convinced that his face portrayed terror, so that everyone knew that he was a coward. He could not bear to go to a barber's, and see his face in the mirror. Since de-mobilization in June 1946 he has felt quite incapable of meeting people, has been almost completely isolated, and made no attempt to find work. He was very ill at ease in the group at first, and showed no inclination to discuss his case. We tried acting out social situations, e.g., that he was one of three patients invited to a tea party by a local woman (played by the nurse). At such a tea-party he sat rigidly staring in front of him, his red face making his protuberant eyes startlingly prominent; discussion of his performance and encouragement by the group seemed to help very little. The nurses' dancing class taught him to dance, but at the routine ward socials he refused to take part. We tried staging a barber's shop in my consulting room, and another patient who was a barber gave him a real haircut in front of a large mirror, with the rest of the group apparently awaiting their turn; but only the familiar inhibition resulted, and we seemed to be no further on after having discussed this scene. But on going over the facts leading up to the acute stage of his illness for a second time, it appeared that his increased self-consciousness dated from two weeks before his first embarrassment in a barber's shop. We now acted out the following scene based on his story. The scene was a Bofor gun-site in Malta: we made a gun-pit by using a corner of the room and a desk and table. Three other patients were on the gun and Hutchins (the ex-Bomb Disposal sergeant) looked after the sound. Parsons was recording on the 'phone just below the gun—20 miles, 10 miles, 5 miles, then suddenly one of the gun team shouted 'there they are.' The gun team swung their Bofor round so that the barrel pointed just over Parsons's head. Hutchins produced his deafening gun explosion, and Parsons dropped to the ground.

(In Malta he had had both ear-drums ruptured by the blast, as the gun was fired a few feet from his head; gasping for breath, with tears streaming from his eyes, he had lain motionless for ten minutes anticipating death.) When, in the acting out, the 'all clear' sounded, Parsons got up looking really dazed, and started to walk with an unsteady gait; the gun team laughed loudly, and Parsons without a word made for the bed in my office and lay down. As he lay on the examination couch, he was told to keep his eyes closed, and continue re-living the situation. He said that in Malta he had felt dazed, overwhelmed, alone, and a coward. He had slowly regained some of his composure during the next few days, but the above episode was never mentioned by his mates. He realized for the first time that the startled face he saw in the barber's mirror two weeks later was to him a coward's face, and it was his own.

The above incident was acted out with intense emotion by Parsons, and was frighteningly real. It was all the more striking as, up to now, Parsons had been almost completely inhibited in talking with the group. Also, ether abreaction had been attempted with no release of emotion. The group now discussed the incident, expressed the view that the gun team's laughter was an expression of relief when the 'all clear' sounded, and they realized Parsons was not killed or seriously injured. They saw no rational grounds for Parsons's feeling of cowardice, and discussed his anxiety that fear was permanently stamped on his features. As the presence of other people immediately evoked this combination of self-consciousness and fear we now returned to acting out social situations which would evoke this response. Progress was slow but definite, and his face actually began to look different as his tension relaxed and he could think and move with freedom.

Davies, aged 31, a pale lean miserable looking man, who always seems to be on the point of running away from the group. He is married, and has three children, but when the Psychiatric Social Worker visited the home, conditions were found to be extremely bad. His intelligence is average (Progressive Matrices: 54th percentile). Although a bricklayer by trade, he has done only occasional short periods of work since being discharged from the Army in January 1942 with a neurosis. He was too dispirited to apply for a pension, or to seek help from any social agency. His failure to get even public assistance was more the result of apathy than pride. When they were near to starving he forced himself to work for a short time, but always felt unwanted by his mates, and gave up his work.

Davies came from an unhappy home, was in terror of his father, and never learnt to make friends. When he was at school a friend told his father that if he persisted in treating his son so brutally, the son would inevitably turn on him one day; to this the father replied: 'I'll break his bloody spirit first,' and Davies thinks he did just that. The Army accentuated the old feeling of helplessness and terror which he had had in childhood, and he preferred the 'shelter' of the detention camp to the dangers of his unit! His attitude to the group was part apathy and part open hostility. He took longer than any other member to become absorbed by the group. In individual interviews he was tense and hostile, and I felt we had reached an impasse. On 8 January 1947 he got drunk when on pass from hospital, and on returning to the ward at 11:00 p.m. he attacked his ward mates verbally, telling them how they'd ignored and slighted him, that in future he was going to get tough and so on. The next day he discussed the episode in the group, and found that the group approved of this self-assertion. He appeared to be much better for a few days and then (surprisingly) disappeared—he had gone home (100 miles distant) and stayed away for almost a week. On return to the group the old hostility was there, and Davies made no attempt to explain his disappearance, and change of attitude. The group was certainly disheartened and resentful, and a marked split occurred. Resentment, normally directed towards me and worked out by the group as part of an individual's attitude towards authority or whatever it might be, was now, for example, directed towards the presence of the two girls. Davies was joined by Parsons, and because of their defeatist attitudes, they were resented by the group, which was sensitive to the idea of failure. The need to *do* something was strong, although there was no clear idea as to what was needed. To meet this mood the two girls were asked to absent themselves from the next meeting, and all visitors to the group were barred. The group now concentrated on Davies, who luckily agreed to talk about his difficulties at work and socially. His lifelong struggle against isolation, his unwillingness to accept help, his set-back in the Army, and feeling that he was overwhelmed by circumstances since discharge were all gone into. A change of attitude occurred, and Davies began to feel that he might be helped. Needless to say the challenge immediately reunited the group, and without exception they wanted the two girls back in the meetings. Davies and Parsons now showed much more willingness to act out embarrassing situations, and began to show real improvement. Davies even managed to show some anger when an imaginary row with his wife was created. The scene showed Davies returning home on week-end pass a day later than was arranged. His wife (acted by the secretary) was not satisfied by his explanation that he'd missed the last train, and her cross-examination and reproaches made him flush and get angry. He said to his wife: 'Have you ever known me to apologize for anything?' and in the discussion afterwards explained that his wife never did question or reproach him. The group stressed the advantages of an occasional row, which they thought much preferable to the complete suppression of all hostility which Davies imposed upon himself.

I have attempted to give some idea of the movement that occurs in a group. It will be apparent that almost any form of psychotherapy can be adapted and introduced into group therapy technique: moreover, the personality of the psychiatrist and his own beliefs together with the selection of the patients forming the group, will probably for some time to come be important factors in the development and direction of the group. What I have described is a purely experimental group. I purposely avoided selecting patients and took what was virtually a random sample. As a group they were much less intelligent than previous groups I have selected (four of the six were below the 65th percentile), and much more mixed from the clinical standpoint: this may explain why there has been less tendency to sit and discuss, and much more action (acting out) than in previous groups. Certainly acting 'loosens up' the group, and is quite a good way of opening the treatment hour. Catharsis in the group is, I think, valuable therapeutically, but difficult to achieve; it would be interesting to contrast this technique with ether abreaction and alcoholic release, but space does not permit. It is clear, however, that in catharsis in the group, consciousness is fully retained, which is not the case with ether abreaction; for this reason the group catharsis may give the patient more insight into his problem. Also, the presence of the other members of the group representing reality or public opinion may have therapeutic advantages.

The meetings themselves represent a social situation, and difficulties of social adaptation which may easily be lost sight of in individual interviews are shown up in sharp relief, particularly when the individual's own particular social difficulties are re-enacted.

Finally, I want to stress that our small group of six is always being studied in relation to the larger social life of the ward. We believe that education should form an important part of the treatment of most neurotics. In practice the whole ward of seventy male patients, with nurses and doctors meet every morning, 9–10 a.m., and once a week the Psychiatric Social Worker, the vocational psychologist, and the Disablement Rehabilitation Officer attend. The aim of these meetings is primarily educational: to teach the men to think about their emotional problems, and other people's viewpoints besides their own, to know what help psychiatry can offer, and where to turn for such help, to understand the workings of the Ministry of Labour, particularly from the viewpoint of the disabled man, and to grasp the rudiments of vocational guidance and selection. To help in achieving these objectives we try to make problems as live and realistic as possible. The D.R.O.'s weekly talk is preceded by a film on training for farmwork, bricklaying, engineering and so on. The function of the P.S.W. is clarified by creating a mock out-patient session with a nurse playing the part of a patient, and the doctor playing his proper role. The case is usually based on a true problem presenting some difficult social situation which calls for a social visit. The theme is elaborated in front of the patients, and when the interview terminates the P.S.W. is called in and asked to make her visit. The P.S.W. then describes to the patients what her findings actually were and how in collaboration with the psychiatrist the situation was dealt with. The whole problem is then discussed by the group.

The patients themselves write and produce a weekly play based on a social problem which they feel to be important; the play presents the problem but leaves it unanswered, and it is in the group discussion after the play that the main value of meetings becomes apparent. This group projection technique has been described elsewhere (Jones, 1944) as has the more detailed description of the ward social organization (Jones, 1946).

References

Jones, Maxwell (1944). Group treatment with particular reference to group projection methods. *Amer. J. Psychiat. 101*, 292.

Jones, Maxwell (1946). Rehabilitation of Forces neurosis patients to civilian life. *Brit. Med. J. 1*, 533.

The Unique Social Climate Experienced in Group Psychotherapy

RUDOLPH DREIKURS, M.D.
Chicago Medical College

Rudolph Dreikurs (1897–1972) worked with Alfred Adler in Vienna where an extensive system of child guidance clinics had been established during the 1920s to deal with the social disruptions following the First World War. Adler maintained that the influence of social and political pressures was underestimated in the psychoanalytic approach. This had led to a split with Freud. The egalitarian atmosphere of group therapy was seen as the natural environment for psychotherapy. In the group such interpersonal issues as inferiority over social status, discrimination, and isolation could be effectively addressed. In this paper, democratic social concepts are applied directly to therapeutic technique.

Dreikurs settled in Chicago in the 1937 and became the leading proponent of Adlerian ideas in America. This work was focused more on educational settings and the training of mental health workers and social service personnel than in more formal treatment programs. Dreikurs collaborated with Rogers' Counseling Center at the University of Chicago in some early psychotherapy research. He is also credited with being the first to use group psychotherapy in private practice. Raymond Corsini, represented elsewhere in this volume, was also a student of Dreikurs. Other Adlerian contributors to the American group literature include Helene Papanek and Asya Kadis.

Dreikurs was President of the American Society of Group Psychotherapy and Psychodrama; this paper was presented at their ninth Annual Conference in New York, February 17, 1951. —Editor

Dreikurs R: The unique social climate experienced in group psychotherapy. *Group Psychotherapy* 3:292-299, 1951.

The process of group-psychotherapy can be viewed from three aspects. Characteristic dynamics which operate in any form of group-psychotherapy and make it an effective tool for influencing individuals, can be observed on three levels: within the patient, between the members of the group and within the total group situation. There is a constant interaction between these three dynamic processes; yet they can be distinguished and separated in their significance. The analytic approach emphasizes the dynamics operating with the patient. Psychodrama and sociodrama are more concerned with the second aspect—the interaction between patients and sub-groups taking place in the total situation of the group in therapy.

The third aspect, namely the characteristic and unique group formation, is often neglected. It is the purpose of this paper to draw the attention to the need for clarification, for exploration, analysis and proper evaluation of the total situation in which the group operates, which distinguishes it from other group situations.

Let us review briefly the dynamics which we recognize as therapeutic agents within the patient and between the members of the group. In group psychotherapy the individual patient is observed in his attitude and behaviour to others. Faulty attitudes are recognized and dealt with through the group procedure. Some assume that the group provides an outlet for aggression, permitting the abreaction of hostility, the formation of new identifications and ego satisfactions. Others see the therapeutic effect in new concepts which the patient develops about himself in regard to others, in his learning to cooperate, to become willing and able to accept the give and take necessary for social living, to reconsider his approaches which he had developed toward social interaction, the goals he had set for himself as an idea of security. Others again may see in the group the opportunity for the patient to develop his spontaneity, to free himself from the distance in which he had kept himself previously. This is not the place to analyze whether these various frames of reference describe the same process from various angles or whether they present a distinctly different type of dynamics. They all have in common their concern with psychological processes occurring within the patient in group-psychotherapy.

Less variety of opinions exists in the second aspect of inter-group relationships. The psychoanalytic approach neglects this aspect almost deliberately, as all social relationships are considered the result and consequence of "intra"-personal dynamics. It is the contribution of Moreno to have pointed out the dynamics which operate between the various members of the group. Since then we have learned to deal in group-psychotherapy directly with the group medium, structuring inter-group relationships for the purpose of helping the individual patient. So far, there is relatively little difference of opinion about the significance, the procedure and the evaluation of inter-group dynamics, regardless of the theoretical frame of reference in which these processes are viewed. The recognition of the group structure and its deliberate manipulation permits each member to warm up, to come closer to the others, and to find his place in the group.

It is the totality of the group which we want to examine here, and which in our opinion deserves more attention on the part of group-psychotherapists. Each group has an organization. It is more than the sum-total of all its members and sub-groups. It has its own dynamics, as it is a unique configuration, a Gestalt. Any group is characterized by its specific social climate. This term is widely used to characterize various group settings, particularly in education. Most discussion on the social climate in classrooms is centred around the person of the leader, the teacher. Moreno[1] found characteristic differences in various group structures, be they authoritarian, democratic or of the laissez-faire type. They appear to depend on the attitude of the group leader. There can be no doubt that the group leader is responsible for the type of relationship which exists in the group. For this reason we will have to focus later upon the role of the therapist in establishing and maintaining the group atmosphere which we may recognize as being most desirable for effective group-psychotherapy. But first we must clarify some of the dynamics operating in a therapeutic group.

It seems that one does not do justice to the significance of any group, particularly a therapy group, unless one recognizes that each group is identified by the values which it represents and with which it affects each of its members. Our therapy groups are a natural testing ground for observation and experimentation with the phenomenon of group values. Relatively few people realize that by joining a group they are effected by values which the group establishes, unnoticed by most. We have to distinguish values from morals. Morals, expressing social conventions, do not vary to a large extent throughout our present American culture. But as most people belong to a variety of groups, their values are rather confused, because the various groups to which they belong do not engender the same value systems. The values characteristic for any family group differs not only from those in any other family, but also from those characteristic for each job situation. Again, different values characterize the church group to which the individual may belong, his political association or club activities. The same moral concepts permeate all of them. Decent behaviour is considered the same way in all of them. But value is different from general conventional behaviour. It sets a yardstick for superior-inferior orientation. The term value implies a quantitative and qualitative judgment; certain qualities provide higher or lower social status and desirability. The degree to which an individual possesses these qualities are measured quantitatively, while the evaluation of good and adverse qualities implies a qualitative judgment. The differences in group judgment give any individual with his personal qualities a different status in the various groups to which he belongs. The child is judged differently at home, in school, amongst his friends and again on the ball-team. The same quality which gives him a high status in one group may place him low in another.

If we regard the therapeutic group as a value promoting agent, we may come to a formulation of the values which are best suited for the therapeutic process This would provide us with a yardstick to measure various therapy groups, and permit us to consider deliberate methods to obtain the desirable group atmosphere or social climate conducive for therapeutic values.

At the present time we find a great variety of methods and group structures in the reports of group-psychotherapists. It may be a lecture and classroom situation, an analytic group session, a discussion or a psychodramatic action-group. It is obvious that the social climate in these various therapy groups is different. However, we witness a tendency away from an autocratic didactic group-therapy to a more permissive group organization, which today characterizes most forms of group-psychotherapy. It may be difficult, therefore, to recognize a common denominator, distinguishing all therapeutic groups from other forms of groups. Nevertheless, an analysis of the social climate found in most therapeutic groups may provide us with the recognition of such characteristic elements.

It is obvious that the permissive group atmosphere is the most distinctive group organization in the field. Nowhere else in our society can an individual fully behave as he wishes without losing status. For this reason our examination should start with this form of group-psychotherapy. Its characteristic significance will be interpreted differently by a therapist who is mostly concerned with the intra-personal dynamics of each member, differently by one who is considering the inter-personal group relationships, and again different by one who examines the total group climate with its characteristic values.

For an analyst the permissive group situation may provide an outlet for aggression without the threat of punishment, so that a new homeostasis may be established, more suitable for a stable emotional equilibrium. In this way the attitude of the individual to others and to social living may be improved, his castration fears diminished, his defensiveness and inner tensions eliminated. For the therapist concerned with group dynamics, the permissive group situation permits a closer integration of each individual, a better mutual understanding, greater friendliness and warmth and consequent increased cooperation. While the analyst tries to free the patient from his inner tensions, the socially oriented therapist tries to remove group tensions, affecting and improving thereby the attitudes and emotional reactions of each individual member.

Looking at the total group situation, other aspects become apparent as distinguishing the permissive therapy group from other groups. The most outstanding aspect seems to be the fact that in this group each member has his place regardless of his personal qualities, his deficiencies and assets. Nowhere else is this true in our society. In any other field of action, the individual is constantly judged according to his abilities and deficiencies, his accomplishments or mistakes. Not so here. One may say that the values which make a person higher or lower anywhere else in society, are discarded here. But no group can exist without definite values. For this reason, the therapy group cannot be identified by its lack of otherwise existing values, but only by the values which it tacitly implies itself. Such values may be recognized if we examine the factors which give each member status in the group. The first and most obvious is the "existence" of the member. Mere regular participation provides him with status. Only if he does not come regularly does he lose status. This is of extreme importance. It implies that full value is granted to each member by his mere existence, regardless of what he is or what he is doing, regardless of personal qualities, achievements or deficiencies. In this regard, the social climate of the group resembles a non-competitive, homogeneous primitive group, where the full worth of each member is taken for granted, merely by his being a part of the group.

Another criterion of positive value is the ability of the member to reveal himself as he really is. Holding back his true emotions, covering up his intentions and hostilities, restraining himself and putting up a front are of low esteem in the therapy group, while they constitute highly valued qualities anywhere else. This stimulates each member to display himself just as a human being, without any pretence or shame.

That does not mean that such behaviour is easy for anyone raised in our present cultural atmosphere. But these values for which the group stands present an intrinsic part of the therapeutic process, particularly if we recognize the patient's fears for his status, his inferiority feeling, his sense of inadequacy and failure, his over-concern with his faults and deficiencies as the causes for his tensions, anxieties and maladjustment. As he learns to accept the values operating in the therapy group, his concepts change, permitting a solution of his emotional problems. Psychotherapy in general leads in the direction of self-confidence, self-respect, certainty of one's social status and its concomitant emotional and action behaviour. In individual therapy the therapeutic influence is limited to the relationship with one person, the therapist, and to the verbal expression of new and therapeutically effective values. In contrast group-psychotherapy provides a much more convincing and impressive experience. Here the patient "learns" by actual experience, not merely on the verbal level. For this reason group-psychotherapy is particularly effective for very disturbed patients who often cannot be reached at all through an individual approach. This is true, for example in cases of severe compulsion neurotics, psychotics and particularly for psychopathic personalities. The latter category is characterized by its defiance of the values accepted within society at large. It is almost impossible to reach such a person individually as the therapist and the patient talk a different language and have concepts and values which are incompatible. The value-producing group gives the patient an opportunity to be affected directly by new values, often without his own awareness that his mere association and existence subjects him to new values which he cannot escape. He discovers that he has value in the eyes of others just because he is a human being, while his previous social contacts made him believe that he never can belong in the adult society because of his deficiencies and faults. The psychotic can be drawn into a close human relationship which may affect and disrupt his isolation within his own "private logic" so that he again can share his thinking and his concepts with others. As soon as he establishes that, the psychotic state is fundamentally dissolved.

This emphasis on a person's unquestionable status in the group, without regard to quality and achievement, seems to characterize all the different approaches and forms of group-psychotherapy. It is equally evident in a completely permissive activity group, in a non-directive activity group, in a psychodramatic action group, in a discussion or in an analytic group and even in some form of didactic groups, provided that the members of the group participate in the program and are not limited to passive listening. In each case an attitude of mutual understanding and respect develops, giving each member the realization of his status as an equal. In almost all cases the admission to the group already represents a fundamental deviation from any other social participation. Admission to a social group is usually based on some kind of accomplishment or asset. Most groups accept as a member only one who comes up to the standards they have set for themselves or who fulfils their value requirements. The child is accepted only in a class after he fulfils the age and scholastic requirements. He has a chance for participating in a social or athletic group only on the strength of his assets. This is equally true for adults. Only in therapeutic groups is the qualification for admission overtly based on some recognized and admitted deficiency. Alcoholics Anonymous, for example, will not accept anyone unless he admits to being an alcoholic. Then he can request understanding and help. One realizes immediately the profound change in the value system whereby a defect which normally provides extreme social degradation becomes a social asset. This is equally true for children who realize their social ostracism due to their unmanageable anti-social behaviour and suddenly find themselves "privileged" to participate in a specially interesting group activity where they receive special attention and respect. Similarly, the adult patient who previously had been ashamed of his shortcomings and deficiencies, suddenly finds himself accepted by others on the strength of these traits which previously had been only a source of social embarrassment.

This unique social climate characteristic for group-psychotherapy does not only explain some of the therapeutically effective dynamics of this form of therapy; it also accounts for the tremendous fascination which it has provoked in our population. The practice of group-therapy not only enjoys an increasing interest and popularity amongst therapists; it also transcends the limitations of psychiatric practice and invades the community at large, leading to experiments in group-psychotherapy on levels heretofore not within the realm of either psychiatry or psychotherapy. Schools, community agencies and churches have become interested and experiment with group-therapeutic procedure. All these tendencies can be well understood on the basis of the specific values provided by group therapy. Once it began within the field of psychiatry and psychotherapy a new social organization started within our culture, forming almost a foreign body in the value systems of our society. It must be said that religious experiences had provided similar group organizations which permitted each individual to have his full place as a "sinner," belonging to his congregation on the strength of his human frailty. But religion has lost for many its appeal, its efficiency of integrating the individual into the group. Fifty percent of all Americans do not belong to any church, and many who do, do it not for their religious faith, but for social and other reasons. It seems that many can no longer accept the authoritarian structure of a religious group and have not yet found a democratic and humanist religious organization which would fill the gap. Consequently, they live in emotional isolation, under constant tension of putting up a front so that nobody will know what they really are and how they feel. Otherwise, they would lose status, would endanger their prestige and might incur ridicule and contempt. Such a condition keeps everyone in fear and anxiety, in tension and uneasiness. People want to get out of this uncomfortable condition, but do not know how. The experiences of those who participated in group-therapy became an incentive for others who heard about it and sought it. This became a focal point for public demand. The rapid spread of group-psychotherapy is not only due to the increased recognition of this new medium by therapists and group leaders, but it also reflects public interest and request. The social values promulgated in group-therapy are in line with man's search for equality. At a time when society as a whole is rapidly moving toward democracy, the recognition of man's fundamental equality is of tantamount importance. In our competitive culture the full implication of human equality, irrespective of personal differences, qualities and achievements, is difficult to comprehend for most people. The spread of group-therapy implies more than assistance to individuals; it becomes a social factor in our culture which is a transition from an authoritarian to a democratic society. For this reason it is more than mere therapy, more than adult education. It is a living experience, a dynamic factor promoting a new social concept and fortifying cultural trends.

Group-psychotherapy has not only its effect on the patients participating in it, but also on the therapist and group leader himself. A social organization in which each member has the status of an equal is not only difficult to accept for patients who have been conditioned to other values; it presents also a tremendous challenge to the leader, even more so as the individual therapist, both by tradition and by the requirements of his function, is inclined to take on an authoritarian position. It is difficult for him to function as an equal amongst equals, and great confusion is created amongst group-therapists as to the best approach to a truly democratic performance. All the complexities characteristic for an era which tries to establish democracy without sufficient precedent and clear techniques is evident here. Many therapists confuse democracy with anarchy, laissez-faire. They try to restrain themselves from directing, from answering questions, as this would imply the assumption of an autocratic role. Many pride themselves that they never answer questions which come up during the therapeutic session; they rather let the members find their own answers. They think that this is democratic. Little do they realize that such procedure not only sets them up as an autocratic ruler who decides not to divulge what he knows, despite the request of the group; it also indicates a lack of respect if one refuses to participate and holds back some knowledge which everybody in the group knows he possesses. Such behaviour is artificial and contrary to the basic principle in group-therapy that each member, including the therapist, is himself without pretence and cover-up. It is not important what the leader does, but in which spirit he is doing it. He cannot deny that he is superior in knowledge. After all, he studied dynamics and knows more about them than the other members of the group. As long as he does not feel superior to them he can let them benefit from his information without setting himself up as an authority. The training of group-therapists would require the ability to function as an equal, to feel humble enough, to be just human without either feeling superior or inferior to anyone else in the group, irrespective of the individual differences which exist here as well as anywhere else in the world. Under these conditions the therapist can benefit from the group as much as any other member. Actually, every good group-therapist learns from this experience, which provides also for him a social climate which he cannot find anywhere else.

Note

1. *Sociometric Review*, Hudson, 1936; see also Moreno's *Sociometry, Experimental Method and the Science of Society*, Beacon House, 1951 (see the Laissez Faire Test, The Autocracy Test and the Democracy Test pp. 46–49).

YEARS OF
THEORETICAL EXPANSION
1952–1967

Notes on Psychoanalytic
Group Therapy:
II. Interpretation and Research

HENRY EZRIEL

The Tavistock Clinic, London

HENRY EZRIEL
The Tavistock Clinic, London

Henry Ezriel received his medical education in Vienna and worked at the Tavistock Clinic in London after his Northfield placement during the war. Under the directorship of J. D. Sutherland, the Tavistock responded to the expectations of the newly created National Health Service by modifying analytic ideas for use in groups so that a larger population could be treated. The Tavistock became the focal point of psychoanalytic work in Britain, an isolated position in a country where analytic practice was actively shunned by the psychiatric establishment.

Ezriel recognized the fact that common group tensions arise through the free associations of group members as they try to address interpersonal needs. This is closely associated with Bion's "basic assumption" states, as well as with Stock's idea of "group focal conflict" (both represented in this volume). The classical Tavistock therapeutic technique is one of relative therapist uninvolvement, and while the theory relates to group themes little use is made of the supportive and interactional features of a group.

This paper by Ezriel is one of a pair appearing in an issue of Psychiatry, *the journal of the Washington School of Psychiatry. The other paper was written by J. D. Sutherland (Notes on psychoanalytic group therapy: I. Therapy and training. Psychiatry 15:111–117, 1952) but unfortunately, space precluded including both in this volume. News of Dr. Sutherland's death was received as this book was going to press.* —Editor

Ezriel H: Notes on psychoanalytic group therapy: II. Interpretation and research. *Psychiatry 15*: 119–126, 1952.

In this paper, I shall outline some suggestions for experimental research which have emerged from our experience in developing what we consider to be a strictly psychoanalytic approach to group therapy. These possible lines of research apply just as much to individual psychoanalytic treatment, but it will become apparent in what follows to what extent they have been stimulated by work with groups.

"Here and Now" Interpretations

My starting point is the development which has taken place in the use of transference interpretations in recent years. A comparison of the technique of interpretation as practiced by various psychoanalysts shows considerable differences. Almost all analysts, however, feel that it is necessary to link up *in their interpretations* the patient's present unconscious conflicts with his past, especially with his infantile experiences.

With regard to this point, the application of psychoanalytic therapy to groups presented to us a certain problem: When interpreting the unconscious common group tension, to what infantile experiences are we to refer? A therapeutic group is an artifact created by us which has, of course, no common infantile history with which we could link the unconscious common group tension.

If it is not the tracing back of present behavior patterns to the patient's past, especially to his infantile history, what is it then that forms the content of such "here and now" interpretations as those mentioned by Dr. Sutherland in his present paper? This issue may become clearer if I reproduce for you the train of thought I had when I started work with groups in 1945.

Freud's original view was that the patient's unconscious *memories* of conflicts concerning persons of his infantile environment acted as a dynamic source for his thoughts during a session, his so-called free associations. Further, Freud considered that psychoanalysis is a method which enables us to make use of these thoughts in order to reconstruct the historical genesis of the patient's symptoms and that the putting before the patient of such historic reconstructions removes these symptoms. Freud himself altered this hypothesis when he discovered two facts which he described as "psychical reality" and "transference." By psychical reality[1] he meant the fact that the so-called "memories" of forgotten events uncovered in psychoanalysis were not necessarily memories of *real* events, but were often phantasies. Nevertheless they were psychologically as effective as if they had been memories of real events. This meant, however, that what the analyst uncovered was not an objective reproduction of the patient's past but *unconscious structures active in the present*, though formed in the past out of phantasies and out of correct or distorted memories of past events.

The second discovery which led to the modification of the genetic theory of psychoanalytic therapy was the phenomenon of transference[2]— that is, the fact that patients who had set out with their analyst to study the genesis of their symptoms by unravelling the history of their past experiences, very soon reproduced, or as Freud called it, "transferred" the conflicts they had had with the persons of their early environment to their therapist in the here and now of his consulting room. While patient and analyst had started their work like two friendly archaeologists trying to dig up the patient's past, they had now become two human beings interacting with one another in the here and now, and the analyst represented to the patient—according to the latter's unconscious phantasies—something different in each session, friend or foe, victim or persecutor, and many other things.

However, once analysts focused their attention on the transference phenomenon, it became apparent that transference is not something that gradually appears in the course of an analysis, but that it is active from the patient's first meeting with his therapist.

Since then the vast majority of analysts have—from the first session on—used the material produced by a patient partly as transference material—that is, as the expression of the patient's *attempts to establish* in the here and now certain kinds of relationships with the analyst—and partly as extra-transference material—that is, as communications in which the patient *reports* to the analyst his present-day or past relations with others (openly or in a disguised form) and which the analyst then tries to interpret as expressions of the patient's unconscious conflicts with others, especially with persons of his infantile environment. Many analysts who employ a more rigorous transference technique still feel a need to combine, in their transference interpretations, explanations of the here and now with comments on the patient's past.

However, it seemed to me a logical step to extend the transference hypothesis—to treat *all* material and hence to use it for here and now interpretations. This means that everything the patient says or does during a session—movements, gestures, phantasies, dreams, correct memories, and even deliberate lies—is considered as the *idiom* used by the patient to give expression to his need in that session for a specific relationship with his therapist. In other words, even the patient's reports to the analyst about his relations with others, past and present, are taken as attempts to *involve* the analyst as an active participant in relations which the patient entertains with his unconscious objects as they seem to exist here and now and with their representatives in external reality. If this extension of the transference hypothesis were justified it would, of course, solve our difficulty with groups which have no infantile history to which we could refer.

Let us return to Dr. Sutherland's example to test this assumption. When I am listening to patients' discussions, I always put to myself the question, What makes these patients say and do these things in front of me at this moment? I make my interpretive comments as soon as I think that I can distinguish in the material *three kinds of object relations*: one, an object relationship which they try to establish within the group, and in particular with myself, and which I should like to call the *required* relationship; another, which they feel they have to *avoid* in external reality, however much they may desire it; and a third, which depicts a *calamity* which the patient seems convinced would follow inevitably if he allowed himself to give in to his secret desire of entering into the avoided object relationship. This conviction could be explained by making the hypothesis that the calamity *does* occur in the psychical reality of his unconscious phantasies, his inner world where he does establish the avoided relationship.

A detailed description of the operational rules which would enable us to recognize these three object relationships in the manifest material will have to form the subject of a separate paper. I do wish, however, to point out here that in *individual* sessions the most important of these rules consists in abstracting the common features of the total material verbalized or enacted by the patient in that session. For instance, if a patient enumerates various experiences in each of which a man appears who is either "disappointing" or "weak" or "not as good as I had thought" or "a rogue," the common dynamic feature may be a relationship with a man towards whom he feels critical. In the same way we try to abstract from the total manifest material three common denominators which correspond to the three object relationships already described—namely, the *required*, the *avoided*, and the *calamitous*.

In a group an additional analytic task is the finding of the common group tension. This is done in a similar way to that just described in regard to the unconscious tension in individual sessions. That is to say, the total material produced by *all* the members of the group is treated as if it had been produced by *one* patient in an individual session, and the object relationships that correspond to the common group tension are abstracted as the common denominators of this material.

For instance, in Dr. Sutherland's example, the calamity the group feared was their expectation of his rejecting them or even being angry with them. It was this fear which made them avoid giving in to their secret and largely unconscious wish to break up the supposedly intimate relationship between Dr. Sutherland and the two observers. You can recognize what they avoided if you consider, in conjunction, Mr. B's dream in which he injured the two men behind the counter and Mr. A's wish to establish an intimate nickname relationship with Dr. Sutherland's substitute, the officer Sutherland, to the exclusion of the two observers. The relationship they required in order to be able to suppress their desire for the avoided relationship was to comfort themselves with an intimate Christian-name relationship among themselves. This ostensibly excluded Dr. Sutherland and the observers, but in fact implied that they put up with the intimacies between the analyst and the observers—intimacies which, as their remarks after the interpretation show, represented to them sexual intimacy between a couple who excluded them and made them jealous. Another outlet which helped them to suppress the avoided relationship in external reality was to give expression to it in their dreams.

In previous papers[3] I quoted case material in an attempt to show that every interpretation, to be effective, must contain a "because" clause: Even if not actually couched in such words, an interpretation must—in my opinion—demonstrate to the patient that he is adopting one course of behavior and avoiding another *because* he fears the supposedly disastrous consequences of the latter. It is at this point that reality testing begins. Thus Dr. Sutherland's patients were able to compare their expectation of the officer Sutherland's becoming angry, with the behavior of the real Dr.

Sutherland who showed to them, through his interpretation, that he knew about their wish to separate him from the observers but that he did not get angry.

It is this reality testing which enables patients to give less disguised expression in external reality to the hitherto avoided behavior pattern, and to integrate the experience gained in that session with experiences outside the analytic situation—experiences both in their present environment and in their past, especially also in their infantile past.

Dr. Sutherland's patients could suddenly recognize that the wishes expressed in their dreams were in fact directed towards him and the observers, and they could follow it up by thinking and speaking about past experiences concerning couples in sexual relationships of which they were jealous. As you see, the analyst used only here and now interpretations in this session. Both this session and a number of group and individual sessions of which I have been able to make electrical recordings confirm the view that whatever effect interpretations referring to the past may have, the specific effects attributed to such interpretations can certainly be achieved by confining oneself to interpretations along the lines discussed by Dr. Sutherland and myself in these papers.

The Psychoanalytic Session as an Experimental Situation

It is not, however, to consider the most effective kind of interpretation that I have raised the subject of a here and now approach in psychoanalysis. I have done so because I think that the recognition of transference as the driving force behind *everything* a patient does during his session has important implications for the use of the psychoanalytic method as a research tool. As long as analysts focus their attention on the patient's behavior *outside* the consulting room—for example by trying to explain what made him behave in a certain way in his past—such conjectures, however near the mark they might be, cannot be tested within the psychoanalytic session and have to rely for scientific validation on other methods, such as confirmation by outsiders, behavioristic studies of children, statistical correlations between behavior in childhood and corresponding personality traits of adults, and so on.

If, however, the psychoanalytic method is one that permits the study of the dynamics underlying the interactions between patient and analyst as they take place in each session—that is, if this method examines events occuring in the here and now—then it ought to be possible to state the dynamics of these events in the form of hypotheses that can be tested, validated or falsified, through direct observation of the patient's behavior during his sessions. In other words, the psychoanalytic session thus becomes an experimental situation and we ought to be able to state the conditions, necessary and sufficient, to produce a predictable event during that session; in fact, we can formulate, as I have done elsewhere, a law of behavior derived from such situations as were reported in Dr. Sutherland's group sessions.

If we set up a field by putting together a group of patients in need of treatment and a therapist presumably able to satisfy this need, and if the therapist assumes a passive nondirective role, then these patients will display in their words and actions a manifest form of behavior from which three kinds of object relationship can be inferred: (i) the avoided relationship, (ii) the calamity they fear, and (iii) the required relationship which they have to adopt because of this fear. If then the analyst gives an interpretation—that is, points out these three object relationships in the here and now—the subsequent material will contain the hitherto avoided object relationship in a less repressed form.

Such a law can even be expressed quantitatively if we use, like Lewin, a nonmetricized topological approach, for instance, by taking as one of our yardsticks the distance of an avoided object relationship from the here and now relationship with the analyst. Thus, as a result of Dr. Sutherland's interpretation, the officer Sutherland turned into the Dr. Sutherland; Mr. A's avoided object relationship had thus moved from the army unit in which he had served during the war into Dr. Sutherland's consulting room.

Analysts will, of course, realize that what is expressed in this law is nothing but the well-known fact which underlies all analytic theory and practice—namely, that analytic interpretations enable the patient to become conscious of his hitherto unconscious needs. A here and now approach has, however, made it possible to formulate this fact as a proposition which can be quantified and tested experimentally in the analytic situation.

The objection has been raised that psychoanalytic sessions cannot be regarded as experiments since the data collected cannot be examined by other observers. This is no longer true. Before analysts saw patients in groups they were convinced that the intrusion of a third person into this most intimate relationship would make analysis impossible. In the group, however, we soon discovered that by using here and now interpretations, which deal effectively with patients' persecutory fears stimulated by such intruders, analytic investigation and therapy *could* be carried out in the presence of seven or eight observers—namely, fellow patients. It was the utilization of this fact which led us to introduce colleagues as additional observers into such groups, and later on we openly suspended microphones as objective means of recording, both in groups and in individual sessions.

I have now collected electrically recorded sessions which provide a means of subsequent examination by other observers—naturally with due precautions to preserve the patients' anonymity—and which have confirmed in every case the law I have already stated.

Another objection is that phenomena observed in psychoanalytic sessions are unique and that only events which can be repeated can be made use of in experiments. I think this view is based on two misunderstandings. One is the clinging to the view that psychoanalysis is a method which reconstructs the unique history of an individual. I have in this paper tried to prove to you the opposite—that psychoanalysis is a method to study events in the here and now.

The second misunderstanding concerns what has and what has not to be observed repeatedly in order to form the basis of experiments or of scientific statements in general. Logicians will tell us that every event in the universe is unique if we take into account *all* its features—that is, if our observations are subtle enough. Every analyst knows that what we are wont to call the Oedipus complex, or any other analytic concept for that matter, manifests itself in a unique way in each session of the same or of different patients. In spite of that we can make scientifically valid statements if we abstract the common dynamically significant features from the dynamically insignificant historically unique differences of these sessions. We can thus—on a certain level of abstraction—arrive at the formulation of the dynamics of the Oedipus complex with as much justification as the physicist has to formulate the laws of gravitation from such manifestly different phenomena as the movements of planets, of a pendulum, or of a freely falling stone. The physicist is well aware that no two experiments he repeats with a pendulum, for instance, are identical in all their features. However, what matters is not that two experiments should be identical in every respect, but that they should have in common those properties which are dynamically significant for the particular kind of event we study. An individual's history is unique; whatever a patient reports in his session about his experiences, his remote or recent past, is always unique. However, the psychodynamically significant elements of this unique history are by no means unique, and it is these elements which allow the formulation of scientifically valid statements as well as the observation of phenomena under experimental conditions.

Perhaps you may feel by now that although this may be a legitimate experimental study of the effects of interpretations, it is of interest only to the psychoanalyst and to no one else. However, if we realize that hidden behind the desire for cure lie those most vital needs which an individual has not been able to satisfy, then we can see that the analyst's *comments* in the analytic situation, his correct as well as incorrect interpretations, represent to the patient *actions* of people who assume different kinds of attitudes towards the ways in which he can satisfy his basic needs. In other words, the analytic situation is a prototype of what underlies human behavior in general; it is a need situation, and the experimental study of an individual's behavior in this situation allows the formulation of laws underlying *all* human behavior.

The Therapeutic Group as
a Medium of Study

Our interpretive technique at present is very much more refined for individual therapy than for group psychoanalysis. I am therefore trying to study the main kinds of unconscious object relations and their role in the structure of personality from the records of individual sessions as well as of group sessions. Such studies should enable us to formulate basic laws of behavior. There are, however, specific problems which can only be investigated in groups.

Perhaps I may refer briefly to one recorded session. In the preceding sessions a man in this group, Mr. X, had tried to escape from various unconscious difficulties by making numerous attempts to oust me, the recognized leader of the group, and to gain the women's admiration. He had been rebuffed by the group on all those occasions. The group as a whole had become increasingly aware of their sexual jealousies and of the aggressive impulses aroused by them. They had also been able to give clearer expression to these impulses within the analytic sessions, but especially outside of the sessions, according to their own statements. The session I wish to report started with a short silence followed by a few remarks which betrayed the uneasiness of the group at things to come. One woman then concluded this initial period by saying that they would probably go on dealing with the same problems as in previous sessions but on a more real level.

Another silence followed, this time broken by another woman who started putting relations in the group on a more real level by turning to a very practical problem. She asked me, "Do you think the fire could be switched off, Dr. E?" When I tried to turn this question back to the group with my usual remark, "What do you think?"an uproar started in the group. Several members expressed unconcealed anger with me, and one of them, a pregnant woman, looked so flushed and upset that I feared something might happen to her. I therefore gave in to the group's request by switching off the fire without seeing clearly what the upheaval was really about. Shortly after that the expression of hostility towards me fizzled out, and the group started speaking about teacher-pupil relations. In particular a teacher was ridiculed who kept on looking out of the window at the playgrounds while depriving his pupils of this pleasure.

Very soon a discussion developed on the benefits one might derive from attending the group and on the kind of discussion which would prove most helpful. At this time, a split occurred in the group. Up to now there had been a more or less cooperative discussion to which various members contributed; but suddenly Mr. X, the male patient mentioned before, became the center of critical remarks from the rest of the group who seemed to line up against him.

The issue under discussion seemed rather confused. Although Mr. X had stood up for the usefulness of psychoanalysis, against another group member's initial doubts that group treatment could help her beyond the point she had already reached, the other group members, reacted towards Mr. X as if he had attacked psychoanalysis. The discussion then veered towards semantics. Here again the implication was that Mr. X was attacking and the rest were defending psychoanalytic therapy; yet this was in fact not true. While the rest of the group insisted that he was trying to avoid psychoanalysis by turning emotionally charged discussions into an intellectual semantic hair-splitting, he insisted that the separation between the intellectual content of a discussion and its emotional tone was an artificial one.

I must point out here that in previous sessions I had said much the same thing on those occasions when I tried to show the group that their ostensibly intellectual discussions were the expressions of emotional conflicts within the group. This time Mr. X had fully accepted the basis of here and now interpretations and was in fact standing up for what he had attacked on previous occasions, under the pressure of feelings of rivalry and jealousy towards me.

A significant point in this discussion was when Mr. Y, a most submissive patient who had consistently played in the group the part of a pacifying and soothing agent, suddenly became the spearhead of the attack against Mr. X and insisted on "having it out" with him with regard to the issue of intellectualizing the emotional content of psychoanalytic sessions. When this happened, the irony of the situation became obvious to the whole group; in fact this attempt to fight Mr. X on the issue of intellectualizing emotions led the group as a whole into the most intellectual hair-splitting discussion, for which, this time, not Mr. X but the rest of the group were responsible. Mr. X pointed this out to the group at the beginning of his contest with the others when he put the teasing remark to Mr. Y, "Are you starting an intellectual discussion?" and provoked laughter in the whole group. In spite of that, Mr. X and the rest of the group did not desist from engaging in what all group members pretended they were so much against—namely, a hair-splitting intellectual discussion.

If we ask again what were the underlying forces motivating the trend of the discussion in that session, it seems clear to me that from the moment I switched off the fire, the group started repeating the pattern which they had tried to enact before towards me. Apparently the reason for this repetition of pattern was that my giving in to their request to switch off the fire had resulted in their *not* being frustrated with regard to an issue which they would have liked to imagine was the cause of their frustration and of their wish to attack me. My behavior had therefore only shelved their problem. I had deprived them of the channel through which they tried to express their piled-up resentment towards a frustrating person. I had, however, not removed—by means of interpretation of the underlying motives—their need to adopt this kind of aggressive object relationship with me. The result was that they felt the same compulsion as before to attack some kind of leader on a displaced issue which allowed them to conceal the real cause of their anger—that is, their sexual frustration. By switching off the fire I had done what reassuring therapy usually does—namely, I had temporarily withdrawn myself from the patients' attempts to transfer their unconscious object relationships to the therapist. Thus, while this had established peace between us for the moment, it left the group with an undiminished need to find a leader whom they could attack.

What then developed between Mr. X and the rest of the group may serve as a good illustration of what is meant by unconscious collusion in interpersonal relations, one of the problems which can only be studied in groups. All members of this group seemed driven by forces beyond their control into what *they* considered to be a useless discussion. The group, for reasons they were not aware of, needed a leader whom they could attack, and they found such a scapegoat in Mr. X. Mr. X, on the other hand, by offering himself as a scapegoat for me achieved his equally unconsciously determined aim of becoming the central figure of the group round whom everything revolved. For this, he was prepared not only to waste a session, but even to become the most unpopular member of the group on that occasion.

This session shows how different unconscious needs of two or more individuals may interact and complement one another and lead to the kind of interpersonal relations which all of them deplore; further, how unconscious tensions may prevent a group from getting on with their job. (In this therapeutic group the apparent not-getting-on-with-the-job became, of course, the subject of interpretation.)

It may also serve as an example for the emergence of various group structures with different roles, such as leader, scapegoat, confronter, and so on, as an attempt to cope with unconscious tensions.

Another problem we can examine here is to consider what kind of personality will be pushed into what particular role which the group requires at that moment, in view of its need for a certain group structure. Further, we can study more lasting attitudes, likes and dislikes, which develop between certain group members who are persistently pushed into certain group roles and therefore become identified with these roles.

The advantage of the therapeutic group over the usual kind of task group in studying such problems is that in the therapeutic group, though it too has as certain preformed structure, this group structure is of comparatively small influence as compared with the unconscious forces within each group member. This therefore allows us to investigate the particular kind of interpersonal relations that develop under the influence of these unconscious factors. However, in principle these unconscious factors are in no way different from similar forces within the conscious sphere; clashes of interest over real issues and the methods which individuals and groups adopt to solve them do not differ basically from the conflicts with unconscious objects which we can observe within an individual personality, or within a therapeutic group in which such *intra*personal conflicts express themselves in *inter*personal relations.

In addition, in a task group, as in a factory, office, or school, real clashes of interest within a group and such unconciously determined conflicts as we study in our therapeutic groups are hopelessly intermingled and react upon one another. The therapeutic group, therefore, seems an excellent opportunity for studying such problems in a comparatively simple field.

The detailed examination of every remark patient and analyst make by what might be called "microanalysis" of recorded sessions and, in addition the development of a set of dynamic concepts seem promising approaches for the formulation and testing of hypotheses about the dynamics of human behavior.

Notes

1. Sigmund Freud, *Introductory Lectures on Psycho-Analysis* (Riviere, tr.), 2nd ed.; London: Allen and Unwin, 1949, pp. 307–309.
2. *Ibid.*, pp. 367–372.
3. (a) Henry Ezriel, "A Psycho-Analytic Approach to Group Treatment," *British J. Med. Psychol.* (1950) 23:59–74.
   (b) Henry Ezriel, "The Psycho-Analytic Session as an Experimental Situation," *British J. Med. Psychol.* (1951) 24:30–34.

Group-Analytic Dynamics with Specific Reference to Psychoanalytic Concepts

S. H. FOULKES, M. D.
President, Group-Analytic Society (London)

S. H. Foulkes (1898–1976) came to London in 1933 from Frankfurt where he practised as an analyst. He had worked at one time with the renowned neurologist Kurt Goldstein who emphasized the importance of understanding not the function of the individual neuron, but rather the communicating network of neurons, using the term "gestalt psychology." Foulkes came to emphasize the individual as a nodal point in the communication matrix of the group, just as another student of Goldstein's, Fritz Perls, adopted the term "gestalt therapy" for his ideas about integrating the parts of the whole person. Foulkes was also influenced by the school of sociologic thought in Frankfurt that was attempting to integrate the ideas of the two great theoreticians of the late nineteenth and early twentieth century: Marx's socialist ideas about the importance of society and Freud's psychoanalytic approach to the individual.

Foulkes formed the Group Analytic Society in 1952 in London, which came to be the major force in the training of British group therapists and has also been influential in the development of continental European group therapy. He published an early group text (Introduction to Group-Analytic Psychotherapy. London: Heinemann Medical Books, 1948) and successive editions of his soft-cover text were widely used throughout the world (Foulkes SH, Anthony EJ: Group Psychotherapy: The Psychoanalytic Approach. Baltimore: Penguin Books, 1957, 1965, 1968).

This article demonstrates Foulkes's interest in the here-and-now group experiences and how these are molded by each person's expectations of how others will respond—the "hall of mirrors" in which the individual can see himself/herself reflected in others. Foulkes's emphasis on both the individual and the group provides a middle ground between group-as-a-whole concepts and the psychoanalysis of the individual in the group.
—Editor

Foulkes SH: Group analytic dynamics with specific reference to psychoanalytic concepts. *International Journal of Group Psychotherapy* 7:40–52, 1957.

Group analysis is concerned with the total field of mental dynamics, whether these be better studied in an individual or group situation. In this paper a selection will be made and particular attention paid to psychoanalytic equivalents, in which connection some personal remarks may not be out of place.

In view of the fact that I am a practicing and teaching psychoanalyst of long standing, surprise has been expressed at my upholding the claim of group analysis to be considered as a therapeutic method valid in its own right and with its own specific theoretical concepts and contributions to make.[1] This does not imply that its practice and theory are at variance with psychoanalysis, indeed without psychoanalysis my particular approach could not have come into being. Incidentally, I would mention here that calling the method I use group analysis and not group psychoanalysis, I am in fundamental agreement with Miss Anna Freud, whose orientation I share closely in the psychoanalytic field. Psychoanalysis is in my view essentially confined to patient and therapist in the individual situation.

Why have I not taken Freud's own specific study of group psychology as the basis on which to form my concepts? Freud's contribution to group psychology was actually based on the findings of individual psychology, although he occasionally showed surprising insight in favor of the reverse procedure. He tended to see group processes merely as extensions of those activities going on in the individual mind which had led him to formulate the concepts of psychoanalysis. Moreover, in his book on this subject,[2] he studied groups of an entirely different nature to those investigated by the present writer. He used two large, highly organized groups—the army and the Catholic church—as models from which to illustrate such concepts as for instance the ego ideal and identification. He did not attempt to explain the dynamic processes taking place in these groups as germane to them, but rather to show how the internal forces characteristic of individual life sought their expression through the group medium.

Classical psychoanalytic concepts can be used with advantage in a group setting to facilitate the process of therapy, but the processes corresponding to them are equivalent to and not identical with those observed in the individual psychoanalytic situation. The wholesale transfer of psychoanalytic concepts to a new field would be particularly inadvisable at the present time when they have lost a good deal of original precision and meaning and are exciting controversy in their own field of origin. Even such vital concepts as transference and identification are in process of revision, or tending to become confused.

Our psychotherapeutic groups are in principle transference groups, in the sense that members can use each other and the therapist as transference figures, as it occurs in psychoanalysis between patient and analyst. However, the pattern of relationships develops with much more complexity in the group situation and cannot be explained by applying to it the term transference. On the contrary, the observation of classical transference processes within the group setting throws new light upon them as they are seen in the individual setting. In psychoanalytic literature, the term transference is increasingly used to cover all interactions between therapist and patient. This development applies equally well to the corresponding concept of countertransference. The group-analytic situation could of course be termed a transference situation in this sense, but it would be more correct to apply to it the symbol "t," meaning therapeutic.[3] Thus we can speak of a therapeutic, or "t," relationship, situation, etc, and reserve the term transference situation for its more specific and legitimate application.

Similar considerations obtain in the case of other terms, such as identification. Here again the group reaction seen as a whole cannot be understood simply on the basis of the psychoanalytic concept, whereas the understanding of the dynamics of the situation in which identifications germinate, precipitate or mature, helps us discern those aspects of the process which escape observation and explanation in the psychoanalytic situation.

Group analysis views man's social nature as basic to him and makes the group or community rather than the individual its primary basis for conducting therapy. Individuals emerge as the result of developments in the community, whether this phenomenon be viewed in historical perspective—a comparatively recent affair[4]—or in its current aspect of the individual personality emerging from and formed by his family, as is the case in psychoanalysis. Conceiving the social nature of man as basic does not deny or reduce the importance of the sexual instinct in the sense of psychoanalysis, nor of the aggressive instinct. The infant-mother relationship is the first social relationship in the same sense as it is the first sexual and love relationship.

In this way the psychoanalytic tendency, more specifically Freud's tendency, to look upon the social instinct as a deployment of the sexual or life instinct is quite acceptable, provided this is not held to be the explanation for the social nature of the species Man. The point we wish to make clear is that we hold man's social nature to be an irreducible basic fact. Therefore the group, originally the community, its cohesion and the currents moving in it are primary elements not to be *explained* in terms of the interactions of individuals. We conceive all illness as occurring and originating within a complex of interpersonal relationships. Group psychotherapy is an attempt to treat the total network of disturbance either at the point of origin in the root—or primary—group, or, through placing the disturbed individual under conditions of transference, in a group of strangers or proxy group.

When people are brought together in a psychotherapeutic group a struggle of conflicting tendencies asserts itself, but in spite of impulses to withdraw, the need of the individual to be understood by and related to the group finally and overwhelmingly prevails. This fundamental need to *relate* shows itself with particular clarity even in our groups. (I add "even," because our artificial groups are in effect conglomerations of isolated individuals.) The social basis at once asserts itself, and thus relatedness viewed within an all-penetrating group matrix is the corner-stone of our working theory. The idea of the group as the mental matrix, the common ground of an operational basis for relationships, comprising all the interactions of individual group members is central for the theory and process of therapy. Within this frame of reference all communications take place. A fund of unconscious understanding, wherein occur reactions and communications of great complexity, is always present.

A principle which can be illustrated and supported from observation in therapeutic groups is that every event, even though apparently confined to one or two participants, in fact involves the group as a whole. Such events are part of a gestalt, configuration, of which they constitute the "figures" (foreground), whereas the ground (background) is manifested in the rest of the group. We have described as *location* the process which brings to life this concealed configuration; it is, however, not always a simple matter to locate this pattern of the group's reactions. Other important concepts specific to group analysis and essential for understanding the group-analytic process are those termed *mirror reaction, occupation* and *translation*, which we can only describe briefly here.

Mirror reactions are characteristically brought out when a number of persons meet and interact.[5] A person sees himself, or part of himself—often a repressed part of himself—reflected in the interactions of other group members. He sees them reacting in the way he does himself, or in contrast to his own behavior. He also gets to know himself—and this is a fundamental process in ego development—by the effect he has upon others, and the picture they form of him.

By *occupation* is meant that which is the group's reason for coming together.[6] In everyday life this may be for the purpose of study or work, to play bridge or golf. Such a declared, manifest occupation is deliberately absent from a group-analytic group. In this it differs from a "free discussion" group. Observation of the group-analytic group makes it clear that such an "occupation" acts as a defensive screen to keep at bay intimate interpersonal reactions, thoughts and fantasies. This defensive or screen function makes the concept of "occupation" important for the understanding of the dynamics both of the group-analytic group and, by implication, of any type of group. There is a tendency for analytic groups to behave as if they had an appointed *occupation*, such as "discussing our problems." An occupation can also be latent, and the group may not be conscious of it. This might be called its *preoccupation*.

Translation is the equivalent of the making conscious of the repressed unconscious in psychoanalysis. The whole group participates in this process, which ranges from inarticulate symptom to verbal expression, understanding and insight, from primary process to secondary process (in the psychoanalytic sense), from primitive to logical, rational expression.

Interpretation in psychoanalysis, refers by contrast only to a special contribution on the part of the psychoanalyst to this translation.

This concept of translation and that of the mental matrix of the group are closely allied to our ideas on *communication*. Group-analytic theory recognizes communication as a process of fundamental importance to the study of behavior and the practice of psychotherapy. In a group-analytic group, all observable data are held to be relevant communications, whether thay take the form of conscious or unconscious, verbal or nonverbal communications.

Characteristic nonverbal communications are those made in the form of behavior, either on the part of individual members or by the group as a whole. Appearance and dress may be communications; an exuberant tie or conspicuous shoes, provocative disorder or meticulous neatness may excite comment and lead to insight in the same way as verbal exchange. One person will press for more light to be put on in the room where the group meets, while another will prefer to sit in near darkness, or mislay his spectacles in order not to see. The group as a whole may communicate tension in the shape of silences, or fitful, disjointed conversation. It may express a cheerful mood of relief, or group gloom in which everyone sits and glowers darkly, some on the point of tears.

At one end of the scale is the inarticulate symptom: it may be nail biting, excessive blushing, palpitation of the heart, or migrainous headache; at the other lies its representation in verbal imagery. Between these two must be cut an intricate sequence of steps leading to verbalization. Many complex processes have to play their part before the mute symptom of a fellow member can attain linguistic expression and its meaning be grasped by the others.

It is the *process of communication* rather than the information it conveys which is important to us. In a group-analytic group, communication moves from remote and primitive levels to articulate modes of conscious expression and is closely bound up with the therapeutic process. The therapeutic group establishes a common zone in which all members can participate and learn to understand one another. Within this process members of the group begin to understand the language of the symptom, symbols and dreams as well as verbal communications. They have to learn this through experience in order for it to be meaningful and therefore therapeutically efficient. The "conductor" strives to broaden and deepen the expressive range of all members, while at the same time increasing their understanding of the deeper, unconscious levels. The zone of communication must include the experience of every member in such a way that it can be shared and understood by the others, on whatever level it is first conveyed. This process of communication has much in common with making the unconscious conscious and altogether with the concepts of unconscious, preconscious and conscious in their topographical and dynamic sense. We will discuss these later.

Ego, Id and Superego in the Group Model

Here we may pause to glance for a moment at the group-analytic group as a model of the mental apparatus. In what way do the psychoanalytic concepts of ego, id and superego reflect in the group? The group is like a model of the mental apparatus in which its dynamics are personified and dramatized. A process analogous to this may be seen in the theater where the characters not only represent themselves but also stand proxy for the audience both in their individual and community reactions. A very good illustration of the way in which this happens can be found in Friedman's and Gassel's study of the Sophoclean tragedy *Oedipus Tyrannus*.[7] Their paper is of no less interest to us because of the fact that it was not intentionally concerned with the dynamics of the group in relation to group psychotherapy.

Oedipus, having committed patricide and incest, had to be punished in order to assuage the guilt feelings aroused in the audience by the activating of their forbidden wishes. The tragedy is played out between Oedipus, representing one wish, and the Chorus representing the other. The authors write: "The chorus by remaining detached absolves itself from responsibility . . . actually the chorus maintains a driving demand on the hero to fulfill what the community expects . . . Oedipus accepts fully the responsibility which the community is so eager for him to assume . . . The chorus is not unlike a helpless community in the habit of throwing responsibility to the leader." The hero, Oedipus, here represents the id, in that he stands for wishes and impulses inherent in everybody. He also embodies a kind of collective ego for the community (see Rank's description of the heroes of mythology as embodying "collective egos" who reflect the forces at work within the society which creates and projects them). Furthermore, he has to be punished for the crime he has committed in the name of the community and is thus in some sense a scapegoat. The conflict within the audience, within any given human being, is given expression by the conflict between Oedipus and the Chorus. The Chorus which in present terms could delineate our group, plays the part of the superego; it remains detached and objective, but exerts a driving pressure on the hero to fulfill his destiny.

In another paper by the same authors, also of interest to us, on the Orestes drama,[8] the Chorus incites and drives on Orestes to murder his mother. Orestes is tried and acquitted by a jury which gives its verdict equally for and against him, thus expressing the ambivalence of the community toward its wish to be rid of the maternal tie through matricide.

We find in our own group similar configurations to those instanced above in the form of Sophoclean drama, notwithstanding the fact that very often the leader or conductor is felt to be in the role of the superego. Group members may also play the part of superego, ego and id in relation to each other. A good example of the latter role occurred in one of my groups, when an older, married woman registered considerable apprehension of a younger, single woman in the same group. Later it transpired that this younger member symbolized the maturer woman's fears of loss of control and impulses of an erotic nature. In other words, here was an incarnation of her own id functioning independently of her control and hence provoking anxiety. The group also manifests something in the nature of a collective ego.

I have repeatedly observed members functioning as scapegoats in place of the conductor. The group, angry with him but not daring to attack him directly or to show open hostility, will relieve and displace its emotion and fury onto one of themselves, usually a weak or absent member. The scapegoat thus chosen bears the brunt of a vicarious attack on the conductor. It therefore very often proves correct in the scapegoat formation for the conductor to look for latent and repressed hostility directed against his own person under guise of the scapegoat. Here is an interesting example of one variation of this process. One of my groups at various times repeatedly accused me of bias against a certain member. In such instances, I assume in principle that the group must have its reasons, however dormant my own awareness. I did not succeed in this case in finding any evidence of bias either in my behavior or unconscious attitude. At a later stage, I had to defend the same patient against strong hostility on the part of the group. This made what had happened clear to me. The group, unconsciously wanting to make a scapegoat of the member in question, defended themselves against this tendency by first projecting it onto me and then accusing me of bias. This brief illustration of clinical importance is valuable for defining how personalization, displacement and location take place in our groups.

Multiple Dimensions in the Group

I will now proceed to enlarge somewhat on concepts which may be helpful for orientation in studying the multiple dimensions operating in the group. In this connection I would like to draw attention to some old and very interesting concepts of Wernicke who thought the most important spheres in which psychosis could be placed were those of (1) the external world, or allopsyche; (2) the *Körperlichkeit*, corporeality or somatopsyche; and (3) the *Persönlichkeit*, or autopsyche.[9]

A similar recent classification of interest in the present connection is that used by Erikson, who envisages three stages of childhood development which can be said to persist in some degree in adult life.[10] The first he called the "autocosmos," wherein the world is experienced and reacted to exclusively in terms of the child's own body. This stage is replaced by the "microsphere." Here object relations are formed, but the child endows the object with his own feelings and wishes, as for instance when the sofa becomes a boat, or the doll an angry mother. Eventually the stage of the "macrosphere" is arrived at, object relations being now experienced in a world genuinely shared with others. Among levels leading from surface to deeper and hidden aspects, four can be discerned in the group.

1. *The Current Level*. This is analogous to Erikson's "macrosphere." Here the group would be experienced as representing the community, public opinion, etc., and the conductor as a leader or authority.

2. *The Transference Level*. This second level corresponds to mature object relations experienced in the "macrosphere." It is the level most often envisaged by group psychotherapists of analytic orientation, on which the group represents the family, the conductor father or mother, and the other members siblings.

3. *The Level of Bodily and Mental Images (Projective Level)*. This level corresponds to primitive, narcissistic inner "object" relations in psychoanalysis. Here other members reflect unconscious elements of the individual self. The group represents as outer what are in truth inner object relations. The closest analogy here is with the concept of play analysis and its resultant psychopathology much associated with the name of Melanie Klein. This is the level of the "microsphere" and also corresponds to Wernicke's allopsyche. Not only may individuals embody a part of the self, but the group as a whole may do so (autopsyche). The group often represents the mother image, as pointed out by Schindler.[11] The body image is reflected and represented in the group and its members. This phenomenon would correspond with Wernicke's somatopsyche, although the concept of a body image, owed in the main to Schilder,[12] was in no way thought of or familiar to Wernicke's generation.

4. *The Primordial Level*. This fourth level is the one in which primordial images occur according to the concepts of Freud and those particularly formulated by Jung concerning the existence of a collective unconscious.

Further illustration of the functioning of all these levels is provided in the table (page 124).

The conclusions arrived at by Schilder as to the close interrelationship between ego and outside world, the social nature of consciousness and the relation between outer world and self as a fundamental human fact, come very close to our own. Schilder writes: "It is our contention that every experience not only refers to these fundamental spheres of self and world, but also to the spheres of the body. Human existence consists in living at once in these three spheres which form an inseparable unit. We may call the fact that experiences are experiences in the outside world, the body and

Levels and Spheres in the Group-Analytic Group

MACROSPHERE	(1) *Current Level* Group = community, society, public opinion, etc. (2) *Transference Level* Mature object relations. Group = family, father, mother, siblings	
MICROSPHERE	(3) *Projective Level* Primitive, narcissistic, "inner" object relations Other members personify (a) part(s) of self	allopsyche autopsyche
AUTOCOSMOS	(b) part(s) of body (-image)	somatopsyche)
	(4) *Primordial Level* Collective Images	

the self, an a priori insight. I would prefer the more modest expression that here we deal simply with an experience which so far has been proved correct."[13]

Arriving now at even closer equivalents of psychoanalytic concepts in the group than those already shown, we will first of all examine the unconscious, conscious, and preconscious in a group setting.

Unconscious, Preconscious, and Conscious

We have already spoken of the *systematic unconscious* as used in psychoanalysis. This primary language in symbolic or symptomatic form, the language of the dream, operates in the group context. We do not merely see the distinction between primary and secondary processes as in psychoanalysis, but also many transition stages, and our process of communication and translation is closely linked with the construction of an ever widening zone of mutual understanding within the group. The concept of unconscious understanding, familiar in psychoanalysis,[14] is one on which we build continuously. Every communication is understood unconsciously on some level and has to negotiate many levels before it can be grasped and shared in its full meaning.

Group Consciousness. Group equivalents of the *topographical* idea of consciousness, unconscious and preconscious, can also be clearly shown. To demonstrate this, we must recall Freud's metapsychological hypothesis that the process of becoming conscious is closely allied to or essentially characterized by the cathexis of word representation. This Freudian concept is of great importance for understanding the meta-psychology of hysteria, schizophrenia and various neuroses. The group equivalent of consciousness in terms of the group entity thus consists in any one member's *saying something in so many words*. If the group is ready and able to understand and assimilate what he says, the particular matter at issue can be said to be fully in its consciousness. The word cathexis assumed by

Freud would here exemplify in the act of verbal expression on the part of any one individual.

The *preconscious* could be defined as something that remains unspoken and the group is in no way conscious of it. But potentially anyone could give utterance to this particular matter at any time and it would meet with no dynamic resistance or lack of understanding on the part of the group. It is easy to see on these lines the group equivalent to the *unconscious* or *repressed*, but for this to be of use more detailed illustration is needed than can be given in this paper.

Free Group Association

An equivalent of prime importance is that which corresponds to free association in individual psychoanalysis. "Free group association" evolved through my own approach, although it may possibly also have been used independently in the 1920's by Trigant Burrow and his circle.[15] An analytic approach to groups was made by Schilder and Wender, but my own differed from theirs in proceeding straightaway to a spontaneous handling of the group situation.[16] I instructed the patients who had had previous psychoanalysis to associate freely in the same way as in the individual situation. As expected, the associations which patients were able to produce were modified by the group situation. I then waited and observed developments over a number of years, eliciting the process to which I later gave the name of "free-floating discussion." Only at a much later date consequent on my studies in analytic groups did it become clear to me that the conversation of *any* group could be considered in its unconscious aspects as the equivalent of free association.

Today I am beginning to fathom what elements in the situation of any given group of people approximate their conversation to free group association. Naturally the group-analytic situation itself is devised to encourage an optimum degree of freedom from censorship. The group association here is therefore the nearest equivalent of free association in psychoanalysis and plays a similar part. More concisely this can be expressed as follows. The more the "occupation" of the group comes to the fore, the less freely can group association emerge; if the occupation is a pretext, or can be completely scrapped as in our own technique, group association can emerge freely. Social groups can stand further or nearer one or the other of these extremes. For example in a casually thrown together social group, such as is seen in a railway carriage, or on conducted motor tours, though there is nobody to interpret, the ongoing conversation approximates to "free group association," the unconscious meaning readily shows itself to my own observation in such contexts.

In the group-analytic group, the manifest content of communication, broadly speaking, relates to the latent meaning of this communication in a similar way as the manifest dream relates to the latent dream thoughts. This matter is so important and so bound up with our concept of a *group matrix* that I shall once more take occasion to stress the group matrix as the operational basis of all relationships and communications. Communications use this network, and the individual is conceived as a nodal point. An analogy can be made with the neuron in anatomy and physiology, the neuron being the nodal point in the total network of the nervous system which always reacts and responds as a whole. As in the case of the neuron in the nervous system, so is the individual suspended in the group matrix.

Looked at in this way it becomes easier to understand our claim that the group associates, responds and reacts as a whole. The group as it were avails itself now of one speaker, now of another, but it is always the transpersonal network which is sensitized and gives utterance, or responds. In this sense we can postulate the existence of a group "mind" in the same way as we postulate an individual "mind." Whereas it is difficult for us to abstract from the concept of an individual in a physical, bodily way, it should not be so difficult to do so in the mental field, and to perceive that the matrix of response is indeed an interconnected whole. In the mental matrix individuals also emerge, but the boundaries of these (perhaps they should be called by some other name such as "psyche-individuals") do not run parallel with the boundaries of their physical person.

Equivalents of Mental Mechanisms

We have already exemplified *displacement* in a group. Suffice it to add here that the group equivalent is seen when repressed tendencies in individuals emerge in the roles of others. The process of displacement should be strictly viewed in this context as occurring between individuals inside the group, not simply as a function of the individual mind.

Isolation occurs when an individual within the group is assigned tendencies, forces or characteristics which are shunned in a phobic way by others. Isolation in the group is also manifested by punctuating silences, or by its abruptly turning from one theme to another at a certain point.

Splitting is another process clearly shown in the group. It takes the form in this context of subgroups, splitting into pairs, etc.

These few illustrations are given to underline the fact that even the processes akin to psychoanalytic ones should be seen as configurations in the group context. Clearly the processes of *personification* or *impersonation* and *dramatization* are particularly stressed in the group and play a much bigger part than in individual psychoanalysis. All the models of processes we have elaborated in this article incorporate this particular group feature, namely dramatization and personification, in this as in other instances reminiscent of the dream process itself.

In conclusion, I would like to stress the difference in emphasis between psychoanalysis and group-analytic psychotherapy.[17] Psychoanalysis, at any rate in its historical aspect, has laid great emphasis on the psychogenesis of illness. In group analysis we are more concerned with the outlook for change and the direction and means whereby to ensure it. We therefore work with operational concepts, formulated and applied in the therapeutic process itself and derived from immediate clinical observations. In our view a dynamic science of psychotherapy is needed which will incorporate and turn to good account the revolutionary idea that therapy is research and research in this field is therapy.

Group analysis as a method will then automatically fall into correct perspective as a powerful therapy, a stimulating theory and a fertile source of information and discovery in the psychosocial field.

References

1. Slavson, S. R.: *Analytic Group Psychotherapy*. New York: Columbia University Press, 1950; Scheidlinger, S.: *Psychoanalysis and Group Behavior*. New York: Norton, 1952.
2. Freud, S.: *Group Psychology and the Analysis of the Ego* (1921). London: Hogarth Press, 1947.
3. Foulkes, S. H. and Anthony, E. J.; *Group Psychotherapy—The Analytic Approach.* London: Pelican Books, 1957.
4. Elias, N.: *über den Prozess der Zivilisation*, Vol. I; Prague: Academia Verlag, 1937; Vol. II; Basel: Verlag Haus zum Falken, 1939.
5. Foulkes, S. H. and Lewis, E.: Group Analysis. *Brit. J. Med. Psych.*, 20:175–184, 1944.
6. Foulkes, S. H.: Group-Analytic Psychotherapy: A Short Account. *Acta Psychother.*, 3:313–319, 1955.
7. Friedman, J. and Gassel, S.: The Chorus in Sophocles' *Oedipus Tyrannus. Psa. Quart.*, 19:213–226, 1950.
8. Friedman, J. and Gassel, S.: Orestes. *Psa. Quart.*, 20:423–433, 1951.
9. Wernicke, C.: *Grundriss der Psychiatrie*. Leipzig: Thieme, 1906.
10. Erikson, E. H.: *Childhood and Society*. New York: Norton, 1950.
11. Schindler, W.: Family Pattern in Group Formation and Therapy. *International Journal of Group Psychotherapy*, 1:101–105, 1951.
12. Schilder, P.: *The Image and Appearance of the Human Body*. New York: International Universities Press, 1950.
13. Schilder, P.: *Mind, Perception and Thought in Their Constructive Aspects*. New York: Columbia University Press, 1942.
14. Fenichel, O.: Concerning Unconscious Communication. *Collected Papers, I*. New York: Norton, 1953.
15. Galt, W.: *Phyloanalysis*. Psyche Miniatures. London: Kegan Paul, 1933.
16. Foulkes, S. H. and Lewis, E.: Group Analysis. *Brit. J. Med. Psychol.*, 20:175–184, 1944; Foulkes, S. H.: On Group Analysis, *Int. J. Psa.*, 27:46–51, 1946.
17. Foulkes, S. H.: Some Similarities and Differences between Psycho-Analytic Principles and Group-Analytic Principles. *Brit. J. Med. Psychol.*, 26:30–35, 1953.

The Deviant Member
in Therapy Groups

DOROTHY STOCK, ROY M. WHITMAN,
AND MORTON A. LIEBERMAN

Dorothy Stock Whitaker (known under both Stock and Whitaker in the literature) took her Ph.D. in clinical and social psychology at the University of Chicago and then worked in the Chicago VA Hospital. She later moved to Britain where she is now Professor of Social Work at the University of York. Stock first became interested in groups under the supervision of Herbert Thelen, who in turn had been influenced by the work of Kurt Lewin at the National Training Laboratories. Thomas French, also in Chicago, had developed the idea of "nuclear conflict," which pervades the way an individual structures relationships. Stock combined these two influences through intensive process analysis of groups in order to explore the evidence for "group focal conflict" themes. In this work she came into contact with fellow graduate students, William F. Hill (the founding editor of Small Group Behavior, now Small Group Research) and Mort Lieberman.

Roy Whitman is currently Professor of Psychiatry at the University of Cincinnati. He and Stock developed their ideas about applying the "focal conflict" ideas to groups in collaboration. Whitman has contributed further to the group literature in the area of self psychology.

Morton A. Lieberman collaborated with Irv Yalom and Matthew Miles in the Stanford Encounter Group study of the late 1960s. One aspect of the study is presented in Yalom's article in this volume. Lieberman later provided provocative findings about how different self-help systems use different techniques matched to the needs of the members (Lieberman MA, Borman LD: Self-Help Groups for Coping with Crises: Origins, Members, Processes, and Impact. San Francisco: Jossey-Bass, 1979). Lieberman is now working on a project regarding psychological adaptation of the elderly at the University of California, San Francisco.

Whitaker and Lieberman collaborated in writing "Psychotherapy through the Group Process" (New York: Atherton, 1964). This was the first major American publication to employ the group-as-a-whole approaches already well established in Britain. The article printed here introduces the idea of group focal conflict. In addition, it applies the theory to an understanding of group deviancy. This is an example of the manner in which these authors creatively applied the focal conflict theory to all aspects of group phenomena. The paper, originally presented at the American Psychological Association meeting in 1957, was written while the authors were participating in a research program funded by the National Institutes of Health, Public Health Service.
—Editor

Stock D, Whitman RM, Lieberman MA: The deviant member in therapy groups. *Human Relations* 11:341–372, 1958.

A deviant member in a therapy group is one who consistently behaves in a way that is different from and unacceptable to the other patients. He is likely to annoy the others, to be paid an unusual amount of resentful attention, to be seen as 'interfering' or 'obstructing,' and to be, in general, noticeably out of step.

Although deviancy is easily recognized, it is not always easily explained. One kind of behavior may be perceived as deviant by the members of a therapy group; while another behavior, which seems equally irritating, is not. A particular kind of behavior may be acceptable in one therapy group but not in another. A particular behavior may go unnoticed at one point in a group's development, and be angrily rejected at another. The members of a group may be evenly matched with respect to such factors as extent of illness, intelligence, and background, yet one person may not fit in. Certain general characteristics such as age, race, or extent of illness do not seem to explain a member's deviant status adequately.

In studying a series of therapy groups (composed of in-patients in the Psychiatric Service of a Veterans Administration hospital) the authors have come upon a number of patients who clearly seemed to be deviants in their groups. Their behavior seemed best understood when viewed against the background of the shifting character of the group interaction. This paper will consider the problem of deviancy from within the framework of a particular set of theoretical concepts. The larger research of which this study is a part has been concerned with developing a theoretical approach to therapy groups that utilizes the concept of 'focal conflict.' This paper explores the usefulness of this theoretical framework in understanding deviant behavior.

The following questions will be considered: what kind of behavior is perceived as deviant in a therapy group? How does the group deal with the deviant member? How is individual personality related to the production of deviant behavior? The main portion of the paper will consist of the presentation of three case studies of deviant members, followed by a discussion of the above questions. As background for this material a brief overview of theory and procedure will be presented.

Theoretical Background: 'The 'Focal Conflict'

Thomas French (6) originally formulated focal-conflict theory as an approach to understanding individual psychoanalysis and dreams. The assumption is that although many diverse and seemingly unrelated elements appear in an analytic hour or in a dream, an underlying coherence and relatedness are present. All of a patient's associations can be seen as relevant to a particular pre-conscious conflict which can be considered 'focal' for that session. Such a conflict involves three major elements: (i) a disturbing motive (usually a wish), (ii) a reactive motive which thwarts the wish (usually some feeling of fear or guilt but occasionally a reality factor), and (iii) some attempts toward a solution of the conflict. These elements of the focal conflict can be diagrammed as follows:

$$\textit{disturbing motive} \times \textit{reactive motive}$$
$$\textit{solution}$$

Part of our research effort has involved testing whether the concept 'focal conflict' can also be useful in understanding group interaction. Here, the attempt is to account for the diverse content of a group therapy session in terms of a slowly emerging and developing conflict situation and varying attempts to solve this conflict. Here, too, the focal conflict occurs on a preconscious level. The patients in a group therapy session are not specifically aware of the underlying theme they are expressing in their comments.

To illustrate briefly, in one group therapy session, led by an inexperienced and aggressive therapist, the patients exchanged many stories about foremen and Army sergeants who had been hard on them and couldn't be pleased. They speculated as to what can be done about such people: grin and bear it, wait till they are in a better mood, etc. One patient said that one such Army sergeant ended up with a bullet in his back. This content could be understood in terms of the following focal conflict:

wish to please the therapist and   ×   *anger that he is pushing*
maintain a good relationship with him   *them too hard*

The dilemma facing the group was that they were experiencing both a wish to please the therapist *and* anger at him, but could not express both these impulses. If they expressed their anger, they felt their good relationship with the therapist was threatened. If they worked on pleasing the therapist, their angry feelings would remain but have no outlet. In this case the group did not arrive at a stable solution, but various possibilities were suggested in the content: accept the situation and say nothing, hope that things will get better, and punish or eliminate the therapist.

In one of the group situations described in detail later in this paper, a focal conflict developed in which the reactive motive was a reality factor. A six-member therapy group had been meeting for some time when five new members were added to the group. This sudden addition of five new 'siblings' led to the following focal conflict:

wish to be unique and be singled   ×   *realization that other patients*
out for special attention from the doctors   *won't permit this*

In this case the wish to receive special attention from the doctors was thwarted, not by an internalized feeling of fear or guilt, but by the awareness that every time a patient demanded attention from the therapist, another patient interfered.

Specific meetings rarely fall into the neat pattern of disturbing motive vs. reactive motion, with a solution. The first illustration presented above demonstrates one pattern that may occur: the emergence of a particular focal conflict together with suggestions as to various solutions, but without the general acceptance of any single solution. At other times a group may fix on a particular solution which is acceptable to the group as a whole. Sometimes the group finds itself in a state of 'solutional conflict,' in which one solution is acceptable to most of the members, but one or two patients fight against accepting it. Since a series of therapy meetings has continuity, a particular meeting may deal with only a fragment of the process which includes focal conflict and solution. For example, an entire meeting may be devoted to the working through of a solutional conflict. One meeting may include the development of a particular focal conflict but end before a satisfactory solution is found. The next meeting may continue the process, or may develop a new conflict which is perhaps an expression of the group's feeling of frustration at the previous unsatisfactory meeting. In some sessions a group focal conflict does not appear but instead diverse individual problems are expressed.

The discussion so far has concentrated on understanding total group interaction in focal-conflict terms. French also defines individual personality dynamics in terms of these same concepts. An individual can be described in terms of a limited number of basic conflicts, called 'nuclear' conflicts. A nuclear conflict is a persisting intra-psychic conflict which operates on an unconscious level and influences much of an individual's overt behavior and perceptions. Over a long period of years the individual may have developed certain 'solutions' to his nuclear conflict which he utilizes habitually in many situations. That is, in a particular situation he may experience a 'focal' conflict which is a derivative of his nuclear conflict but whose specific character is influenced by the particular interpersonal context in which it occurs.

For example, the following nuclear conflict was formulated for a patient who will be described in greater detail later in this paper:

need to be dependent on his mother x *shame about not being a man*

In the setting of a specific group therapy session, the patient's behavior could be understood in terms of the following derived focal conflict:

need to be dependent on   x   *shame about his weakness, especially*
the group for help   *about having been psychotic*

Since the same concept—focal conflict—can be applied to an understanding of both intra-psychic and group phenomena, this approach offers a way of understanding the relationship between individual personality and group events.

Procedure

Before presenting the case material, the method used in analysing group therapy sessions will be described. Typically, our therapy groups include from six to ten patients. Our practice is not to introduce content but to permit the conversation to flow as freely as is permitted by the patients' feelings and fears. Such discussion takes on the character of free association. The topics which are taken up and the shifts in content can be seen as relevant to an underlying concern.

In early attempts to formulate the underlying concerns (i.e. the pattern of focal conflicts and solutions) we worked from tape-recordings and from verbatim protocols of the meetings. As our experience increased we found we could work satisfactorily from fairly detailed content summaries. Two-and-a-half typewritten pages were found to summarize adequately a session lasting an hour and a quarter. In order to minimize possible individual biases the analysis of a meeting is worked out by two or three persons working together rather than by a single individual working alone. The first step involves each person's reading over the summary in order to get a general impression of the session. The therapist provides information about the mood of the group, the tone of voice of various key contributions, and so on. Following this general familiarization with the meeting, each paragraph is discussed separately and some agreement is reached as to 'what was really happening,' i.e. the theme of the part of the meeting. In this way a series of 8 or 10 or 12 brief statements of successive themes is produced. A formulation is then made of the entire meeting in focal-conflict terms. As a final check the detailed content is again reviewed. Details which do not seem to fit in may lead to modifications or elaborations of the formulation.

Although somewhat condensed, the case material which follows will provide further illustrations of both the theory and the method.

******

The first two case illustrations have been omitted.

******

Third Illustration: Max

Since this patient has been described in some detail in earlier papers (10, 11) only a very brief summary will be presented here.

Max belonged to an eight-member therapy group. At first he participated very little, but as the meetings went on he gave the others to understand that he didn't like the meetings and wasn't going to say anything about himself because the group couldn't help him anyway. At first this behavior did not seem to bother the other members, but during the seventh meeting they indicated their concern by arguing with him that the group really could help, and by focusing all their attention on him. The background for this seemed to be that during the fifth and sixth meetings the group had slowly been building some shared conviction that group therapy could be beneficial. By the seventh meeting Max was the only hold-out. The following group focal confiict was formulated to account for the interaction during the seventh meeting:

disturbing motive:		*reactive motive:*
wish to be dependent on the doctor and the group for help with their problems	×	*shame about needing to depend on others for help*

The members were moving toward the solution: 'Everyone agrees he is sick, and needs help.' This solution would adequately deal with both sides of the conflict. No one need feel shameful about his dependency since everyone would be in the same boat. In contrast to the rest of the patients, Max continued to insist that he was strong and self-sufficient and had no need of anyone. At this point the group was in a state of solutional conflict:

group's solution:		*Max's solution:*
everyone agrees that he is sick and needs help	×	*insists that he doesn't need the group and that the group can't help anyway*

The group was faced with the dilemma of having arrived at a solution which would only work if it were unanimously accepted. That is, if everyone would agree that he needed help, the shame about dependency would be more tolerable because it was shared; no one would be in a position to shame anyone else. In holding out, Max created a difficult problem for this group and was perceived by them as recalcitrant and disruptive.

Direct attempts to get Max to admit that he really needed and liked the group failed, and the patients then chose another way out of their solutional conflict. They developed the idea that Max had had a very hard time as a child and in the Army and couldn't be expected to react as other people did. They agreed, 'No wonder he has a chip on his shoulder. No wonder he expects no one to help him.' This idea amounted to a fantasy based on no information about Max's earlier life and denied by Max himself. Yet the group held fast to this notion. This fantasy constituted a way out of their solutional conflict, since, if Max could be seen as an exception, it did not matter if he could not accept the group's solution. It was not enough simply to observe that Max could not see things their way. The group had to justify his holding-out behavior. The members also agreed that Max really liked the group but would not admit it. There was some evidence for this, since Max continued to attend although there was no direct pressure on him to do so.

In the course of developing this fantasy, a number of positive feelings were expressed about Max. At first Max distrusted the group and could not see these feelings as really positive. However, under persistent expressions of liking and understanding Max could see that the others were on his side. While he never admitted verbally that he needed help and valued the group, his behavior changed noticeably. He was, with some lapses, less hostile and more constructive in his behavior. It is assumed that the experience of being liked, a rather unusual one for this patient, was of therapeutic benefit to him.

To summarize, the group members were able to maintain their solution by (i) changing their perception of the deviant in a way which justified and excused his violation of the solution, (ii) perceiving that he really agreed with their solution but couldn't admit, and (iii) behaving toward him in a way which led him to modify his behavior so that it was less threatening to the solution.

Again, the question arises as to why Max could not accept the group's solution. From information gained from his individual therapist the following nuclear conflict was formulated for Max:

disturbing motive:		*reactive motive:*
need to be dependent on his mother	x	*shame about not being a man*

Max's habitual solution to his conflict involved a hostile protest that he didn't need anybody. In the context of this particular therapy group, Max's behavior could be understood in terms of the following derived focal conflict:

disturbing motive:		*reactive motive:*
need to be dependent on the group in order to be helped with his interpersonal difficulties	x	*shame about his weakness, about having been psychotic*

Thus, Max's individual focal conflict was very similar to the one formulated for the group as a whole. It was with respect to a possible solution to the conflict that Max and the rest of the members diverged. In the group setting, Max's habitual hostile protest took the form of insisting that he disliked and could do without the group.

Discussion

A Definition of Deviant Behavior

In the three illustrations presented here, the content of the deviant behavior included depreciating the group (Max), describing a personal problem (Clifford), and talking about a Utopia in which policemen would not be necessary (Simon). Clifford's and Simon's deviant behavior also involved monopolizing the group discussion. At first glance, monopolizing and depreciating behavior might be thought of as inevitably arousing the resentment of the other members. Yet there are times when such behavior is accepted in a therapy group. For example, at times the members of Clifford's group invited Paul, a great talker, to take over the meeting; there were times in Max's group when most of the members were in a depreciating mood. Specific behaviors, then, are not inevitably or consistently deviant.

The deviancy of the three patients discussed in this paper could only be understood when the group context in which the behavior occurred was also examined. In every case the patient was reacted to as a deviant because he did not accept certain implicit agreements which were acceptable to the rest of the group. In terms of a focal-conflict approach to group interaction, the group as a whole had been struggling with some conflict and had arrived at a solution which was acceptable to most of the members. One member was unwilling to accept this solution and instead adhered visibly to some incompatible way of behaving. The deviant behavior consisted of interfering with a solution which most members of the group found acceptable. This can be summarized as follows:

group focal conflict: ×   *reactive motive:*
  disturbing motive   ↓

              group solution   × *active interference with the group*
                                    solution on the part of one
                                    member (= deviancy)

When a member does not accept an otherwise generally acceptable group solution, the other patients seem to find this intolerable. The situation becomes something they feel compelled to do something about. This strong reaction can be understood if one bears in mind the function the solution serves for the group. An adequate solution binds the tensions aroused by two incompatible needs or motives. As long as the solution is in effect, the anxieties involved in the conflict are allayed. When the solution is challenged or violated, the anxieties re-emerge and the group is again in a state of discomfort and tension. It is the function that the solution serves in dealing with conflict which gives it its forceful quality and which makes deviancy from the solution so intolerable to the other members.

If a particular behavior is intolerable because it violates a specific group solution, it follows that the same behavior may occur at other times and not be intolerable, simply because in another context it is not a violation of a group solution. For example, Max rather consistently displayed a certain kind of behavior, but he was not perceived as deviant by the other members until the seventh meeting.

To summarize, the point of view developed here states that deviant behavior emerges when a focal conflict develops in a group, when a solution is found which is acceptable to most of the members and would adequately bind the tensions aroused by the conflict, and when one of the members interferes with this solution. The group can be described as being in a state of solutional conflict. The person who does not accept or who interferes with the group solution is reacted to as a deviant by the others.

Dealing with Deviant Behavior

The preceding discussion has pointed out that when deviant behavior occurs in a therapy group it cannot be ignored. The members must do something to relieve the tension and anxiety which has been aroused by the deviant's behavior. This anxiety develops because a previously satisfactory solution has been challenged, and the associated conflict reactivated for the group. The reaction on the part of the group to deviant behavior can be seen as attempts to deal with the re-opened conflict. In our sample, three kinds of mechanisms can be observed; usually some combination of these is employed.

First, the group may try to get the deviant to change his behavior so that it conforms with the group solution. For example, Max's group directly tried to get him to admit that he needed help. Clifford's group indirectly punished his deviant behavior by depreciating his problem.

Second, the group may re-perceive the deviant behavior or the deviant in such a way that the solution is no longer threatened. For example, Simon's group came to see his confused and symbolic talk as really relevant to the group discussion, and therefore less threatening. The other members of Max's group agreed that he had had a hard time as a child and could not be expected to behave differently. In both cases the deviant behavior did not change, but the group shifted its perception of the behavior so that the previous solution could be maintained.

Third, the group may shift its solution so as to encompass the deviant behavior. For example, in dealing with the threat presented by Simon, part of the members' effort was to assure themselves that the old solution ('maintain control by talking about impersonal matters') was no longer necessary and a new solution ('know when to stop') could adequately deal with the conflict. In Clifford's group the members eventually shifted their solution from 'all be alike superficially' to 'all be alike basically.' This modification seemed to occur, not directly in response to Clifford's behavior, but because the original solution was inherently unrealistic. Nevertheless, by shifting the solution in a direction which included Clifford's behavior, his previously irritating behavior became more tolerable.

All three mechanisms fulfil the same function—that of dealing with the anxieties associated with the group focal conflict. The first two mechanisms involve maintaining the old solution; the third involves finding a new solution to the same focal conflict.

In all cases the patients paid a great deal of attention to the deviant, and worked on him either directly or indirectly. A question arises as to whether, for example, a group could deal with their anxieties entirely on a symbolic level without mentioning the deviant at all. This is a question which is still unanswered. However, in our experience thus far the patients have always eventually specifically dealt with the deviant. The reasons for this may lie in the need to make certain, in a very explicit way, that the mechanism will be effective.

The specific ways in which these three general mechanisms are utilized or expressed vary from group to group. The particular mechanism or combination of mechanisms, and their order and content, seem to be dependent on many specific factors. One such factor is the past history of the group. For example, it was easy for Simon's group to perceive that he was really not basically different from the other members, because this perception was consistent with a solution which had played an important part in their past history ('everyone is basically alike').

One way out—that of expelling the deviant—was consistently rejected in these therapy groups. The members were undoubtedly aware that neither the therapist nor the hospital policy would permit this. Yet there also seemed to be an intrinsic unwillingness on the part of the patients to expel a member. For example, although Max was grossly disruptive and taunted the group by saying, 'Kick me out, I don't care,' there was no suggestion that the group even considered this. Simon's group considered expelling him in a very tangential way, but immediately rejected the idea. It is possible that one reason expulsion was not tolerated in a therapy group is that the patients are unwilling to permit this to become a part of the culture of the group. They may feel 'If I let it happen to him, it may happen to me.' Since, in the course of a therapy group, members are likely to express feelings about which they feel ashamed or guilty, it is essential that they feel firmly assured that they will not be punished in this drastic way for such feelings. A second point is that expulsion may be more readily tolerated by a group when it can be justified in terms of a partial characteristic and does not involve a rejection of the total personality. For example, in secondary groups such as a club or an office staff it is not so difficult to expel a member because he has not paid dues or has failed to fulfil job requirements. In a therapy group no such impersonal criteria exist, and if a member is to be expelled he must be rejected on a very personal basis.

It has been pointed out that the group's efforts in dealing with the anxieties aroused by the deviant behavior seem to involve some direct attention to the deviant himself. For two of the three patients discussed here (Simon and Max) this resulted in some therapeutic benefit to the patient. It is probable that the experience of being unaccepted, disliked, or misunderstood was not new to Max or Simon. Simon was schizophrenic and had had several previous episodes; Max's hostile and rejecting attitude made it difficult for others to like him. It is reasonable to suppose that in most ordinary circumstances people would be unwilling to make the considerable effort required to get along with these two persons. In both cases, however, the other members of their respective therapy groups were willing to struggle long and hard to find a way to accept Max and Simon. They were willing to do this not because of an altruistic wish to help these patients, but out of a compelling need to deal with the solutional conflict which had developed in the group. In this sense the therapeutic benefit to these patients was a by-product of the members' need to deal with certain group problems.

The role the therapist may or should have in dealing with deviant behavior is an interesting issue. Possible ways in which the therapist may intervene are by blocking, supporting, or suggesting certain ways of dealing with the situation.

Occasionally a group wishes to deal with a deviant in some way which requires the active cooperation of the therapist. For example, they may wish the therapist to punish the deviant. In an instance of deviant behavior not specifically studied here, the deviant behavior involved tattling, and the group members wanted the therapist to make a general and anonymous ruling against tattling. By refusing to do so the therapist blocked this way of dealing with the problem and forced the group to discuss the situation more specifically. In these circumstances the group must revise its solution. A therapist may lend his support to certain ways of dealing with the deviant by pointing out more explicitly to the group a particular approach which is already latent in their discussion. More direct suggestions on the part of the therapist may be contraindicated for several reasons. First, in so complex a situation the therapist may suggest a way of dealing with the deviant only to find that for some reason not apparent at the time the group cannot act on his suggestion. He then has risked creating a new problem for the group—that of coping with a situation in which the therapist is pressuring the group in a direction in which the members are unwilling or unable to go. Second, direct suggestion is not likely to be effectively translated into behavior unless the motivation comes from within the patient group. Third, dealing with a deviant member arouses much affect for all the patients. If the therapist provides a shortcut solution a variety of therapeutic benefits, sometimes unanticipated, may be missed.

To summarize, deviant behavior threatens a group solution which otherwise adequately deals with a particular group focal conflict. Because the solution is threatened, anxieties involved in the conflict are re-aroused in the group. In order to deal with the so re-aroused anxieties the group members may (i) reinstitute the original solution by influencing the deviant to conform to it; (ii) reinstitute the original solution by reinterpreting the deviant's behavior in such a way that it no longer threatens the solution; and/or (iii) modify the solution or find a new one which encompasses the deviant behavior. In the course of dealing with the situation certain therapeutic benefits may occur for the deviant. The therapist may influence the process by blocking or lending support to certain ways of dealing with the situation.

Individual Personality and the Production of Deviant Behavior

The discussion so far has considered why a certain behavior is reacted to as deviant at a particular time in a therapy group, and how the group deals with such behavior. The question remains as to why a particular patient produces deviant behavior of a certain type at a certain time. This paper offers the hypothesis that this can be understood in terms of the relationship between the focal conflict and solution which develops in the group and certain persisting nuclear conflicts characteristic of the individual. Our suggestions in this area must be considered quite tentative, since the personal history available for the patients was limited and since the non-deviant members were not studied from this point of view.

It seems reasonable to think of the group situation as the stimulus for individual behavior of all sorts—including deviant behavior. The general task is to examine in each case the individual characteristics which led the patient to react as he did to the group situation. For the two patients for whom personal-history data were available, the group situation seemed to have special relevance to certain deep-lying and persistent individual conflicts. Max's group became concerned with a problem having to do with shame over admitting weakness and a need for help; Max's past history suggested that a problem involving shame over dependency was of central importance for him. Clifford's group became preoccupied with fears of being punished for their wishes for an exclusive relationship with the therapists: Clifford's personal history suggested that this was an important area for him. Because of this relationship the group situation seemed to constitute for both these patients another setting in which a nuclear conflict was experienced in a derived form. In focal-conflict terms, one might say that a state of 'resonance' existed between the individual and the group focal conflict. 'Resonance' may be understood as a state in which the focal conflict which develops for the group as a whole is close to, although not necessarily identical with, an important nuclear conflict of the individual. The specific character of the resonance may vary. For example, in Max's case both the disturbing and the reactive motives corresponded. For Clifford, only the disturbing motive was similar.

Both Max and Clifford had developed certain ways of dealing with these habitual conflicts. That is, they had developed certain habitual solutions. These might also be thought of as well-entrenched defensive reactions which functioned for the patient to ward off anxieties involved in a particular conflict area. In the group setting these habitual solutions were again elicited. When the individual's personal solution was incompatible with the solution toward which the group as a whole was moving, the other patients perceived this behavior as deviant. This can be summarized schematically as follows:

All the patients studied were quite fixed in their deviant behavior and did not yield easily to the pressures of the group to get them to accept another solution or to change their behavior. This is understandable if one bears in mind the function the habitual solution serves for the member in binding the anxieties involved in a persisting nuclear conflict.

A patient in a therapy group may express disagreement without becoming a deviant. For example, in the course of arriving at a generally acceptable solution to a focal conflict, the members of a therapy group can be expected to suggest a variety of solutions. As the group is moving toward agreement, one patient may challenge a solution momentarily but then give in to the pressures of the group. In such a case we would assume that the group focal conflict is irrelevant or tangential to this patient's central individual concerns. If it were related more centrally, the patient would not be able to shift as readily in response to the other members.

There also are times in a therapy group when a patient behaves in a way which to an outsider seems deviant but apparently is not perceived as deviant by the other patients. For example, in Max's group there was another patient, Earl, who was like Max in that he also rejected the group. However, Earl was not considered a problem by the other patients. They knew that his dislike of the group did not stem from a refusal to admit that he needed help, but from a fear that he would 'go too far.' The group was able to distinguish between differing motivations for the same behavior. Earl's behavior did not threaten the group's solution and was tolerated; Max's behavior *did* threaten the group's solution and was not tolerated.

To summarize, for the two patients for whom some early history is available, the specific relationship between the group setting and the individual personality is as follows: a focal conflict develops in the group which is resonant with the individual's nuclear conflict. As a result the individual experiences, in the special setting of the group, a derivative focal conflict—that is, a conflict which is related to his nuclear conflict, but influenced in its specific form by the current interactive circumstances. In an attempt to deal with this derivative focal conflict, the individual repeats in the group setting certain habitual solutions which have been useful to him in the past in dealing with such a conflict. When his individual solution is inconsistent with the group's solution, his behavior is threatening to the group as a whole and he is perceived as a deviant. The deviant clings tenaciously to his habitual solution, because it functions to bind the anxieties involved in his individual focal conflict.

******

A more technical section that discusses deviancy in relation to group norms and pressure to conform has been omitted.

******

Summary

Three patients were studied who were deviant members in their respective therapy groups; that is, their behavior was different from that of the other patients and unacceptable to them. A theoretical approach was adopted in which both the group interaction and the individual personality of the deviants were formulated in focal-conflict terms. In each case the group setting, the deviant behavior, the way the group dealt with the behavior, and the personality characteristics of the deviant were examined. This examination led to the following formulation of the character of deviancy:

1. Deviant behavior emerges when a focal conflict develops in a group, when a solution is found which is acceptable to most of the members and would adequately bind the tensions aroused by the conflict, and when one of the members interferes with this solution. The person who does not accept or interferes with the group solution is perceived as a deviant by the other members.

2. When deviant behavior occurs, the anxieties previously held in check by the solution come to the fore and must be dealt with by the group. In order to deal with these re-aroused anxieties the patients may (i) reinstitute the original solution by influencing the deviant to conform to it; (ii) reinstitute the original solution by reinterpreting the deviant's behavior so that it no longer threatens the solution; and/or (iii) modify the solution so that it now encompasses the deviant behavior.

3. The therapist may influence this process by blocking or lending support to certain solutions or certain ways of dealing with the deviant.

4. A specific individual may produce deviant behavior when the focal conflict which develops in the group is in resonance with certain of his persisting personal (nuclear) conflicts. In these circumstances the individual is likely to repeat in the group setting certain habitual solutions which he has found useful in the past for dealing with such a conflict. He becomes a deviant when his rigidly maintained habitual solution interferes with the solution the group as a whole wishes to adopt.

Implications of this point of view for understanding the development and maintenance of group standards, conformity, and pressures toward conformity are discussed and related to previous studies.

References

1. Cartwright, D., and Zander, A. 'Group Pressures and Standards.' In D. Cartwright and A. Zander (Eds.), *Group Dynamics*. Evanston: Row, Peterson, 1953; London: Tavistock Publications, 1954.
2. Festinger, L. 'An Analysis of Compliant Behavior.' In M. Sherif & M. O. Wilson, *Group Relations at the Crossroads*. New York: Harper and Bros., 1953.
3. Festinger, L., Gerard, H. B., Hymovitch, B., Kelley, H. H., & Raven, B. 'The Influence Process in the Presence of Extreme Deviates.' *Hum. Relat.*, Vol. V, 1952, pp. 327–46.
4. Festinger, L., Schachter, S., & Back, K. 'The Operation of Group Standards.' In D. Cartwright & A. Zander (Eds.), *Group Dynamics*. Evanston: Row, Peterson, 1953; London: Tavistock Publications, 1954.
5. Festinger, L., and Thibaut, J. 'Interpersonal Communication in Small Groups.' *J.*

Abnorm. Soc. Psychol., Vol. 46, 1951, pp. 82–103.

6. French, T. M. *The Integration of Behavior.* Vols. I, II. Chicago: University of Chicago Press, 1952 and 1954.

7. Gorden, R. L. 'Interaction between Attitude and the Definition of the Situation in the Expression of Opinion.' *Amer. sociol. Review,* Vol. 17, 1952, 50–8. Also in D. Cartwright and A. Zander (Eds.), *Group Dynamics.* Evanston: Row, Peterson, 1953; London: Tavistock Publications, 1954.

8. Schachter, S. 'Deviation, Rejection, and Communication.' *J. abnorm. soc. Psychol.,* Vol. 46, No. 2, 1951, pp. 190–207.

9. Schachter, S., Nuttin, J., de Monchaux, C., Maucorps, P. H., Osmer, D., Dujiker, H., Rommetveit, R., and Israel, J. 'Cross-Cultural Experiments on Threat and Rejection.' *Hum. Relat.,* Vol. VII, 1954, pp. 403–39.

10. Stock, D., and Whitman, R. M. 'Patients' and Therapist's Apperceptions of an Episode in Group Therapy.' *Hum. Relat.,* Vol. X, 1957, pp. 367–83.

11. Whitman, R. M., and Stock, D. 'The Group Focal Conflict.' *Psychiatry* 21:269–276, 1958.

Mechanisms of
Group Psychotherapy:
Processes and Dynamics

RAYMOND J. CORSINI
BINA ROSENBERG

Raymond Corsini, currently Professor of Psychology at the University of Hawaii, published extensively during the 1950s in the group psychodrama literature including an early group text (Methods of Group Psychotherapy. New York: McGraw-Hill, 1957). Corsini was a student of Rudolph Dreikurs in Chicago. His focus on therapeutic factors is very much in keeping with the Adlerian views on the importance of the group as a vehicle for personal and social change. Corsini has continued to make important contributions to the psychotherapy literature (Corsini RJ, Wedding D: Current Psychotherapies, 4th ed. Itasca, Illinois: Peacock Publishers, 1989). This book is dedicated to Dreikurs, Moreno and Rogers.

The present paper is commonly cited as the first major review of what have since become known as "group therapeutic factors." While the authors do not explicitly make reference to the broader social psychology literature, they are clearly operating in line with Lewin's concerns regarding the characteristics of group systems. This paper also moves away from theoretical explanations for group events to descriptions of mechanisms observed to be operating. More recent reviewers of this literature confirm most of the dimensions identified by Corsini and Rosenberg (Bloch S, Crouch E: Therapeutic Factors in Group Psychotherapy. Oxford: Oxford University Press, 1985). Perhaps their greatest contribution occurred indirectly when the "therapeutic factor" literature was adopted as a principal organizing feature in Yalom's influential text.

—Editor

Corsini R, Rosenberg B: Mechanisms of group psychotherapy. *Journal of Abnormal and Social Psychology* 15: 406–411, 1955.

Scientific progress in psychotherapy is dependent to a large extent on the ability of psychotherapists of different schools of thought to communicate. Lacking the universal language of mathematics which has enabled the rapid and orderly development of the natural sciences, social scientists may find that the medium of verbal communication sometimes actually forms a barrier to understanding and progress. The question of semantics and syntactics in psychotherapy is an important one and needs to be explored.

Group psychotherapy has expanded greatly in the past two decades and has already developed a considerable literature. But as may be expected, no differently from individual therapy, it has generated a number of special concepts couched sometimes in esoteric language. While diversity of language per se is not to be deplored, it does seem necessary to find means of effecting maximal communication between people exposed to different frames of reference. The question arises as to whether it is possible to come to semantic generalizations. This paper is devoted to an attempt along these lines.

The Problem

A central issue of psychotherapy is the nature of the dynamics that lead to successful therapy. What within the group therapeutic situation is of the essence?

A simple way to find the answer is to examine the literature. This is perhaps the best way since it must be expected that those who have written on this subject, having gained their knowledge from clinical experience, should have at least partially valid opinions. However, the inquirer finds so much, stated so variously, often so convincingly, and mostly without reference to anyone else, that it is not to be wondered at that one often retires from the literature sadder but not wiser. This can be illustrated in miniature. Three articles are searched for the answer to the question of the dynamics of group therapy.

The first writer lists five dynamics: relationships, catharsis, insight, reality testing, and sublimation.[1] This list seems to make sense and the author's contention that these are the dynamics may assure the reader that the answer has been found. In the second article the reader finds five dynamics. This time they are transference, catharsis, abreaction, loss of isolation, and ego support.[2] The comparison is interesting. Only one dynamic, catharsis, is mentioned by both authorities, and between them they have listed nine mechanisms. Going to the third article, once again five mechanisms are listed: reassurance, reeducation, desensitization, catharsis, and transference.[3] The three writers each have contributed five mechanisms, of which only one, catharsis, is mentioned by all three; transference being mentioned by two. Each of the other ten mechanisms is mentioned by only one of the three experts.

How can this be explained? Have the authorities had different experiences and so found different mechanisms? Are there really 12 different mechanisms, and has each expert recognized only some of them? Or is it possible they are saying the same things in different ways? This problem, here illustrated in miniature, extends throughout the literature on psychotherapy. Had samples been taken from ten or from one hundred writers the list would have been longer and still more puzzling. What is needed is to find some way of arranging, classifying, and synthesizing these separate elements into an orderly and meaningful system. It is this that we have attempted to do.

The Method

The procedures used were based on two assumptions. The first was that all writers on the question of the dynamic mechanisms of group psychotherapy are correct in their opinions, no matter how unusual or how unique their observations. The second assumption is that it is possible for the authors to make certain unifying classificatory judgments about concepts.

The procedures involved four steps:

Step 1: The literature on group psychotherapy was searched for expressions of dynamics. Data were sought in approximately 300 articles, amounting to about one-quarter of the entire literature on group therapy.

Step 2: More than 300 statements were abstracted from the literature and then examined critically to determine whether they could be considered dynamics rather than results, or something else. Eliminating doubtful items left 220 statements to be analyzed.

Step 3: All identical statements were combined. This resulted in 166 different mechanisms.

Step 4: The 166 statements were put on cards and examined to find combinatory hypotheses. For example, it was noted that some of the statements indicated that an often-occurring concept was one that involved a person doing something for another, being philanthropic or altruistic. All cards were then examined to locate statements such as "patient is a therapist to other patients,"[4] "advice by patient," [5] "patients help each other."[6] All cards involving "altruism" were isolated to form a cluster. In this manner hypotheses were suggested and the remaining items searched and combined until a number of cards remained that could not be placed in any established category but yet did not seem to form other categories.

Results

Ten classes of mechanisms were finally isolated by this procedure, nine of which could be assigned specific labels. A tenth group, consisting of items not otherwise assignable, was also formed. The nine chief mechanisms will now be defined. The actual statements will also be listed to show the diversity of opinions in this field and to permit further independent research on this problem.

Mechanisms

Acceptance: This statistically most frequent concept was taken to mean respect for and sympathy with the individual. Acceptance implies belongingness, a warm, friendly, comfortable feeling in the group.

Altruism: Closely related to acceptance, but in addition involving wanting to do something for others, is the mechanism of altruism. The essence of this mechanism is the desire to help others.

Universalization: This concept refers to the realization that one is not unique, that there are others like oneself with problems either identical with or very similar to one's own.

Intellectualization: This is a process of learning or acquiring knowledge in the group. Intellectualization leads to insight, which itself we considered not a mechanism, but a result of intellectualization.

Reality testing: This concept means that the group situation is one where real and important things happen; it is not only a temporary artificial environment. It assumes reality and in it the patient can test himself in a safe and unthreatening atmosphere.

Transference: This concept implies the existence of a strong emotional attachment either to the therapist, to separate members of the group, or to the group as a whole.

Interaction: Perhaps the most difficult of the mechanisms to understand and classify is the one which relates to relationships of unspecified nature within the group. What this process seems to amount to is that any interaction engaged in by a therapeutic group manages to have beneficial results.

Spectator therapy: Through this mechanism people gain from listening to and observing themselves and others.

Ventilation: As in individual therapy, one of the important mechanisms in the group is the release of feelings and the expression of ideas usually repressed in other nontherapeutic situations.

Miscellaneous: A number of statements remaining after classification are listed separately. It must be understood that the concepts in this set of statements need not be considered any less important or any less universal than others that have been either more frequent or easier to combine. Classification is not intended to be value-forming.

The Statements

Below are listed the original data from which the classifications were made. In many cases statements were compressed or reworded to get the essence of the authors' ideas. They are listed according to their classifications in order of statistical frequency, with bibliographic notations to the original articles.

Acceptance. Group identification (23), (40), (58); Group status (25), (55); Esprit de corps (5), (33); Friendly environment (54); Communal feeling (7); Unification of the group (31); Group socialization (33); Loss of isolation (27); Emotional acceptance (63); Feeling of belonging (25), (31); Acceptance by the group (64); Cohesiveness (61); Identification with others (32), (62); Togetherness (16); Strength through belonging (6); Group is tolerant of the patient (52); Protection of the group (52); Ego support (27); Security of the group (52); Conviction of social approval (17); Friendly relations between patients (28); Permissivism (12); "No longer feel alone" (33); Security in a nonthreatening environment (6); Supportive relations (54); Therapist tolerant of patient (37); Therapist is accepting of patient (37); Loss of feeling of isolation (27); Permissive environment (53); Feeling of reassurance (25); Group support (6); Group cohesion (15); Emotional support (4).

Universalization. Universalization (47), (5); Patient recognizes his behavior has been duplicated by many of his mates (48); Realization others have the same problems (28); "People fighting what I am fighting" (26); Realization others similarly affected (26); Demonstrative universality of problems (51); Recognize similar problems in others (13); Illness not individualized (13); Recognize other patients have same difficulty (60); Resonance (36); Realize others are in the same boat (41); Realization of similar problems (34); Knowledge of others with same problems (57); Discovers he is not unique (55).

Reality testing. Testing reality (4), (35), (40), (45), (55), (56); Working through (31), (33), (35); Relive old family conflicts (60); Put patient where he cannot fail (14); Experience for personal interaction (53); Recapitulation of family relationships (32); Practice field for social relations (23); Provides a testing forum (9); Living out of ego frustrations (64); Outlet for aggression (18); Patient finds a setting where he can re-evaluate his concepts (8); Test social reality (4); Recreate family setting (49); Surrogate family (64); Reality of hostilities (33); Revival of conflicts (51); Defenses can be tested (25); Field where one can relate self to others (54); Catharsis-in-the-family (63); Substitute family (55); Appropriate targets for hostility (55).

Altruism. Encouragement (10), (66), (34); Advice by patient (44); Direction by patient (44); Sense of being important in the lives of others (26); Interpretation by patient (23); Suggestion by patient (44); Altruism (24); Patient a therapist to other patients (21); Patient sacrifices personal interest to group (39); Patients help each other (44); Reassurance by compassion (33); Giving love (3).

Transference. Transference (5), (15), (16), (27), (31), (46), (49); Transference to therapist (19), (20), (38), (40); Transference to group (15), (20), (22), (32), (63); Continued flow of emotional support (4); Patient-to-patient transference (63); Countertransference (31); Attachment to therapist (58); Identification to therapist (28).

Spectator Therapy. People patient can imitate (54); Testimony of members (28); Patient listens to himself objectively (19); Passive participation (19); Spectator therapy (42); Example of others (44).

Interaction. Interaction (38), (49), (56); Contagion (39), (61); Relationship (55), (56); Group interaction (34), (63); Relationship to leader (46); Relationship pattern (2); Interaction atmosphere (67); Contact with others (26); Relationship of patient and therapist (34); Experience for personal interaction (53); Interstimulation (51).

Intellectualization. Interpretation (4), (19), (31), (55); Intellectualization (19), (29); Awareness of interpersonal relations (1); Learning common thoughts of others (50); Explanation (57); Understanding defenses of others (1); Understanding (18); Intellectual comprehension (63); Learning (61); Reeducation (15); Analysis of dreams (31); Analysis of resistance (31); Proper evaluation of symptoms (30); Relearning (21); Subject evaluates symptoms in others (48).

Ventilation. Catharsis (15), (21), (25), (27), (33), (35), (40), (43), (55), (56), (59), (63); Abreaction (27), (62); Ventilation of hostilities (9), (63); Ventilation (33), (35); Animosities abreact (20); Verbalization of fantasy (40); Emotional release (2); Release of hostilities in a socially acceptable way (66); Relief of guilt through confession (33); Ventilation of guilt (11); Release of hostilities (66); Activity catharsis (56); Ventilation of anxiety (21); Attitude of verbal expressions (52); Release of unconscious material (63); Expression of unconscious tendencies (2); Activate emotional release (4); Release of repressed drives (4); Releases emotional tension (55).

Miscellaneous. Sublimation (65), (66); Spontaneity (43), (61); Rivalry for improvement (28); Suggestion (10); Authority of the therapist (31); Suggestibility of the group (28); Heightening action (61); Closure of tension systems (21); Therapist's confidence in the patient (37); Substitution (5); Facing the traumatic past (6); Inspired by others to greater effort (26); Social coercion to think rationally (33); Sharing mutual experiences (17); Sharing (62); Relief of isolation through sharing (51); Reinforcement (61); Integration of contradictory tendencies (6); Shock (42); Relaxation (61); Desensitization (15); Sharing difficulties (41); Reassurance (15); Rivalry (39); Intensification (56); Emotional infection (56).

Discussion

The process of combining separate elements into general classes is known as taxonomy. Whether the reductions here effected are the most efficient possible, and whether others operating on other premises or even using the same procedures would have come to the same conclusions, is open to question and to further research. In any case, a rational beginning has been made in the combining of elements into general classes and in the providing of a series of relatively independent factors. This process can be utilized for more effective communication through the reduction of terms.

The nine classes found appear to reduce to three still more general factors. An intellectual factor consisting of universalization, intellectualization, and spectator therapy appears. Also, an emotional factor including acceptance, altruism, and transference evolves. And, there is an actional factor of reality testing, interaction, and ventilation.

From this arises the possibility of evaluating any method of group psychotherapy in terms of these three factors. For example, it seems that Klapman's textbook-mediated therapy and Dreikurs' group counseling have a high component of the intellectual factor; that Rogers' nondirective group counseling and Schilder's analytic group therapy have a relatively high degree of the emotional factor; and that Moreno's psychodrama and Slavson's activity group therapy have a large amount of the actional factor.

Summary

Some 300 articles in the literature of group psychotherapy were examined to locate expressions referring to effecting dynamic processes of therapy. Some 200 items were obtained and reduced by inspection to nine general classes and a miscellaneous class. The nine general classes appear to reduce to three factors: an *intellectual* one, consisting of universalization, intellectualization, and spectator therapy; an *emotional* one, consisting of acceptance, altruism, and transference; and an *actional* factor, consisting of reality testing, interaction, and ventilation.

It is believed this reductionism can be useful in providing better communication between group therapists and can be the basis for further research in the basic components of group therapy.

References

1. S. R. Slavson, "Advances in Group Psychotherapy," *Int. Congr. Ment. Health*, 24–26, 1948.
2. S. B. Hadden, "Dynamics of Group Psychotherapy," *Arch. Neurol. Psychiat.*, 65:125, 1944
3. J. M. Cotton, "Group Psychotherapy: An Appraisal," in P. H. Hoch (ed.), *Failures in Psychiatric Treatment* (New York: Grune and Stratton, 1948), pp. 121–128.
4. J. M. Enneis, "The Dynamics of Group and Action Procedures in Therapy," *Group Psychother.*, 4:17–22, 1951.

5. H. Mullan, "Some Essentials of Group Psychotherapy," *Group Psychother.*, 5:68–69, 1952.
6. *Ibid.*

Bibliography

1. Abrahams, J., "Preliminary Report of an Experience in the Group Therapy of Schizophrenics," *Am. J. Psychiat.*, *104*:613–617,1948.
2. Ackerman, N. W., "Group Therapy from the Viewpoint of a Psychiatrist," *Am. J. Orthopsychiat.*, *31*:667–681, 1943.
3. ————, "Psychotherapy and Giving Love," *Psychiat.*, 7:129–137, 1944.
4. ————, "Some General Principles in the Use of Group Psychotherapy," in B. Glueck, ed., *Current Therapies of Personality Disorders* (New York: Grune & Stratton, 1946), pp. 275–280.
5. Altschuler, I. M., "One Year's Experience with Group Psychotherapy," *Ment. Hyg.*, 24:190–196, 1940.
6. Bettelheim, B., and Sylvester, Emmy, "Therapeutic Influence of the Group and the Individual," *Am. J. Orthopsychiat.*, *17*:684–692, 1947.
7. Betz, K., "Gruppentraining und Bilderlefen," *Z. Psychother. Med. Psychol.*, *1*:71–76, 1951.
8. Blackman, N., "Ward Therapy—New Method of Group Psychotherapy," *Psychiat. Quart.*, *16*:660–667, 1942.
9. ————, "Group Psychotherapy with Aphasics," *J. Nerv. Ment. Dis.*, *154–163*, 1950.
10. Buck, R. W., "The Class Method in the Treatment of Essential Hypertension," *Ann. Int. Med.*, *11*:514–518, 1937.
11. Caplan, G., "Mental Hygiene Work with Expectant Mothers," *Ment. Hyg.*, 35:41–50, 1951.
12. Coffey, H., Friedman, M., Leary, T., and Ossorio, A., "Social Implications of the Group Therapeutic Situation," *J. Soc. Issues*, 6:44–61,1950.
13. Colthorp, R. W., "Group Psychotherapy in Patients Recovering from Psychoses, *Am. J. Psychiat.*, *104*:414–417,1947.
14. Cotton, J. M., "The Psychiatric Treatment Program at Welch Convalescent Hospital," *Res. Pub. Ass. Nerv. Ment. Dis.*, *25*:316–321, 1946.
15. ————, "Group Psychotherapy: An Appraisal," in P. H. Hoch, ed., Failures in Psychiatric Treatment (New York: Grune & Stratton, 1948), pp. 121–128.
16. ————, "Group Structure and Group Psychotherapy," *Group Psychother.*, *3*:216–217, 1951.
17. Curran, F. J., and Schilder, P., "A Constructive Approach to the Problems of Childhood and Adolescence," *J. Crim. Psychopath.*, *2*:125–142, 305–320, 1940–1941.
18. Curran, F. J., "Group Therapy: Introductory Remarks," *Neuropsychiat.*, *2*:43–47, 1952.
19. Dreikurs, R., "Technique and Dynamics of Multiple Psychotherapy," *Psychiat. Quart.*, *24*:788–799, 1950.
20. Dreyfus-Moreau, J., "A Propos du Transfert en Psychotherapie Collective," *Rev. Franc. Psychoanal.*, *14*:244–257, 1950.

21. Enneis, J. M., "The Dynamics of Group and Action Procedures in Therapy," *Group Psychother.*, 4:17–22, 1951.
22. Glatzer, H., "Transference in Group Therapy," *Am. J. Orthopsychiat.*, 22:499–509, 1952.
23. Golden, M. M., "Some Mechanisms of Analytic Group Therapy," *Int. J. Group Psychother.*, 3:280–284, 1952.
24. Greenblatt, M., "Altruism in the Psychotherapeutic Relation," in P. A. Sorokin, ed., Explorations in Altruistic Love and Behavior (Boston: Beacon Press, 1950), pp. 188–193.
25. Grotjahn, M., "Experiences with Group Psychotherapy as a Method for the Treatment of Veterans," *Am. J. Psychiat.*, 103:637–643, 1947.
26. Hadden, S. B., "Group Psychotherapy: A Superior Method of Treating Larger Numbers of Neurotics," *Am. J. Psychiat.*, 101:68–72, 1944.
27. ———, "Dynamics of Group Psychotherapy," *Arch. Neurol. Psychiat.*, 65:125, 1951.
28. Harris, H. I, "Efficient Psychotherapy for the Large Outpatient Clinic," *New England J. Med.*, 221:1–15, 1939.
29. Johnston, M., "Experiment with Narcotic Addicts," *Am. J. Psychother.*,5:24–31, 1951.
30. Jones, M., "Group Treatment with Particular Reference to Group Projective Methods," *Am. J. Psychiat.*, 101:293–299, 1944.
31. Kew, C. E., and Kew, C. J., "Group Psychotherapy in a Church Setting," *Pastoral Psychol.*, 1:36–39, 1950.
32. Klapman, J. W., "Group Treatment of the Mentally Ill," *Survey Mid-Monthly*, 82:80–81, 1946.
33. Kline, N. S., and Dreyfus, A., "Group Psychotherapy in a Veterans Administration Hospital," *Am. J. Psychiat.*, 104:618–622, 1948.
34. Konopka, G., "Group Work and Therapy," in C. E. Hendy, ed., A Decade of Group Work (New York: Association Press, 1948), pp. 39–44.
35. Krise, M., "Creative Dramatics and Group Psychotherapy," *J. Child Psychiat.*, 2:337–342, 1952
36. Lebovici, S., Diatkine, R., and Kestenberg, E., "Applications of Psychoanalysis to Group Psychotherapy and Psychodramatic Therapy in France," Group Psychother., 5:38–50, 1952.
37. Lipkin, S., "Notes on Group Psychotherapy," *J. Nerv. Ment. Dis.*, 107:459–479, 1948.
38. Lowrey, L. G., "Group Treatment for Mothers," *Am. J. Orthopsychiat.*, 14:589–592, 1944
39. Marsh, L. C., "Group Therapy of the Psychoses by the Psychological Equivalent of the Revival," *Ment. Hyg.*, 15:328–349, 1931.
40. Mayers, A. N., "A Psychiatric Evaluation of Discussion Groups," *J. Nerv. Ment. Dis.*, 111:499–509, 1950.
41. Miller, H., and Baruch, D., "Psychological Dynamics in Allergic Patients as Shown in Group and Individual Psychotherapy," *J. Consult. Psychol.*, 12:111–115, 1948.
42. Moreno, J. L., "Psychodramatic Shock Therapy," *Sociometry*, 2:1–30, 1939.
43. Moreno, J. L., and Toeman, Z., "The Group Approach in Psychodrama," Sociometry, 5:191–194, 1942.
44. Mullan, H., "Some Essentials of Group Psychotherapy," *Group Psychother.*,

5:68–69, 1952.

45. Parrish, M., and Mitchell, J., "Psychodrama in Pontiac State Hospital," *Group Psychother.*, 4:80–84, 1951 .

46. Pederson-Krag, G., "Unconscious Factors in Group Therapy," *Psychoanal. Quart.*, 15:180–189, 1946.

47. Pfeffer, A. Z., Friedland, P., and Wortis, S. B., "Group Psychotherapy with Alcoholics," *Quart. J. Stud. Alchol.*, 10:198–216, 1949.

48. Rome, H. P., "Group Psychotherapy," *Dis. Nerv. Syst.*, 6:237–241, 1945.

49. Scheidlinger, S., "Group Therapy: Its Place in Psychotherapy," *J. Soc. Casewk.*, 29:299–304, 1948.

50. Schilder, P., "Introductory Remarks on Groups," *J. Soc. Psychol.*, 12:83–100, 1940.

51. Shaskan, D. A., and Jolesch, M., "War and Group Psychotherapy," *Am. J. Orthopsychiat.*, 14:571–577, 1944

52. Shaskan, D. A., "Development of Group Psychotherapy in a Military Setting," *Proc. Assoc. Research Nerv. Ment. Dis.*, 25:311–315, 1946.

53. Slavson, S. R., An Introduction to Group Therapy (New York: Commonwealth, Fund, 1943).

54. ———, "Differential Methods of Group Therapy in Relation to Age Levels," *Nerv. Child*, 4:196–210, 1945.

55. ———, "The Field and Objectives of Group Therapy," in B. Glueck, ed., Current Therapies of Personality Disorders (New York: Grune & Stratton, 1946), pp. 166–193.

56. ———, "Advances in Group Psychotherapy," *Int. Congr. Ment. Health*, 24:26, 1948.

57. Snowden, E. N., "Mass Psychotherapy," *Lancet*, 11:769–770, 1940.

58. Sternbach, O., "The Dynamics of Psychological Treatment in the Group," *J. Child Psychiat.*, 1:91–112, 1947.

59. Swenson, W. M., "Round Table Group Psychotherapy at St. Peters State Hospital," *Group Psychother.*, 4:63–65, 1953.

60. Teirich, H. R., "Was Ist Gruppenpsychotherapie?" *Psychother. Med. Psychol.*, 1: 26–30, 1951.

61. Twitchell-Allen, D., and Stephens, F. M., "Some Theoretical and Practical Aspects of Group Psychotherapy," *Group Psychother.*, 4:9–16, 1951.

62. Wender, L., "The Dynamics of Group Psychotherapy and Its Applications," *J. Nerv. Ment. Dis.*, 84:54–60, 1936.

63. ———, "Group Psychotherapy Within the Psychiatric Hospital," in B. Glueck, ed., Current Therapies of Personality Disorders (New York: Grune & Stratton, 1946), pp. 46–58.

64. ———, "Current Trends in Group Psychotherapy," *Am. J. Psychother.*, 5:381–404, 1951.

65. Willner, G. P., "Preliminary Report of the Introduction of Group Psychotherapy on a Chronic Ward in a Mental Hospital," *Psychiat. Quart. Suppl.*, 26:86–92, 1952.

66. Wittenberg, R., "Psychiatric Concepts in Group Work," *Am. J. Orthopsychiat.*, 14:76–83, 1944.

67. Wolf. A.. Locke, N., Rosenbaum, M., Hillpern, E. P., Goldfarb, W., Kadis, A. L., Obers, S. J., Milberg, I. L., and Abell, R. G., "The Psychoanalysis of Groups: The Analysts' Objections," *Int. J. Group Psychother.*, 2:221–231, 1952.

Some Determinants, Manifestations, and Effects of Cohesiveness in Therapy Groups

JEROME D. FRANK, M.D., PH.D.

Department of Psychiatry,
Johns Hopkins University Medical School, Baltimore, Md.

Jerome D. Frank began his career as a graduate student in psychology under the direct supervision of Kurt Lewin. His projects included issues related to self-esteem and the effects of social pressure. Following medical training he joined the staff at the Johns Hopkins Medical School, where he is now Professor Emeritus of Psychiatry.

He had the opportunity to work with Florence Powdermaker at the National Institute of Health on a large study of group psychotherapy. One of the important early group texts resulted (Powdermaker F, Frank JD. Group Psychotherapy: Studies in Methodology of Research and Therapy. Westport, CT: Greenwood Press, 1953). Since that time, Frank's named has been linked to numerous prominent psychotherapy researchers such Morris Parloff and Stanley Imber. Frank introduced Irv Yalom to group psychotherapy and was one of his early group supervisors, producing a continuous group psychotherapy lineage from the mid-thirties to the present.

Frank's work led him to the conclusion that the central therapeutic mechanism of psychotherapy was its effect on combating a demoralized state. This would account for the general effectiveness of psychotherapy but the lack of differentiation between different approaches. This theme was central to his book "Persuasion and Healing: A Comparative Study of Psychotherapy" first published in 1961. A true classic in the psychotherapy literature, it is now available in a new and revised third edition co-authored with his daughter Julia B. Frank (Baltimore: Johns Hopkins University Press, 1991).

Group cohesiveness can be seen as the group analogue of the therapeutic alliance in individual therapy. Current documentation of the links between a positive alliance and outcome provides confirmation of Frank's early emphasis on the importance of a positive, supportive and mastery-focused therapeutic environment. —Editor

Frank JD: Some determinants, manifestations, and effects of cohesiveness in therapy groups. *International Journal of Group Psychotherapy* 7:53–63, 1957.

Group therapy, like all therapy, attempts to foster change in individual patients. Group therapists, therefore, tend to conceptualize phenomena in therapeutic groups exclusively in terms of the influence of personal characteristics and behaviour of the members and therapist on each other, the group itself being merely the arena in which these events occur.

It is clear, however, that a person's responses are determined not only by the other persons with whom he comes in contact but by the properties of the groups to which he belongs. Group standards and codes which a member has internalized may be relatively independent of the particular members of the group. In this sense the group is not so much an arena as a social field. The properties of this field are determined by many factors, in addition to personal attributes of the members composing it at any one time, and each member is influenced by these properties. The attitudes of a professional soldier, for example, are determined to a larger degree by the codes and standards of the army than by the personal characteristics of his fellows. And these standards are only very slightly modified by any individual soldier.

Recent experimental studies of small face-to-face groups suggest that, as with larger, more permanent organizations, certain of their properties which are relatively independent of the personal attributes of the members, may strongly influence aspects of the behaviour of each participant. Since these studies are based on "a face-to-face social organization involving a lasting, personally meaningful communication relationship,"[1] it would seem that they might be relevant to group psychotherapy. One such property is cohesiveness. This is defined experimentally as the degree of the members' sense of belonging to a group or, more simply, as the attractiveness of a group for its members. This concept seems to have special relevance for psychotherapy, because it has been found that the greater the cohesiveness of a group the more influence its standards exert on its members.

While recognizing the indispensability of conceptualization of group therapy in terms of the interplay of the particular personalities of the group members, this paper attempts to explore some implications for therapy of group cohesiveness, viewed as a property of the group in itself. Some well-known phenomena will be looked at as determinants, manifestations, and effects of the cohesiveness of the therapeutic group.[2]

Gregariousness and Its Manifestations

A major source of cohesiveness in therapeutic groups may lie in the fact that man is gregarious and can gain complete self-fulfilment only through harmonious interactions with his fellows. The tendency of groups to maintain themselves is seen in all gregarious creatures.[3] An example of its operation in humans is the way committees and institutions strive to continue their existence after they have fulfilled the purpose for which they were created.

Certain phenomena occur so regularly in therapeutic groups as to suggest that, although they may be convincingly explained on the basis of the psychodynamics of the individuals involved, they may also represent the tendency of all human beings to make those groups of which they are members cohesive. Our patients, like the rest of mankind, seem to strive to make the groups they are in the kind of groups they want to belong to. Thus, in early meetings of a group members try hard to find bases for mutual attraction. They hasten to identify themselves and others in ways which they believe will be acceptable. They search for superficial similarities, but fail to pursue these to the point where important points of difference might emerge. Expressions of hostility are directed toward the environment of the group rather than toward the group itself. In a hospital mutual griping about the conditions of hospitalization occurs universally. In outpatient groups complaints are usually directed toward influential members of the social environment of the patients. This type of activity serves not only to find common grounds on which the group may coalesce, but to displace expressions of hostility from the group to the environment. Attacks on those outside the group may also serve to increase the attractiveness of the group to its members as a source of prestige, as when an attack is based on the failure of the outsider to understand the value of this type of experience or to appreciate his own need for it.

The universal tendency of members to continue interacting outside of the regular group meetings may be viewed as a manifestation of their efforts to become cohesive. Patients chat animatedly before the therapist enters the room or after he leaves, only to freeze up in his presence. Social contacts soon progress to stopping for coffee after the group therapy sessions or sharing rides to and from them. There may develop, even without the therapist's encouragement, meetings of segments of the group or even the total group in members homes, although this seldom eventuates well unless it occurs with his sanction and guidance. In these subgroups patients have a chance to dissipate disjunctive feelings generated at the group sessions and to strengthen mutually attractive forces. In this connection, it has been shown experimentally that the more the members of a group communicate in a friendly way with each other, the more they like the group.

It has also been found that splinter groups tend to disrupt a parent group when their goals are incompatible with it, but strengthen it when their goals are the same as or supportive of the larger body's goals. Many disadvantages of informal subgroup formation outside the therapeutic group have been noted. Hostile patients may utilize such meetings to disrupt the functioning of the larger group. Social meetings may dispel the social incognito which some therapists feel must be maintained if there is to be a free interchange of feeling in the group.[4] Occasionally they intensify the scapegoating of a member who does not participate in any of them. It is, however, my impression that the activities of most informal subgroups are primarily concerned with fence mending; that is, seeking increased intimacy and dispelling hostilities and anxieties which the larger group may have conjured up. As these goals are compatible, though not identical, with those of the parent group participation in sub-groups probably tends to increase its attractiveness. The conflictful attitudes of therapy groups to new members may express one of the problems inherent in a group's efforts to maintain cohesiveness. A group wishes to exclude strangers as threats to its cohesiveness, but if it kept them out forever it would eventually perish by attrition. The initiation rites of organized groups may be viewed as resolutions of this problem. Members are accepted only after they have demonstrated their adherence to the group's code by undergoing suffering for its sake.

Applying this thought to therapy groups, we may note, first, two circumstances under which new members are usually accepted without difficulty. One is in early sessions before much feeling of cohesiveness has developed; the other is when the group is so small that its survival is doubtful. Patients of such a group often request that members be added.

A well established therapy group however, resents newcomers, and the behaviour of the regular members vacillates between attempts to integrate and to exclude them. At one extreme are activities that can be interpreted as efforts to freeze the newcomer out, such as discussion of incidents in earlier sessions or of members who are absent. The flurry of questions about absentees, which the entrance of a newcomer often provokes, may also represent efforts of old members to reassure themselves as to the stability of the group. An intermediate activity is close personal questioning of the newcomer, often maliciously tinged, which may simultaneously express urges to identify and assimilate the stranger as rapidly as possible, to test the strength of his willingness to accept the group, to demonstrate how the group functions, and to drive him out. It often seems somewhat analogous to hazing. Finally, old members may try to facilitate the integration of the newcomer by demonstrating through their own interactions how the group functions, or by offering information about its goals and procedures.

Aspects of patients' management of hostility may also be viewed as related to the need of the group to remain cohesive. Although the group facilitates expression of hostility to the therapist, if the group is at all cohesive, the latter can always count on some members of the group coming to his rescue and on the tone of the group as a whole not remaining hostile for long. This seems related to the fact that the attractiveness of the group depends partly on members' preserving their perception of the therapist as a potential source of help and a figure of prestige, through identification with whom they gain status.

With respect to hostility toward fellow members, the kind of patient who most often receives the group's ire is more easily defined in terms of his effect on the group than his underlying psychodynamics. Common to all patients who are strongly attacked by the group is that their behaviour tends to disrupt the group's cohesiveness or prevent its increase. It has been noted in research groups that members tend to leave when others are felt to be too dominating. In therapy groups, similarly, the compulsive monopolist, who grossly impedes the development of a cohesive interaction network, regularly arouses hostility in other group members. Those members who cannot vent their hostility often leave; and if the compulsive monopolist cannot be brought to modify his behaviour he may disrupt the group. The frequent scapegoating of patients who have a derogatory attitude to the group, even if they are outwardly pleasant, may be related to their being a threat to the attractiveness of the group for the other members.

One of the puzzling phenomena of group psychotherapy is that attacks under certain conditions are therapeutically helpful to their object rather than the reverse. The attacked member may emerge with increased self-confidence and with a beneficial change of attitude. Some of the conditions making for this fortunate result have been considered in another publication.[5] Reviewing this subject in the light of its possible relationship to group cohesiveness, I have been struck by how frequently helpful attacks have been made, as it were, in the name of the group. Criticism of a member because he is behaving in such a way that the group cannot integrate him into their activities seems especially likely to eventuate usefully. When a patient yields to such an attack and modifies his behaviour accordingly, he is promptly rewarded by experiencing a greater sense of acceptance by the group. This may shield his self-respect from the damage that it would otherwise have suffered and also reinforce the new pattern of behaviour.

Other Sources of Cohesiveness

The gregarious drive as a source of group cohesiveness is probably impossible to manipulate experimentally. Experimenters with small groups have distinguished four general sources of group cohesiveness which can be manipulated, and therefore have implications for the management of therapeutic groups. They have found that a member tends to find a group attractive to the extent that (1) he perceives it as potentially meeting a personal need; (2) he likes the other members; (3) he likes the group activities; and (4) he sees the group as conferring prestige or status because of its relation to its social environment. Let us consider some implications of these points for the handling of therapeutic groups.

Satisfaction of Personal Needs

The attractiveness of a group can be increased either by heightening the satisfaction the members get from participating in it, or by increasing their awareness that they can fulfil their needs through it. The therapist can increase members' satisfaction from participation, through his definition of the therapeutic task as discussed below. With respect to the second point, many patients do not see how a group can do them any good. Cultural traditions in our society portray the therapeutic relationship exclusively as a private one between patient and therapist. Furthermore, many patients do not initially perceive the kind of activity that goes on in a therapy group as even remotely useful to them. Thus, to foster the development of cohesiveness the therapist should keep before the members the ways in which the group can help them.

Attractiveness of Members

With respect to the mutual attraction of members, it should be mentioned first that members of a group need not like each other in order for it to be cohesive. Individuals may have a strong sense of belonging to groups in the face of considerable mutual antagonism. Family loyalty, for example, is entirely compatible with dislike of certain members of the clan, and even the healthiest primary groups inevitably contain components of competition, rivalry, jealousy and other disjunctive feelings.[6] Nevertheless, mutual liking is undoubtedly a strong source of group cohesiveness, and in this respect the therapeutic group is initially at a great disadvantage. Mentally ill patients characteristically are contemptuous of themselves and therefore of each other. In line with their rather immature level of functioning they are apt to be self centred and to lack a genuine interest in others. Because of damaging past experiences with people, many of them have little expectancy of gaining anything from close relationships. The normal fear of the stranger is heightened in psychiatric patients and tends to create mutual hostility.[7] Moreover, mutual attractions of patients are often based on transference reactions, "set-up operations," and so on, and are therefore apt to evaporate or change to antagonisms as patients' self-understanding increases.

The group therapist, however, has certain opportunities to facilitate the development of mutual attractions. He can exploit patients' initial attraction to himself as the major source of help by clearly assuming his role as leader, a role which is definite even in the most permissive of groups. Through identifying with him, patients are helped to identify with each other. Moreover, many patients who cannot relate comfortably as peers can do so as help-seekers. Links formed on this basis may afford a starting point for developing more mutually satisfying relationships. The leader can tacitly or openly encourage the "fence-mending" activities described earlier not only in the group but outside it, so long as the material brought up in these situations is regarded as grist for the mill of the group itself. He can help members to see similarities in their problems or experiences which might make them potentially useful to each other. In short, the therapist can foster transient and superficial sources of mutual liking as a temporary scaffolding until sounder relationships develop. A major source of these is patients' eventual discovery that they can be helpful to each other. This does not always increase mutual liking, but it invariably leads to increased self-respect, which makes the group more attractive.

Attractiveness of Group's Activities

Therapy groups as ordinarily conducted pay little attention to this. Often it is not clear just what the activity or the goals of the group are. This contributes to the confusion many patients feel in early sessions. Nor does the group have a goal outside itself which would serve to guide its activities and to minimize personal clashes, as patients work toward a common end.

Whatever the activities of a therapy group, the therapist can help make them attractive to the members by selecting those which are within the patients' competence but sufficiently difficult to be challenging, and by making clear what they are and how success in carrying them out is to be judged. He should do this more by example than precept so as not to intensify the patients' conflicts about submission to authority. In the process of defining the group's activities, he is at the same time implying how they can be expected to meet the patients' needs.

These considerations apply as much to free discussion groups as to therapeutic social clubs or psychodrama, for free discussion is a specific task with definite standards of success. These include the extent to which participants express their feelings honestly and accept responsibility for the consequences, and the skill at analyzing their own and others' motives.

The activities of a therapy group yield two kinds of rewards which help to make them attractive. The first is the approbation of the therapist and other group members for performing successfully in the group. A patient may gain a real sense of achievement by, for example, being the first to recognize a distortion of perception in another patient or himself. The second source of satisfaction lies in the patient's increased success in dealing with persons outside the group as a carryover from his successful performance in it.

Attractive and Restraining Forces in the Group's Environment

A group in relation to its social environment may exert attractive forces on its members or the environment may exert restraining forces impeding members from leaving it. The most common source of attraction is prestige and status that accrues from belonging to it. Initially, therapy groups are at a gross disadvantage in this respect. Most members feel stigmatized at having to come to them. In successful groups, however, patients gradually develop some pride in membership. They come to look down on persons they know who have similar emotional problems but who lack the sense to seek treatment. They come to perceive the values and standards of the group as better than those of the world at large, in that, for example, they are more tolerant and stress the value of self-knowledge.

Restraining forces play a significant part in securing members attendance at many therapy groups. Quite a few patients, especially in the lower cultural and economic class, come to therapy under pressure from family, employer, or social agencies. Obviously a group maintained by outside pressures, although it may obtain overt conformity of behaviour is unlikely to produce genuine changes of attitude and motivation. Not too infrequently, however, patients who come to a group under compulsion undergo a change of heart and find it genuinely attractive. We have seen this phenomenon particularly in alcoholics. An example from daily life is that of a draftee who struggles against being inducted but once in the army wholeheartedly accepts its activities and values.

Group Cohesiveness and the Aims of Psychotherapy

Having considered some of the sources of cohesiveness in therapeutic groups and certain behaviour patterns of members in the light of this concept, I should like to mention some effects on members of attraction to a group as related to the aims of psychotherapy.

All forms of psychotherapy try to help patients achieve beneficial and permanent changes of attitude through resolution of conflicts. Essential to this aim is the maintenance and strengthening of the patient's self-esteem so that he gains courage to face his problems and to try new means of resolving them, and the mobilization of his emotions which supply the motive power for change. A cohesive group with proper standards protects and enhances the self-esteem of its members, fortifies their ability to consolidate and maintain beneficial changes in behaviour or attitudes, helps them to resolve conflicts, and facilitates constructive release of feeling.

Maintaining Therapeutic Change

A cohesive group not only exerts pressure on members to change, but strengthens their ability to maintain the changes it has helped bring about. Allegiance to a group helps members to hold to their decisions. If these decisions arise out of group discussion and have its sanction, the member feels that he cannot let the group down by recanting. It has been shown that group discussion leads to more permanent change of behaviour than individual persuasion.[8] It seems likely that the more cohesive a group is—that is, the more each member feels himself a part of it—the stronger this force will be. Thus, the group helps its members to maintain changes which in the eyes of the group are beneficial to him until they can gain sufficient reinforcement from experiences outside the group. A paradoxical example is that of the submissive member who, in compliance with the group's standards, forces himself to act aggressively; that is, he acts aggressively because he is basically submissive. This pseudo aggressiveness, bolstered by his allegiance to the group, may lead to beneficial changes in his relationships with important persons in his life.

Cohesiveness and Resistance

The cohesiveness of a group might conceivably impede therapy if its standards were such as to strengthen members' resistance. Emotionally ill persons cling to their symptoms and have distorted perceptions of themselves and others; hence groups composed of them might well be expected to develop antitherapeutic norms. Although this misgiving seems plausible, its validity is dubious. Foulkes has suggested that "The deepest reason why . . . patients . . . can reinforce each other's normal reactions and correct each other's neurotic reactions is that *collectively they constitute the very Norm from which, individually, they deviate.*"[9] An important safeguard against a therapy group's becoming cohesively resistant is that it can develop cohesiveness only by incorporating the standards of the therapist. It cannot remain in a stable league against him because the patients come to it in order to get his help. This is seen in the group's reluctance to gang up on the therapist, as mentioned above. If certain members find his terms unacceptable, they will leave. Thus the therapist, provided he makes his expectancies for the group clear, can be confident that, despite forces toward resistance, the group as it develops cohesiveness will incorporate the standards which he considers desirable. In this connection it is worth pointing out that cohesiveness does not necessarily imply pressure toward conformity, which is undesirable in therapeutic groups, because the standards of even a cohesive group may encourage diversity. According to Cartwright and Zander, "Groups may sometimes agree that they will not allow pressures for conformity to develop in certain areas in order for example . . . that freedom of thought may be respected."[10]

Cohesiveness and Members' Self-Esteem

The feeling of belonging to a group is a powerful supporter of self-respect. The self-esteem of a member of a cohesive group rests partly, of course, on the group's prestige in his eyes. One thinks of the family pride of a scion of the upper class as compared to the self-derogatory feelings of some members of slum families. Membership in any group, however, seems to convey more self-esteem than membership in no group at all. It heightens the member's sense of personal importance because each knows that he has an influence on the others, even when absent; that is, they will act differently in his absence than when he is present. In therapy groups, furthermore, each patient gains confidence and encouragement from watching others improve; he then identifies with them, which in turn would seem to be a function of the cohesiveness of the group. Members of a cohesive group come to occupy definite roles and to have clear role expectations for each other. In this way, each is helped to clarify his self-image, at least in respect to those aspects of himself that are relevant to the group's functioning.

Cohesiveness and Resolution of Conflicts

Most mental patients are in deadlocked conflicts with certain aspects of their social environment, reflecting their inner conflicts. Individual therapy attempts to resolve the latter and so facilitate resolution of the former. But the converse also holds; in the process of resolving a neurotically based conflict with another person, internal integration may be increased. In a cohesive group patients can work out such conflicts, if the group standard is that antagonists must continue communicating no matter how angry they become with each other. Mutual hostilities disrupt communications, permitting mutual distortions to develop, which increase the hostility, leading to a vicious circle.[11] A cohesive therapy group increases the ability of patients to tolerate a conflict by protecting their self-esteem. By putting pressure on them to continue communicating, it can often carry them to a successful resolution based on deeper and more accurate mutual understanding.

Cohesiveness and Expression of Feelings

Finally, a cohesive therapy group with the proper code mobilizes and guides the release of emotion in its members in such a way as to be most helpful to them. The code must encourage each member to express his feelings freely and honestly but only on condition that he take full responsibility for them. This implies trying to understand his own motivations and being willing to accept the consequences of his actions in the reactions of other patients. Under these conditions the free expression of emotion can be a powerful aid, if not a necessary prerequisite, to therapeutic changes of attitude.

This leads to another presumed drawback of group cohesiveness, namely, that the more members are attracted to a group, the more they may be inclined to guard expressions of feeling which might be disruptive. This may result in the group's being "too comfortable." Though it is true that in early group meetings members, out of their urge to develop cohesion, may struggle to establish a code of superficial conformity and social politeness, the therapist's attitude and the desire of members to express themselves more freely are usually sufficient to counteract this. In my experience groups seldom become too comfortable. They may become apathetic, but this is rarely an expression of comfort, it is rather an indication that patients are concealing hostile feelings which they do not yet dare express. It should be added, however, that for certain groups of psychotics, alcoholics and aggressive psychopaths the norm should be one of greater control of feelings rather than freer expression of them.

Conclusion

The thesis of this paper is that interactions of members of a therapy group may be understood in part as manifestations of properties of the group per se rather than as exclusively determined by personal characteristics of the members. As an illustration, some therapeutic implications of the concept of group cohesiveness, as used by researchers in group dynamics, are explored. The therapeutic relevance of group cohesiveness lies chiefly in the fact that the more a group's members are attracted to it, the more they are influenced by its standards. If these approve diversity of outlook, nondefensive expressions of feelings and honest attempts at self-examinations; if they reward maintenance of communication no matter how angry patients get at each other; and if they put a premium not on mutual liking but on mutual respect—then the more cohesive the group is, the more likely it is to induce therapeutic changes in its members.

References

1. Libo, L.M.: *Measuring Group Cohesiveness.* Ann Arbor, Mich: University of Michigan, 1953, p.5.
2. The following discussion draws heavily on the following: Cartwright, D. and Zander, A.: *Group Dynamics.* Evanston, Illinois: Row Peterson and Company, 1953; Libo: *op. cit.*; Lippitt, R.: Group Dynamics: 2. Group Dynamics and Personality Dynamics. *Am. J. Orthopsychiat., 21*:18–31, 1951; Bach, G. R.: *Intensive Group Psychotherapy.* New York: Ronald Press Co., 1954.
3. David Levy has discussed this point in a particularly stimulating way. Cf. The Strange Hen. *Am. J. Orthopsychiat., 20*:355–362, 1950.
4. Lindt, H. and Sherman, M. A.: "Social Incognito" in Analytically Oriented Group Psychotherapy. *International Journal of Group Psychotherapy, 2*:209, 1952.
5. Frank, J. D.: Some Values of Conflict in Therapeutic Groups. *Group Psychother., 8*:142–151, 1955.
6. Cooley, C. H.: The Social Foundations and Functions of Thought and Communication. In: *Small Groups: Studies in Social Interaction*, ed. A. Hare, E. Borgatta, and R. Bales. New York: Alfred A. Knopf, 1955.
7. Mann, J.: Some Theoretic Concepts of the Group Process. *International Journal of Group Psychotherapy, 5*:235, 1955.
8. Lewin, K. Group Decision and Social Change. In *Readings in Social Psychology*, ed.

T. M. Newcomb and E. L. Hartley. New York: H. Holt, 1947.

9. Foulkes, S. H: *Introduction to Group-Analytic Psychotherapy.* London: W. Heinemann, 1948, p.29.

10. Cartwright, D. and Zander, A., *op. cit.*, p. 141. See ref. 2.

11. Newcomb, T. M.: Autistic Hostility—Social Reality. *Human Relations,* 1:69- 87, 1947.

Are There "Group Dynamics" in Therapy Groups?

S. R. SLAVSON
New York, NY

Samuel R. Slavson (1890–1981) is the father of group psychotherapy in America. He was born in Russia and immigrated to New York at the age of 13. He first became interested in group methods through his development in 1911 of coeducational groups for adolescents known as "Self-Culture" clubs. These emphasized an introduction to the creative arts as well as group discussions. There is an ironic symmetry that during the same year, Moreno was exploring the use of group methods on the streets of Vienna.

Slavson later became involved in progressive education as a consultant to the prestigious Walden School in New York and the Malting Housing School in Cambridge, England. His early publication (with Robert K. Spear. Science in the New Education. New York: Prentice-Hall, 1934) was chosen as one the Ten Best Books of the Year by the American Publishers Association. During the early thirties Slavson, who in the meantime had acquired training and work as a civil engineer, became involved with the Jewish Board of Guardians as a further extension of his community service. Casual experiments with group activities for troubled young girls resulted in a shift in emphasis from a creative to a therapeutic function. The first formally organized group therapy with children began in 1934. With the support of his brother John Slavson, who was Director of the agency, Slavson actively promoted the use of groups and eventually joined the staff and became head of the new Group Therapy Department in 1939. It was only after the main principles of Activity Group Therapy were well established that Slavson became more conversant with psychoanalytical psychology.

Slavson's first major presentation concerning group methods was at the 1943 meeting of the American Orthopsychiatric Association in New York City. From that time onward he became a prolific contributor to the literature, particularly through the International Journal of Group Psychotherapy, which he founded in 1951 and edited for many years. Slavson was the most dominant leader in the American group psychotherapy movement and the primary sustaining force behind the early years of the American Group Psychotherapy Association. These events are dealt with at more length in the historical chapter of this book.

There was considerable discussion about which of Slavson's 194 publications to include in this volume. For example, his paper on selection is highly regarded (Criteria for selection and rejection of patients for various types of group psychotherapy. International Journal of Group Psychotherapy 5:3–30, 1955). The article printed here was chosen because it highlights a central theoretical divide in the history of group therapy. From the beginning, there has been tension between treating the individual in the group, focusing on the interactions and distortions emerging between the members, or viewing the group as a single entity. Perhaps the strongest statements favoring treatment of the individual in the group context have been made by Alexander Wolf and Emmanuel Schwartz (Psychoanalysis in Groups. New York: Grune & Stratton, 1962). The tension between these viewpoints lies not only in the theoretical literature, but in the daily practice of running groups when decisions must constantly be made regarding which level to address. Slavson, characteristically, comes down strongly on the importance of treating the individual in the group and even goes so far as to suggest that group dynamics get in the way of this process. Some of the background for this position is clarified by Mortimer Schiffer in his Preface to a collection of Slavson's major papers (Slavson SR: Dynamics of Group Psychotherapy. New York: Aronson, 1979): "When one weighs Slavson's background, his social, political, economic, and humanistic roots, his extensive engagement in creative group enterprises of various types, what is discernable is the inevitable transition of his concern for the welfare of mankind to an all-encompassing involvement for more than four decades in group psychotherapy. There is an unmistakable thread of continuity linking Slavson's work with individuals in groups that illuminates a deeper meaning. The common factor was his basic regard for the needs of individuals, his recognition of the creative potentialities of every human, given the opportunities for their actualization, and an overriding conviction that troubled individuals can derive sustenance in constructive group participation" (p. xix). —Editor

Slavson SR: Are there "group dynamics" in therapy groups? *International Journal of Group Psychotherapy* 7:131–154, 1957.

The question whether *group dynamics* in the ordinary sense of the phrase arise in therapy groups of nonpsychotic adults is a pivotal one. Its importance lies in the fact that if such dynamics are operative, much that we understand of group psychotherapy and the intrapersonal therapeutic process would have to be revised, and its practice, which is *clinical therapy* and not a sociological theory or constructs would have to be altered. The question whether we deal in group therapy with the group as a *unitary entity*, or with the individuals, that is, the patients in them, *as individuals*, may well determine the course of its development as a science and as a therapeutic tool.[1] Another problem that will have to be solved is whether patients improve merely by virtue of their *adjustment to a group* or because of its "influence" on them, or because of the relationships they establish with fellow members; or whether the improvement is a result of *personality changes* that accrue from the release of anxiety previously bound up in the neurotic nucleus originating in childhood, the insight they acquire, and the new self image that emerges. In other words, are relationships and group adaptation by themselves sufficient to serve the ends of sound psychotherapy, which is personality change? Many individuals with problems seek out groups and social movements as an escape or as a source of relief, and observation confirms that they do receive a certain degree of comfort and for a time show improvement in behavior. But these improvements are not lasting. In addition, the individual who seeks relief through these means becomes permanently dependent on one or another of these groups or movements. Freud has called attention to the fact that "where a powerful impetus has been given to group formation, neuroses may diminish and . . . *temporarily* disappear."[2]

In order to arrive at some clarity on these and related subjects, it will be necessary to draw upon other experiences and operational systems. To do this, let us define, on the basis of its inherence, nature, and function as we know them, what a "group" is, keeping in mind that not every compresence of persons is a *group*. Because of the differences in numbers, motivation, aims and interpersonal relations, gatherings are variously designated as masses, crowds, assemblies, audiences, congregations, mobs, groups, and by still other terms, all of which imply the existence of different relationships among their constituents.

The definition that most nearly describes a "group" can be formulated as follows: A group is a voluntary gathering of three or more persons in a free face-to-face relation *under leadership*, who have a *common goal* or aim and who interact with one another relative to the common plans or goals, as a result of which personality growth may occur and latent talents and interests may be evoked. The salient features of this definition are: (a) a group consists of a small number of persons so that meaningful face-to-face relationships can take place; (b) it has leadership; (c) it has a purpose common to all (or to the majority) of the participants; (d) the participants and members are in a dynamic interaction with one another; (e) it fosters personality growth.

Assuming this definition as a frame of reference, a definition that is acceptable to professional group workers, let us examine therapy and social groups in the light of it. In respect to (a), both groups are similar; both consist of small numbers, though therapy groups must of necessity be much smaller than social or educational groups. Regarding (b), a therapy group does not have a leader in the usual sense of the term. A leader can be defined as the central person who personifies the conscious and the unconscious (especially the latter) needs, trends and urges of the constituents; who initiates or sets the pace in achieving the common aim or objective of all or the majority of the membership. The ordinary group can survive only if it accepts the leader. In therapy groups, neither the therapist nor any of the patients assume such a role. The therapist does not occupy this leadership position in the group hegemony. In a therapy group, the therapist is the recipient of libidinal and other types of transference feelings and is an object of dependency. He is, therefore, the target of periodic positive, negative and ambivalent feelings. If he functions adequately in the role that psychotherapy demands from him, he does not serve as an initiator, nor does he set the pace for the group, even though he may at times have to help a particular patient or a number of patients to focus their discussion, to garner the significance of their communications and feelings, and to acquire insight.[3]

Perhaps the most important difference between social and educational, and therapy groups, is to be found in the characteristic subsumed in section (c): common purpose or aim. Certainly members of a therapy group do not have a *common* purpose. They are not gathered to discharge a specific community function, to pioneer a cause, to find expression of a talent common to them all, or advance an interest they all share; nor do they meet for the pleasure derived from congenial social intercourse. Patients come together because each hopes to get relief from suffering and to overcome personality deficiencies that prevent or interfere with his enjoyment of life and human relationships. Each is driven most often to a resentful compresence in quest of relief from unhappiness, tensions, fears and anxieties. By and large, the motives for attending therapy groups may be said to be the *same* in all or most of the participants, namely, to improve, but because each seeks *his own* salvation, it does not have the nature of a common motive as understood in a sociological or educational sense. Each seeks to achieve an aim *as an individual* for his own individual ends and not for the benefit or advantage of the group as a unit or for the sake of and in the interest of the common group aim. The patients have the same purpose, but it is not a *common* purpose. In my opinion which is derived from working with several hundred social, educational, business, political and therapeutic groups, it is this factor more than any other that prevents the emergence of the usual "group dynamics."

The basic integrating force that assures the survival and achievement of ordinary groups is what has been described as *synergy*. By synergy is meant the drive, purpose, aim and effort common to and congruent in all the individuals constituting a group or a mass of people. The cementing tie, the coherence in these groups, is the personal homogeneity of their members and/or of their interest or goal, whatever it may be, which is personified or represented by a leader, or cathected idea or ideal. This element is absent in therapy groups. In fact, as we shall show, its presence prevents therapeutic gains for the participating patients. Instead of coherence, essential to social-educational groups, therapeutic groups feed upon interpersonal conflict and overt expression of hostility among the members. They are in positive, negative and ambivalent transference relations with each other and are mutual objects of paratoxic projections and displacement. Essentially, in therapeutic groups, patients are held together by anxiety and not by pleasure-yielding occupations. The urge of each is to find relief from that personal anxiety through talk and acting out, and insight. Obviously no other type of voluntary group could survive under conditions where aggression is so rampant and anxiety so pervasive. It must be noted, however, that in both ordinary and therapy groups, the leader in one, and the therapist in the other, is the center of the emotional cluster of the constituent members. But it is equally important to observe that in order to survive, these emotions must be positive in ordinary groups, while they alternate between the extreme poles of positive and negative feelings in therapy groups.

There is distinct similarity and confluence of the two types of groups in the category (d). In both types there is present "dynamic interaction" among the members, although here, too, one can readily observe differences. In the social-educational groups the interaction is largely in the realm of ideas or comeraderie, even though these are not altogether free from emotional undercurrents. In the psychotherapeutic groups, on the other hand, the interactions are almost exclusively in the realm of feeling and emotions. Even ideational differences and conflicts mask feelings, especially hostility and resentment, which are always present in each participant, for it is the presence of excessive feelings of this nature that makes them "patients."

As to fostering of personality growth and uncovering latent talent, i.e., category (e), there is also seeming similarity, but this similarity proves illusory on closer examination. The aim and results of social-educational groups is to implant and/or activate social attitudes and values, to help acquire tools of social living. In "special interest" groups such as in art, literature and dramatics, the effect is to activate latent talent and interest and bring them to fruition through some form of "self-expression." Under the stimulation of leaders and teachers, powers and talents are uncovered and brought to function. The latter occasionally occurs also in therapy groups as blockings and inhibitions are removed, but the aim of these groups is not uncovering talents but rather personality repair, as a result of which talents become manifest. Analytic psychotherapy does not directly aim to achieve these; they are rather the results of personality improvement, released ego powers, better capacity for reality testing and enhanced self-esteem that psychotherapy achieves.

In order to test the applicability of group dynamics derived from the behavior of voluntary social, educational and action groups to therapeutic groups, let us examine them now from the clinical viewpoint. The operational elements of group psychotherapy, as it is in all psychotherapy, are (a) transference, (b) catharsis, (c) insight, (d) reality testing, and (e) sublimation. As we compare these in the two types of group, we shall find them at even greater dissonance than in respect to the characteristics we have already examined.

We have already touched upon the element of transference and tried to show that its nature and manifestations are quite different in the two types of groups: in one it is almost always positive and largely nonsexual, in the other it is libidinized and bipolar. As to catharsis, it is obvious that no nontherapeutic group could survive long if its members are free to reveal their unmoral and immoral acts, preoccupations and urges, past and present, as they do in psychotherapy. Nor would such groups hold together if their members attacked and abused one another as they do in the latter.

Under the impact of free catharsis no social-educational group could survive. The cross-currents of hostility that result would easily deteriorate and disintegrate it. Nor can a social or educational aim-directed group withstand the uncovering and interpretations of hidden motives and latent meanings, which are not always the noblest or purest in nature. While interpretation (as differentiated from explanation) that leads to insight (as differentiated from understanding) alleviates anxiety in a therapy group, such interpretation would intensify anxiety were it to be offered to a social-educational group. In everyday relations, interpretation and even explanation of basic, unconscious and preconscious motives and meanings generate a high degree of anxiety and resentment because they are essentially attacks on normal and necessary ego defenses.

Since reality testing and sublimation of primitive drives are carried on constantly at every point of the individual's life, they are present in all relations, group and individual, and since they are minor elements in the actual group situation of adult, nonpsychotic patients, only cursory mention of them is necessary here. One fact need be mentioned in this connection however; namely, that the therapy group is a *conditioned* reality, planned and arranged by the therapist with a therapeutic aim in mind and an eye upon its suitability to each of the participants. This conditioning is not inherent to social-educational or action groups, in which membership is self-chosen on the basis of some element of homogeneity.

Although the term "group ego" is usually employed euphemistically, actually there is a group ego which is represented by the leader through the investment in him by the members of the group. One of the tacit demands imposed by cohesive groups upon each of its members is that he modify his ego functioning which reduces its intensity and quantum, for, obviously, were each to act out in full his own drives, plans, preferences and judgments, no group as such could come into being or exist for any appreciable time. The condition of belonging to a group is *partial de-egotizing* of the individual so that a portion of his ego is given up to the group, and especially to the leader as its representative. In other words, the individual has to submit to the group in order that he may be a part of it and groups come into being and survive because of this partial de-egotization of its members. It is out of these "discarded" portions of the individuals' egos that a "group ego" emerges.

******

A series of interactional diagrams have been omitted in the following discussion.

******

A part of the ego of each of the constituent members is given up to form the "group ego." This is part of the process commonly referred to as "socialization" or "assimilation"—a process essential for human survival. The more "individualistic" (neurotic) a person is, the less can he give up of his personal ego and is therefore less capable of becoming part of his social milieu. In mobs, for example, a much larger portion of the individual's ego is given up so that he is guided less by it than in democratic deliberative groups. During the periods of violent mob action, the egos of the molesters are entirely suspended, while the initiator or social reformer possesses a minimal capacity for being assimilated.

The fact must always be kept in mind that all group action, whether deliberative or uncontrolled, is a result of a group's ego functioning which is personified or represented by the leader who is a cathected and idealized symbol. What has been said of the ego is equally true of the superego. Superego judgments are weakened in each member by the group's primary code, its sanctions and approval. The libido thus freed is invested in the leader who becomes the representative of the "group superego." When an individual's superego functioning is at too great divergence from that of the group, he will either withdraw, or the group will reject him. An individual whose superego is either too lax or too strict, as compared with the standards of the group, generates anxiety and guilt and is rejected as a consequence.

By its very nature psychotherapy utilizes ego and superego functioning in quite a different manner. Although it is permissive and is based on freedom of action and expression, it does not divest the patient of individual responsibility. It encourages unimpeded exercise of the id, ego and superego, for only through free expression can they be exposed and corrected. The important tenet of psychotherapy is to give to the patient freedom to act in accordance with the dictates of his superego and the strengths of his ego, but he remains responsible for his conduct rather than having this responsibility invested in the group or the leader. The power for judging must remain with the patient. It is through the unimpeded functioning of the patient's *real* ego and his *real* superego, and not their pretend or feigned character, that the patient discovers the *"reality of himself"* (self-confrontation) which has to be corrected and brought in alignment with outer reality. In effect, the individual in a therapeutic setting is put on his own more severely than he has ever been before, for it is only through this testing of himself against inner and outer reality that he readjusts his psychic forces. Even in activity group therapy of children which is an extremely permissive method, the child is placed in a position where he must take the consequences of his acts. The more permissive an environment is, the more burdensome does one's task become, for freedom is the heaviest load an individual is called upon to carry.

In the differentials of the ego and superego functioning in the ordinary groups and in therapeutic groups lies one of the major contrasts of the two. As a result, the dynamics that operate in one obviously cannot operate in the other.

The factors of *group fixity* of social, educational and action groups and the corresponding *group mobility* of therapeutic groups which I have discussed elsewhere[4] contribute greatly to the emergence of different types of group processes that cannot be considered in a blanket fashion. The solidity of the group formation in which the leader is the center, we designate as *group fixity*. In a therapy group there is fluidity of relations. For example, there might be a bilateral relation between Member A and Member B; a unilateral relation between Members E and D; a peripheral relation to A and B on the part of Member C; Member I is an isolate; Member F is a floater without attachment. A new member in a group characterized by *group fixity* has to cut across many relationship lines to make his way into the group. In a therapy group, he can try to make contact with a number of individuals. This total free and fluid characteristic of the group we designate as *group mobility*. Note that the leader in the former is the center, while in the latter the therapist tends to be outside of the group context with various individuals attempting to make contact with him.

In the one the leader is the central source of security and serves as a guide; upon him are focused positive feelings of the members to varying intensities, kinds and degrees; it is from him that stem the unified impulse of the group members to act, and it is he who in part serves as the group's ego and superego. In therapy groups, the intent is that the therapist play a functionally passive or neutral role and that the interactions occur among the members who serve as targets for each other's hostilities, as objects of identification, as catalysers, as clarifiers, as support. The therapist who functions adequately in his role abrogates the leadership role to various members of the group at different times so as to encourage individuation and emotional maturity. This he can do only to the extent to which his patients will allow it, however, and which varies with their personality evolvement. The maximum viability can be achieved in activity group therapy where the therapist assumes a "neutral" role and no interpretations are offered. In analytic groups in which he interprets, the therapist can only approach this function and relation as a limit, but not fully attain it.

One of the major characteristics of ordinary groups is that each member deals not only with every other, but also *with their relations to each other*. It is for this reason that I have suggested many years ago that a group must have at least three persons. The erroneous, though often repeated idea that two persons make up a group does not conform with the nature of groups. A definition that stipulates two as a group confuses interpersonal and group reactions as being one and the same. They are distinctly different, however. Two persons are in a direct bilateral person-to-person relation which must be differentiated from multilateral or group interactions. In a bilateral relation the individuals interact with one another without incursion or interference from others. Their relations and interactions are, therefore, comparatively simple.[5] The bilateral relation is vastly complicated and the multiplicity of reactions and possible tensions are greatly increased by the addition of one or more persons because they impinge upon that relation in a variety of ways and affect the existing and constantly arising interpersonal and group equilibria or disequilibria.

This intragroup dynamic can best be illustrated in family constellations. The interpersonal equilibrium that emerges from the relation between husband and wife is disturbed by the arrival of a child and a new group equilibrium has to be established.[6] This becomes necessary because the relation between the man and his wife is no longer a direct, simple and linear one, as it had been. The husband no longer relates to the wife as an individual only; he also has to relate to her as mother in relation to their child. His acts and behavior, as well as his feelings, have to take into account the feelings and needs of the child and mother as individuals as well as the relation between them. At the advent of subsequent children, or the addition to the intimate family circle of a relative such as a grandparent, an aunt or an uncle, a new complex of group and interpersonal relationships emerges. Readjustments have to be made by other members of the family as well; that is, the wife and the child and the relatives deal with the relation that exists among the other members of the family group. The wife and mother, for example, adapts her reactions and responses to accord with the requirements of the father-child relation, and the child with that of the father-mother relation. These are rendered still more complex by the presence of other persons in the family.

Psychoanalytic studies have thrown light upon and adequately described the relation of the child to each parent as individuals and to them *as a couple*. This fundamental formulation has made palpable to us some of the most baffling aspects of human personality. The oedipus complex arises from the reaction of the child to the emotional and sexual relations of the two parents. Less attention has been given to the attitudes of each of the parents to the reaction of his or her mate to their child or children. That they exist and are fraught with much potential tension and pathology is evident to everyone engaged in clinical work. It is equally evident that the complexities of family processes and tensions are enhanced with each addition to the family. The addition of a child may occasionally reduce tension, but these instances are rare indeed.

The interpersonal and intragroup dynamics delineated for families hold good for all voluntary groups whose members are in close, intimate, face-to-face relation and interaction, though their emotional significance to each other is less charged with affect than in a family group. Since the emotional investment here is quantitatively and qualitatively of lesser degree and poignancy, tensions are likely to be much less intense. However, the basic patterns are the same and are much more obvious and more intense in therapy groups than they are in ordinary groups—as evidenced in the interpatient transference reactions.[7]

Because of the nature of the group discussions in therapeutic groups, it is inevitable that feelings toward important persons in the early life of each should be aroused and acted out, verbalized, displaced and projected upon fellow patients, especially upon those who in some way resemble the earlier prototypes, either physically, in manner or accomplishments. These are specially chosen as targets of affection, hostility, objects of identification or dependence, rivalry and jealousy. As in families, also in other groups, especially therapy groups, specific feelings may be mobilized toward one person. These may be positive, negative or ambivalent; they may be transient or permanent. However, what is important is that these are not group reactions; rather they are *individual* reactions and assume a form, direction and intensity that is shaped by the history and early experiences of each participant. The pattern of acting out or withholding, the manner of behavior and the nature of the verbalization, stem from the ontogenetic experiences of each. One may or may not arouse reactions in others or he may activate one or only a few of those present. The element of synergy is absent here. Each expresses his transference feelings in his own peculiar way. The fact that there may exist at a given time a common feeling in which all share or to which all are subject does not make it a "group feeling" or a group reaction. The intensity of this feeling, its significance, and the impulse to act upon it are different in each of those present. In fact, what seems at first a "universal" feeling or attitude in a therapy group, actually is not so, for the uncovering of reactions shows that there are those who are affected by it deeply, others only slightly and still others remain indifferent. This is both inevitable and understandable in the light of the individual superego and ego differences, capacity for identification, identity in experience, and especially in the transference and projection mechanisms of each. That there should be emotional contagions is just as inevitable, but still the responses are individual, are felt by the individual and are acted upon by the individual, even though he is a member of a group. The outstanding feature of these reactions is that they are specific to, peculiar and characteristic of each member.

A group of persons in any type of active occupation sets up specific dynamics that are more or less universal. Some of them are discernible in therapy groups as well. Where there is action on the part of a group there is also some type and some degree of *interaction* among either all or some of its members. Such interaction is greater among free-acting, self-directed, voluntary groups, and is largely if not entirely determined by the type of leadership function. In groups where the leader is either authoritarian, directive or assertive, the interaction of the members will be lesser both in frequency and intensity than in a group in which the leader assumes a laissez-faire attitude or one approaching that character. The interaction of a number of people under the latter condition may lead to varying degrees of tension and under specific conditions, due to overstimulation, even to mob violence and disruption.

To be constructive and productive, social, educational and all other aim-directed groups have to set limits to the interaction of their members. At certain periods a common aim or agreement must emerge (group code) that holds the group to a generally accepted or agreed-upon purpose or end. If the tensions in a group prevent movement toward its aim, some means are found to resolve the tension. *Compromise* is the most common and essential mechanism in social, political and aim-directed groups and is the outcome of another process that may be termed *neutralization*. When emotional drives are counteracted or the individual entertaining them is won over by placation or some other ego-gratifying strategy, neutralization of his feelings occurs. Among the chief neutralizing agents in groups is the leader who represents in the unconscious of the members the parental figure, and when he assumes the role of the good parent, the members submit to his expectations. This neutralizing effect of the leader, as we shall presently see, is exerted also in therapy groups by the therapist, though it is accomplished differently and with a different intent.

Compromise is partial and not total neutralization. "It comes about through . . . (a) finding a common ground for agreement or (b) lessening the emotional pressure among the participants . . . This permits at once self-determination (even though a partial one) for all concerned and meets group needs. The group leader's chief function is to act as a catalytic agent in this neutralization process."[8]

Another dynamic that is present in ordinary groups and which is an outgrowth of interaction is *interstimulation*. This is the phenomenon through which persons in close proximity engaged in a common objective which can be achieved through common effort on the part of the participants, activate one another either through their attitudes, specific conduct, acts, emotions or ideas. Interstimulation in constructive effort can produce most desirable results, but when it is exercised to the ends of destruction, it can prove to be devastating in its effect, as in the case of mobs.

Of less obvious nature but equally universal and similar in process and effect is the dynamic of *mutual induction* . This, however, is confined to feeling and emotion, whereas interstimulation occurs largely, though not exclusively, in the realm of action. The term "induction" is borrowed from electrical phenomena in which process a coil placed in the field of another becomes charged without being in direct contact with it. People induce attitudes and feelings in one another without verbal or other tangible or observable forms of communication. The mutually inductive processes are enhanced and individuals grow susceptible to them with closer association and intimacy, as in the case of close friends, married couples and other members of a family. The closer and more prolonged the emotional and physical association among persons, the more responsive they are to the inductive effect of one another, since through it empathy is heightened.

In all associations of people, positive and negative *identifications* occur according to the emotional prototypes of each participant. Identifications take place as a result of constitutional similarity and that of background and experience that makes people feel alike in any situation. Identification is particularly important in therapy groups for it makes possible vicarious catharsis and spectator therapy. It is for this reason that patients assigned to the same group should have, as far as possible, common central or nuclear problems even though their symptoms and clinical diagnoses may be at variance or dissimilar. Identification, however, operates differently in a nontherapeutic group. I am quoting again from *Character Education in a Democracy* to illustrate this point.

"The most cohesive groups that act in concert and with unified purpose are those in which there is mutual identification (commonly designated as sympathy or 'understanding') among their members. In a group where there is a great degree of such understanding there also exists the possibility for concerted action; here the positive elements are intensified. Mutual identification is at once the most potent and the most nearly universal socializing influence on society. The 'homogeneous' groups (common-interest groups, social coteries, economic classes, cultural groups, etc.) are groups in which there is mutual identification. Patriotic organizations and all types of sects originate in identification of their members" (p. 79).

One of the undesirable by-products of interaction and interstimulation is the resultant *intensification* of the emotion involved and the acting out of it. Where a number of persons share a common emotion, especially that of hostility and aggression, their tonus is heightened through (a) removal of ego and superego restraints due to group consent, and (b) the need to be at one with the group, which is an outcome of "social hunger." Because of hostility or anxiety an emotion or a drive generated or induced in a number of persons mounts in intensity. The extreme example of intensification of emotion in its negative manifestation is the behavior of mobs where id impulses are released. In a similar fashion, constructive and benevolent emotions and acts are intensified through group example, pressure and demand. Here the group superego is reinforced and the individual's need to belong to, and be a part of, his social milieu (social hunger) aids the process.

These and other dynamics described are in varying degrees present in all groups and gatherings in which interaction is present, but their utility and significance are vastly different in different types of group and the specific aims and objectives that they have. This difference is especially marked in the case of therapy groups. Whereas in all groups except the latter, the dynamics are directed toward socially approved ends by a leader, other effective members, or by the culture, in therapy groups they are permitted to run their course and their psychologic and interpersonal roots are explored and their significance to each person uncovered. The pivotal difference in the operation of psychotherapeutic and ordinary groups lies in this: *group dynamics in the latter remain the operational instruments of the synergy of a group; in therapy groups individual reactions are explored and interpreted in terms of intrapsychic determinants in each of the participating as well as the nonparticipating patients.*[9] Thus, even the most common group dynamics described are not permitted to operate, for it is the task of the therapist, which is often discharged by fellow patients, to uncover the underlying, most often the hostile feelings, from which reactions flow. Thus, dynamics in therapy groups are "nipped in the bud," as it were, for just as soon as responses are analyzed and related to their emotional sources, they no longer operate. It is this process in therapy groups that prevents the operation of the dynamics manifest in nontherapeutic groups. Therapeutically directed exploration, uncovering and insight prevent the emergence of group synergy and the resultant intrapsychic accommodation of each participant so that unitary synergic effort cannot emerge. Thus, *the therapeutic aim in its very nature is antagonistic to group formation and group dynamics.* The reinforcement of feelings and intensification that periodically set in may result in specific dynamics if permitted to take their course. In analytic therapy groups, however, this development is prevented through the intervention of the therapist and his and other members' interpretations which tend to dissipate the building up of group patterns and group effort.

In discussing synergic or collaborative activity of a number of people, Freud says, ". . . experience has shown that in cases of collaboration libidinal ties are regularly formed between the fellow-workers which prolong and solidify the relation between them to a point beyond what is merely profitable. . . The libido props itself upon the great vital needs, and chooses as its first objects the people who have a share in that process."[10] As will be shown later, in a therapy group collaboration is not a virtue. At most times it is entirely absent, at others it is present to a minimal degree and is fleeting. Patients in groups do not collaborate, in the sense employed in the quotation, for any length of time. They *react* to each other and at times help one another, but are not engaged in a *common* (collaborative) project or process, and therefore no ties among them are, or should be, established. The libido cathexis among patients in a therapy group emanates from transference projections which have to be analyzed. When emotional ties arise among patients, that is absence of negative transference, the therapeutic effectiveness of the group is diminished and even vitiated as a result.[11]

Another dynamic manifestation of groups is polarity. In my *Character Education in a Democracy* to which reference has already been made, I said: "Group polarity, . . . the center around which a group gathers, be it a person or an issue, is always more or less definite. Nearly all groups are polarized around some such center . . . the most stable; and most vital groups are those that have very sharp and emotion arousing poles or centers . . ." (p. 89). Obviously in this regard as in others, therapy groups are vastly different from ordinary groups in the community. Polarity produces rigidity and fixity; while therapy groups must be fluid and mobile. Interaction must be mobile and each patient's role in the group has to alter with his personality integration and emerging ego strengths. A rigidly determined, unaltered place in the group and relation to fellow patients would prevent inner change. As the individual changes, his functions and reactions also change. If this cannot occur, the corrective and re-educational process of therapy is prevented. To assure personality change, freedom and flexibility are essential in interpersonal relations for reasons already indicated, and also because it is part of self- and reality testing.[12] Polarity, as understood in sociologic and psychologic terms, would prevent this essential flexibility in the role and function of each member of the group since it generates group fixity.

There is nonetheless polarity of a sort in therapy groups. To begin with, the therapist serves as a pole on which the patients are centered. Each patient comes because of the therapist's importance to him as an object of cathexis and of dependence. But the attitudes toward him are ambivalent and because he is not a representative of an idea or aim common to all, his hold on the patients is dissimilar to that of a leader of a movement or of a special-interest group. Even though he is a cathected object, the cathexis is felt by each member separately and differently from all the others. Another emotional pole in therapy groups is each patient who serves as a special and separate pole of his own, namely, his interest in changing and improving that brings him to the group. Still a third pole of cathexis are the other members of the group.

One of the inevitable behavioral dynamics that is not preventable because of the inherent nature of human interaction (which is also observable in stocks and herds of animals) is the phenomenon of what I have described elsewhere as *nodal* and *antinodal* behavior. It occurs in all gatherings of three or more persons, and the larger the number and the freer they are, the more intense is the acting out (nodal) and more prolonged are the period of silence or comparative inactivity (antinodal). The periods of the nodal aspect of group behavior are characterized by mounting animation and communication, rising noise and a general atmosphere of interaction and conviviality. When the noise and chaotic atmosphere reach a high level of intensity, sudden quiet sets in. This alternation is observable in all free gatherings, such as parties and other types of assemblies. Even mobs finally spend their energies, bring themselves under control and quiet down. In activity groups of children nodal and antinodal behavior appears in an almost steady rhythm. Although no time study has been made of the frequency and, duration of the changes in the pattern, observation suggests that there may be a mathematical relation in this phenomenon.

The rise to the nodal level obviously stems from interstimulation. However, a state of tension is engendered in all the participants due to the physical and emotional exertion expended. Also organic anxiety is activated by the overstimulating and almost chaotic state into which the gathering falls and which produces a reaction in each. As a result, silence (rest) sets in. The alternation between nodal and antinodal behavior occurs also in therapy groups. There are periods of considerable interchange among the patients as well as interaction, interstimulation and intensification. There may even be present mutual induction and reinforcement of hostility and aggression toward a single target, usually one of the patients. In activity therapy groups this is allowed to run its course so that the ego and superego may become involved in the behavior and thus personality growth and integration can occur, as the children bring themselves under control on their own. But in groups of adult patients, this type of acting out of feelings is checked at the appropriate time by the therapist who attempts to help the patients to recognize their behavior in the light of therapeutic "understanding." His move in this direction at once brings the nodal state of the group to a halt. As the patients investigate their actions and underlying feelings in the light of current or past emotional experiences and attitudes, the behavior is changed to that of an antinodal character.

Similarly, silence by a group (extreme antinodal behavior) is allowed to continue only to a permissible extent. One of the patients, usually the most anxious and insecure, breaks the silence. When this does not transpire, the therapist asks the group to examine the silence and helps bring into the open feelings that hold the patients in check. Here again the course of group dynamics is not allowed to run unhampered; the therapist's or a patient's intervention prevents it.

The nodal-antinodal group pattern can be understood in terms of *group homeostasis*. Just as an organism naturally seeks to establish equilibrium, human groups (as well as animal herds or flocks) are prone to this basic natural trend or law. Groups, as do also individual organisms in a state of tension or agitation, generate counterirritants to the excessive activation and hypertenseness which they find in the antinodal period. This process is analogous to rest and recuperation.

******

A clinical vignette has been omitted.

******

The preceding episode illustrates the fact that there is no synergic or common effort present. Each of the participants acts out according to his own character organization, ego functioning, and transference projections. The center or focus is Mrs. S. who at the moment holds the stage, the others reacting to her as individuals, some in a positive, helpful fashion; others with hostility and attack. The reactions also vary. At times a patient is friendly, at another time she turns antagonistic. Mrs. G. remains uncommunicative throughout this episode. The topic under discussion may not have activated her either because it was alien to her own experience or because she found it necessary to remain defensive.

There are no "group dynamics" in evidence. Rather they are replete in interpersonal stimulation and activation. These are basically different in their nature. The therapist's focusing his questions upon individuals in the group, their feelings toward each other and the meaning of these feelings, prevent the emergence of common dynamics in which all participate or are involved for a common, unitary aim or purpose.

Summary

It is essential to differentiate between "group dynamics" and interpersonal interactions. The first arises in groups with a goal common to all members who act by the consent of the majority. Synergy then arises and various activities are evolved to attain the common aim. At this point group dynamics arise, such as conflict, compromise, agreement, domination and submission. These processes are characteristic of educational, social, and action groups.

A "group ego" and "group superego" are evolved in this process of group cohesion which can come into operation only when each of the participants relegates part of the functions of his ego and superego to the group and especially the central person or the leader. Active leadership is essential in groups operating on the basis of synergy.

In the therapy groups, on the other hand, no common aim is in evidence, even though the aim in all is the same, namely, to overcome intrapsychic difficulties and social maladjustments. Group cohesion has to be prevented so that each can communicate his problems and work them through. This requires freedom and the retention of one's own ego and superego functioning. This process of individuation prevents synergic effort and in consequence also the dynamics that arise in ordinary groups. In therapy groups there constantly occurs verbalized and nonverbalized interpersonal action and reaction, partly as a result of transference projections and partly because of the inevitable effect persons have upon one another, such as contagion, mutual induction, inter-stimulation, intensification of emotions, sympathy, empathy and others. These cannot be considered, however, as "group dynamics," but rather as "interpersonal interactions."

Notes

1. Slavson, S.R.: Current Trends of Group Psychotherapy. *International Journal of Group Psychotherapy*, 1:7–15, 1951; Common Sources of Error and Confusion in Group Psychotherapy, *Internationl Journal of Group Psychotherapy*, 3:1–28, 1953.
2. Freud, S.: *Group Psychology and the Analysis of the Ego*. New York: Boni and Liveright, 1940, p. 124 (my italics) (original work published 1922). See my discussion of this passage in "Freud's Contributions to Group Psychotherapy" (*International Journal of Group Psychotherapy*, 6:349–357, 1956) where it is pointed out (1) that "group formation" is the pivot, and (2) that improvement is "temporary." Neither is suitable for therapeutic ends.
3. I have suggested four main functions for a group therapist: directional, stimulative, extensional and interpretative. See my *Analytic Group Psychotherapy*. New York: Columbia Universities Press, 1952, pp. 108 et seq.
4. Common Sources of Error and Confusion in Group Psychotherapy, *op. cit.*, as well as in *Analytic Group Psychotherapy, op. cit.*
5. This is an oversimplification of the complexities of human relations. Actually, all relations, including those of two persons, are complicated by the internalized urges and each one's attitudes and feelings toward them. I like to refer to these as "phantoms." Chief among the phantoms is the mother, with other important traumatogenic individuals added.
6. See the discussion on "equilibrium under tension" in my *Child Psychotherapy*. New York: Columbia University Press, 1952, pp. 68–70.
7. The requirement of three persons constituting a group cannot be met in therapy groups by including the therapist. Three patients are a minimum since the therapist should not be drawn into the emotional complex of the patients.
8. Slavson, S. R.: *Character Education in a Democracy*. New York: Association Press, 1939, p. 78. See also discussion on "Group Dynamics," Chapter IV in that volume.
9. There are rare exceptions to this when all the patients are involved. At any rate the intent is always to work through individual reactions.
10. *Group Psychology and the Analysis of the Ego, loc. cit.*, p. 57.
11. It is conceivable that a therapy group may become a cohesive, collaborative group as a result of prolonged treatment and near its termination.
12. This is one reason why it often becomes necessary to involve members of a patient's family in treatment. Their unbending attitudes and rigid insistence of patients' roles in the family and elsewhere prevent improvement in the latter.

Toward a Common Basis for Group Dynamics: Group and Therapeutic Processes in Group Psychotherapy

HELEN E. DURKIN, PH.D.
Postgraduate Institute for Psychotherapy
New York City

Helen Durkin grew up in Brooklyn and received her advanced education at the New York School of Social Work and Columbia University. She worked first with John Levy who practiced "relationship therapy," a psychoanalytically oriented Rankian approach that emphasized the ongoing relationship between therapist and patient. The impact of this early experience is evident in her later work. Durkin's first paper appeared in 1939 when she was working with children and families in the Jewish Board of Guardians in New York City with Henrietta Glatzer and Samuel Slavson. She later worked as a Training Analyst for many years at the Postgraduate Center for Mental Health.

Durkin has been an active member of AGPA throughout her professional career. Her inquisitive mind has always sought new ways of conceptualizing how groups can best be understood. She was one of the prime forces behind the emergence of the General Systems Task Force in AGPA. It was a difficult choice between the article printed here and her later general systems paper (General systems theory and group psychotherapy: An introduction. International Journal of Group Psychotherapy 22:159–166, 1972).

Durkin's book "The Group in Depth" (New York: International Universities Press, 1964) is a classic group psychotherapy text that remains in print to this day. In this book, she devotes a major introductory section to findings from the social psychology literature regarding the dynamics of small groups. This was a major shift in the clinical group literature, which had tended to exist in almost complete dissociation from other scientific inquiry. The paper included here forecast the nature of the book that was to follow. It also laid the foundations for her later interest in general systems theory. —Editor

Durkin HE: Toward a common basis for group dynamics: group and therapeutic processes in group psychotherapy. *International Journal of Group Psychotherapy* 7:115–130, 1957.

Extensive material has been produced in recent years by a large number of sociologists, social psychologists, and group psychotherapists who are interested in the nature of groups. A review of the literature presents an impression of confusion if not chaos because of the widely diverse methods and the contradictory results described. But a closer scrutiny reveals two general trends consisting of the clinical presentations of the group therapists, and the experimental findings of the social scientists. Until recently little has been done by either side to understand its relationship to the other. The proverbial visitor from Mars would have thought it very peculiar indeed that two groups of scientists interested in the same subject had seemed to be working as if there were an invisible barricade between them. The truth is that a serious problem of communication must be solved before mutual understanding and integration between the two approaches are possible. And it is of paramount scientific importance that such an integration be made of their findings and their theoretical implications.

Since 1950 a beginning has been made in this direction. The work of Bach (1) is an example. He attempts to fuse the group dynamics viewpoint with analytic group therapy in his clinical work and theoretical papers. However, he does not attempt to clarify the taxonomic foundations of the subject before he proceeds to use the sociological findings as if they were of established clinical value on a par with known therapeutic process. My own view is that mixing these findings on a clinical level is less important than a more discriminating integration on the level of knowledge, and that it leaves the danger of clinical misapplication. At the Postgraduate Institute for Psychotherapy, Deutsch, Kadis, and Durkin gave a course (1955–56) which attempted to integrate these approaches in a meaningful and more systematic way for students of group psychotherapy.

When I made my first attempt to review the literature in the middle of the 1940's, I came up against one very puzzling situation which forced me to recognize the lack in communication I speak of and to search for its causes. I found that the social scientists had not only used different terms than the group therapists but seemed to be operating on a different wave length altogether. (Quite apart from the fact that they used different kinds of groups—a subject which I shall discuss in detail later.) To illustrate, the word "dynamics" conjures up concepts to the analytically oriented group therapist which are connected with the motivating forces of individual human interaction—emotions, drives, conflicts, defenses, etc. Such concepts, however, are conspicuously absent in the writings of the social scientists. Instead, they use terms referring to group behavioral phenomena such as leadership, status, role, structure, climate, standards, pressure, communication, contagion, and so on. Conversely, these terms are rare in the writings of the group therapists, although few, if any of them, would deny their validity as part of group process. This verbal "by-pass" highlights the gap between the two approaches. What does it signify?

The easy and obvious answer is that they were studying different types of groups. The clue to the deeper understanding of these disparities and to making any sort of integration possible lies, it seems to me, in comprehending the goals and the "mental set" of the researchers, for their differences grow out of their "mental set" and their omissions occur as the result of their respective professional lacunae. This hypothesis leads inevitably to certain pertinent observations. Psychotherapists in working with groups were primarily interested in therapeusis and only secondarily in knowledge about groups. From a research point of view, however, they were interested in whether or not the basic principles of group psychology are the same as, or different from, those of individual psychology. They worked clinically, continuing to use the same research tool they had found so productive in individual psychoanalysis. They analyzed transference and resistance. The only difference was that now they were studying many transferences in process of interaction. Social scientists, on the other hand, were interested only in the nature of groups as such, not at first in their clinical value, nor in comparing group with individual functioning. They too applied their traditional tools of experimentation. Out of these disparate purposes and methodologies came another factor that made the findings of one side almost incomprehensible in terms of the other. Group therapists focused on the latent meanings of the interaction among the members, while the social scientists dealt only with their overt manifestations. The latter were not interested in or trained to observe or deal with the latent content behind the overt behavior. As Robert Bales (2) puts it, "all our relevant empirical generalizations must refer sooner or later to some aspects of concrete action or the situation of action."

Because of these differences in their purposes, their methodologies, and the "sights" they set to make their observations, the two disciplines interpreted the concept of "group dynamics" differently, or more accurately, concentrated on different aspects of it. By definition "dynamics" refers to "motivating forces." Group therapists interpreted it as the latent dynamic causes of interaction among individual members of the group which produce and shape the group behavior. Social scientists interpreted dynamics to refer to the overt behavioral phenomena of the group and their effect on the individuals in them. Thus one side deals with the dynamic causes of group behavior; the other, with their dynamic effect. It is no wonder, then, that in reporting on their findings they used two different vocabularies; that by and large they failed to grasp the essential significance of each other's findings; that confusion rather than integration characterized the literature. But surely no complete understanding of group dynamics can be achieved without including the causes and the effects of group interaction. The two approaches should be considered complementary, never antagonistic.

Scheidlinger (10), who has summarized the literature in his book *Psychoanalysis and Group Behavior*, made the significant comment that group therapists on the whole reported on the therapeutic process in the group while the social scientists reported on group process as such. This is understandable on the basis that the group therapists wield a powerful dynamic instrument of their own, the therapeutic technique, which cuts boldly across the very group processes which the social scientist is studying per se.

Several authors among the social scientists have attempted to summarize the voluminous experimental literature. Two outstanding books are *Group Dynamics* edited by Cartwright and Zander (5), and *Small Groups* by Borgatta, Hare and Bales (4). Borgatta et al. bring about some unity by organizing the material into topics. Cartwright goes much further in this direction by presenting the chief theoretical orientations among the experimentalists and giving us their different methodological approaches and then giving experimental findings as examples from each group. In his introduction Cartwright (5) explains why there is so much confusion and diversion of opinion among the experimentalists, by saying that many differently oriented students have worked with many different kinds of groups, with many different scientific methods, for many different reasons. He indicates that his attempt to organize the vast material is incomplete because the work is still in its early stages, but he succeeds in illuminating the main trends.

Among the individual authors who have published findings on group functioning, Redl (9) is an exception in that he combines the two points of view. He is a trained analyst who has done a good deal of group work (as distinguished from group therapy) as part of school and camp life in a therapeutically oriented setting. In writing on the group dimension which he calls "contagion," he gives evidence which points in the direction of the conclusion I have drawn above. However, he was concerned only with the single phenomenon of group contagion, and did not at all deal with the interrelationship between group therapy and group dynamics. He lists the causes of contagion under two headings: Under the heading of "the situation" he places factors which account for the how and when of contagion. This seems to me to be the chief concern of the social scientists. Under his heading of "personality factors" fall those which account for the "why" of contagion. According to my way of thinking, this is the chief concern of the group therapists. This seems to me to illustrate one reason why there is such a disparity among the findings of the two approaches.

Once one has understood the reasons for these differences one may raise the scientifically important question of the comparability of their findings. Is the dynamic basis of all groups the same? For only if this is true, is it feasible to compare them. Catell (5) warned that "experimental results are uninterpretable and noncomparable unless they are understood in reference to the taxonomic foundations." The taxonomic foundations in this field are as yet far from established. We must therefore find out whether the basic dynamics are the same in all groups; and if they are, we must examine the specific points of similarity and difference between their situations before we attempt to understand the nature of the therapeutic group in sociological terms and certainly before we apply that information clinically. Only then can different types of groups be compared or the findings based on one type be appropriately modified and applied to another. Unfortunately not all writers on the subject have emphasized or even recognized this basic principle with the result that many misapplications of findings have been made to noncomparable situations. It is imperative that we determine, with much greater exactitude than has heretofore been done, the extent and the limits of the common ground between any two types of groups, and in that way establish a truer measure of comparability.

It will be my contention that at root level the dynamic basis of all groups is the same. Although one of the most frequent and apparently obvious arguments offered against the comparability of therapy with ordinary groups is the fact that the latter are composed of emotionally disturbed people, careful psychological scrutiny disproves its validity. Even superficially this difference in composition is not a valid argument because there will be a good sprinkling of neurotics among the so-called normal groups, and the normal members in them will certainly have a certain number of neurotic character traits. Therapy group members, on the other hand, are by no means entirely neurotic in their functioning. Simply functioning in an analytic group requires a certain amount of ego strength. (I am excepting for the present groups of schizophrenics.) There is, moreover, a more profound argument for psychological comparability between therapy and ordinary groups. Analytic group therapists will agree that members of all types of groups must interact with one another out of the repertoire of their habitual modes and patterns of attitudes and behavior. Group interaction must proceed through that part of the members' ego development that we call character or personality. It is, if you will, ego interaction. Now psychoanalytic research has established the fact that character formation is the same, in principle, for normal and neurotic individuals. Beyond the normally developed ego functions, character structure is developed in an individual's early years as a compromise between the gratification of his inner needs and the demands of his social environment. It is the sum total of the individual's protective devices against too much pain and anxiety from within and without. The sum of such compromises forms his basic behavior patterns, his way of life, and is the basis of his interaction with other human beings. The patterns of neurotics, because of the greater anxiety under which the patterns were established, may produce poorer choices, may be more rigidly adhered to, be less adaptive, and give less gratification or cause more friction with the environment, but they will not be different in kind from those in normal people. Neurotics will, like normal people, interact through their ego defenses. They will, like normal people, often repeat, in present relationships, patterns which were more appropriate in past situations. These common ways of human interaction form the dynamic basis for all types of interaction and will be present in all types of groups. For this reason the composition of groups gives them a common ground. This reasoning will, I believe, serve until experimental proof is established or the hypothesis disproved.

On the basis of it we may amend Bales's appropriately cautious warning. He says in his paper on Phases of Problem Solving, "These results do not apply to groups where the major emphasis is on expressive personality interaction" and again, "They do not apply to groups of seriously disturbed persons" (5). This sound warning may be modified to read, "They do not necessarily apply" to such groups. According to my hypothesis, they *could* apply; but before such application is attempted, they must be evaluated in the light of the specific group situations. For instance, many compulsive neurotics might function just as well in a problem-solving group as normals, although groups consisting of members with neurotic reading problems could not be compared to normal problem-solving groups which require reading as a major function. My contention is that, broadly speaking, all kinds of groups are comparable on a characterological basis as to their composition, but the specific extent and limitations of their situations must be examined before absolute comparability is assumed.

The exceptions mentioned above lead us to the examination of those determinants which most vitally affect my contention's validity and supply us with a sound basis for deciding in how far findings made on one type of group may be safely applied to another. I submit that the purpose for which the group has come together is the most vital of such determinants. It is the group goal which determines the nature of its leadership, its particular composition, its internal structure, its methods of locomotion, and so on. If this is true, then the group goal is that element in the situation that must be most carefully analyzed when the question of comparability is being decided upon.

To sum up: comparability of different kinds of groups cannot be ruled out because the dynamic basis of all groups may be presumed to be the same, nor can it be taken for granted until the specific elements in the group situation are carefully analyzed. It is only when the degree of comparability is established that the findings on ordinary groups may be applied to therapeutic groups.

Now we are in a position to examine some of the major findings of the experimentalists in relation to therapeutic groups. We shall be asking two questions. To what extent can we apply to therapeutic groups findings derived from experimental or field study of other types of groups? And what part does the group-dynamic process play in the movement of the therapeutic group toward its goal—in other words, what is the relationship between group process and therapeutic process?

Since the nature of leadership occupies a rather prominent position in the studies of both therapists and experimentalists, it seems appropriate to begin with some detailed examination of this topic. One important conclusion of the experimentalists, with which the therapists will agree, is the emergence of a new definition of leadership. Leadership has come to be defined in dynamic rather than in static terms. No longer is it considered to be the function of the personality alone, nor of just the situation, but rather of the relationship between the personality and the situation. For instance, Bales (2) contends that leadership depends on an individual's access to the resources necessary to achieve the group goal, his identification with it, and his degree of influence on the other members. The very acceptance of this new definition ties in with our conclusion that when studying any group dimension in different kinds of groups, one must do so in terms of the specific situation of each group (particularly the goal).

Therefore, if we are to study leadership in normal and therapeutic groups we shall want to know in how far the effect of the goal on the specific conditions of leadership differs in the two situations. In ordinary problem-solving groups, for example, the goal is concrete and external, and the members have as much or nearly as much access to the resources for solving the problem as does the leader. For this reason the leader in such groups may be an *ad hoc* appointee or be elected. The goal for therapy groups is internal, emotional, and the resources for reaching it are so complex and technical that the members must choose a professional leader. In fact they choose the therapist, and it is he who decides whether or not they should join a group. Such a difference in the group situation cannot help but have an appreciable effect on the nature of its leadership, so that one cannot unquestioningly apply results from the one to the other. Furthermore, the goals of the therapeutic group are inextricably bound up with the most basic psychological needs of its members, whereas those of problem-solving groups—in fact, of most ordinary groups—are seldom of paramount importance to them. Field study groups are closer to therapy groups in this respect, but their goals pertain usually to only one important segment of the members' needs. Few other types of groups are so intimately, so vitally, and so completely involved with the members' total life situation as are therapeutic groups. These differences have a powerful effect on the responsibilities of the leaders and on the nature of their leadership. We must expect to allow for such differences when we consider applying results from other kinds of groups.

Let us test out some specific experimental findings gained from normal groups to see whether they confirm the principles we have been evolving. White and Lippitt (5), in their well-known study of group atmosphere as established by the leader in problem-solving groups, came to the conclusion that a democratic atmosphere has a better effect in production and interaction than a laissez-faire or an autocratic atmosphere. Preston and Heintz (8) came to a similar conclusion, also using problem-solving groups. They feel that the more distribution without leadership intervention, the better is the production and the interaction. Kahn and Katz (5) in a field study with industrial workers agree.

Can these results be applied to therapy groups? I believe that *they can*, but not *without modifications* based on the group goals. It is true that the contemporary literature on group therapy stresses the importance of the members as adjunct therapists. It is also true that there would be therapeutic effect (though not necessarily therapy) if the therapist simply allowed the normal group-dynamic processes to function without intervening. I do maintain, however, that analytic group therapy with its goal of solving pathogenic conflicts through analysis of transference and resistance would be seriously interfered with if White's and Lippitt's results were applied without modification.

We may leave aside Lippitt's point that production is increased because production in a therapeutic group is obviously of a different nature from that in a problem-solving group. But his finding that interaction is better in a democratic atmosphere, and Preston's and Heintz's finding that distribution of leadership without intervention of the leader makes for better interaction, must be examined most carefully. Interaction is indeed an important factor in goal locomotion in both types of groups. But in the light of the goals, one must define "good interaction" for each if one wishes to compare them. In problem-solving groups, "good interaction" is friendly interaction. Inimical feelings must be avoided if cooperation toward the external goal is to be paramount. In the therapeutic group "good" interaction is free interaction in which the whole range of underlying feelings comes into play. Often this means that the leader must work toward the expression of varying degrees of hostile feelings in order to facilitate self-understanding and the development of sounder relationships. Helping to set aside conscious antagonisms does not require the same degree of technical skill as removing defenses against unconscious hostile feelings. Any member can do it. Therefore the distribution of leadership must be more restricted in a therapy group. The leader must keep his finger on the pulse of every member and be ready to make the interpretations necessary to bring the hostile reactions to consciousness. The same comments might be made with regard to other unconscious feelings. For example, overprotectiveness of one member to another which might well be utilized in a problem-solving group would call for analytic intervention on the part of the group therapist. The leader must be free, therefore, to intervene and to exert his functional authority through his technical skill. The need to do so puts limits on the distribution of leadership in the therapeutic group.

Moreover, the members of the therapeutic group have chosen their leader with the idea of being able to rely on his personal maturity. Treatment principles may prescribe periods of accepting and then examining their dependency needs. They may rightfully be dependent on him for a relatively long period of treatment, even though his aim is to make them independent eventually. The leader cannot relinquish this function, nor other seemingly authoritative interventions, for the sake of group democracy. Leader distribution increases gradually as the members become free enough from their neurotic unconscious motivation to carry on themselves.

It may be worth while at this point to adduce an example from a group therapy session. In the mixed therapy group to which I refer, Jim was perhaps the chief "adjunct therapist." He had the insight and the courage to make many good interpretations. He was more willing than most patients to bring his impulses into the group for inspection, and often insisted that others do likewise. There was no question that he brought lifelikeness and vividness to the group proceedings which helped us "locomote" to our goal. For example, when Alice spoke rather vaguely about a new love relationship, he insisted that she give us the specific details. When she tried to answer she was forced to face squarely and to present to the rest of the group more meaningful material to which they could relate themselves. He also tended to keep the focus of the group talk related to the group experience itself. Once when Grace was telling us about the difficulties she was having with a romantic relationship, he said to her, "Why not you and me go out and fuck?" She had to examine her relationship with him.

In the first situation the leader could encourage Jim's leadership. The second comment, however, illustrates the point that the therapist leader must put limits on a patient's leadership. If the therapist did not intervene and at least momentarily draw the leadership back to himself, Jim would have led the group away from its goal of understanding the meaning of their emotional relationships. He and Grace might have moved toward acting out instead. The therapist, however, drew upon his training and tried to make this experience an insightful one for all of them. He said, "Try to tell us, Jim, just what you think you might do in such a rendezvous." With great effort, Jim who usually talked glibly tried to put impulses he usually acted out into words and feelings instead of plunging into action. This made him very anxious, but it helped him experience the difference between feeling and acting on impulse. It also helped Grace understand the true motivations of the men in whom she was so often disappointed. At one point in this case, a more democratic distribution of the leadership, and in another, reserving leadership for the therapist made for goal locomotion.

In order to clarify this problem of democracy in group leadership it will be necessary to take a small detour, for the problem has been inadvertently complicated by some confused thinking in both camps. Cartwright (5) has pointed out a fallacy of some of the group-dynamics researches which I believe also holds true of some enthusiastically democratic group therapists. He says that ideological considerations have somehow insinuated themselves into scientific matters, although ideology has no place in scientific experiment. It seems to me to have none in clinical matters either. Democracy is hardly the first duty of a doctor to his patient, even though we prefer him to administer treatment in a democratic manner. He has been selected and will be paid to apply his training and skill with due realistic authority. Here we come upon what I believe is a semantic confusion which adds to the misleading effect of the fallacy Cartwright mentions. To be realistically authoritative is not the equivalent of being authoritarian, which, in our culture at least, is rarely realistic. There need be no mutual exclusiveness between authority and democracy as there must be between authoritarianism and democracy.

The problem, although misnamed, does have some subtler implications for the leader of the therapeutic group. Every therapist in a democratic society has been taught a sound respect for the humanity of his partners in the therapeutic relationship. This respect must be evident in his attitude and will show up in the *way he makes his comments*, not in leaning over backward to be on a par with them in the very area in which he must offer superiority. It is just here that the intrusion of ideology plus semantic error has confused the clinical issues, for group therapists sometimes do reveal unconscious authoritarian motivations which stem from unresolved fantasies of omnipotence, or from remaining status conflicts. Such attitudes are undesirable because they are anti-therapeutic, not because they are undemocratic. Every therapist is committed to analyze both his own omnipotent needs and the patient's needs to have him be omnipotent. Group therapists who are too aggressive and controlling and those who suffer from reaction formations to these tendencies fail to live up to their realistic functions. But this is a question of the leader's maturity and his techniques—not one of democracy.

To sum up: if we are to compare normal with therapeutic groups and to consider applying the experimental findings which have been made on the former to the management of the latter, then we must qualify those findings according to the specific requirements deriving from the differences between their separate goals. The present paper attempts to lay the theoretical groundwork for such modifications, but the final solution must come through further experiment with therapeutic groups.

A similar conclusion may be reached for the signally important group function of communication. Let us take Bavelas' findings (3) as an example around which to study the conditions differentiating the therapeutic from the problem-solving group. On the basis of experimental work with task-oriented groups he concluded that freedom of communication makes for better results than communication that is interfered with by leaders controlling the whole system of communication. When we examine the conditions carefully we find that in a problem-solving group verbal communication is largely in terms of ideas and is taken at its face value. There may be evidences of latent emotional meaning, but this remains rightfully incidental as far as locomotion toward the goal is concerned. The leaders and the members operate on the same overt ideational level.

In the therapeutic group the situation is very different. Locomotion toward the integral goal of characterological change requires that latent emotional communication play a central role. Feeling communication is focal; that of ideas, secondary. For a long period the members communicate in their usual way on an overt level, relatively unaware of latent emotional meanings. The leader whose training has taught him the language of the unconscious (and the preconscious) helps translate them. Through his personal analysis he is also cognizant of his own latent feelings and must handle them. Only gradually do the members learn this technique and as they do they can help to interpret their and one another's communications. It is true that certain members, as for example, schizophrenic individuals, may be far keener than the therapist at catching unconscious elements in the members' participations, but they are seldom aware of more than a single segment of such productions, whereas the therapist must keep the total psychodynamic picture of each patient in mind.

Moreover, members are also unable, from lack of experience or because of the intrusion of their own unconscious needs, to time their interpretations correctly. The therapist has to be ready to intervene when a member makes an interpretation which, whether it be correct or not, also reacts an unconscious motive. In uncovering this unconscious motive (let us say, of hostility) the leader will help the interpreter understand himself, and may also help the recipient of the interpretation become willing to accept it instead of reacting to its unconscious hostile purposes. In order further to help the recipient assess for himself the core of truth in another member's interpretation the therapist may have to help the recipient eliminate further resistance stemming from inner sources. The leader-therapist, in other words, must guide the whole system of communication. One might even go so far as to define therapy as the process of changing the basic nature of communication among members. As everyone knows, this is a delicate and intricate task which requires long professional training. Of necessity it puts a greater distance between the leader and the members than exists in most nontherapeutic groups. This by no means contraindicates his leaving the communication to the members, but it does indicate the necessary limits to which the principle of "free" communication can be applied in the therapeutic group. Accordingly, the findings of Bavelas must be rather markedly modified if they are to be applied in therapeutic groups.

To put this another way: the resistance of human beings to understanding the unconscious emotional meaning of their communications creates a formidable difference in the situation of the two kinds of groups. It is a distinction which cannot be ignored by anyone who compares them. Therapists cannot ignore resistance without blocking the road to their goal. They must therefore be much more involved in the whole system of communications than the leaders of ordinary groups. Thus, our study of communication also demonstrates the validity of the principle that comparison between different kinds of groups is feasible only in terms of the specific situations, and that findings made on one type of group often require modification when they are applied to another.

The second question we asked referred to the relationship between the therapeutic process and the group-dynamic processes per se, as these function side by side in the therapeutic group. Careful inspection reveals that on the whole the group processes tend to enhance the therapeutic process, but that in certain situations and at certain times they work against the therapeutic goal. They can never substitute for it.

The analytic therapist tends naturally to focus on the therapeutic process and until recently has often ignored the group-dynamic processes. This neglect has not seemed to interfere seriously with his therapeutic aim. Experience has shown that skilled use of the therapeutic process will achieve his aim. Since the group processes are natural ones, they will function regardless of whether or not the therapist is aware of them, and for the most part they will nevertheless help locomote the group to its goal. In those instances when they work in an opposite direction, the therapeutic process will effectively counteract them.

In one group for example, the therapist had enlisted the natural forces of the group to develop a climate and standards of its own and had guided them toward permissiveness and freedom of emotional expression. In this group there were a number of impulsive characters with a tendency toward acting out and one rigid compulsive character. It soon became the fashion to use four-letter words indiscriminately. This habit was interpreted by the majority to fit in with the free atmosphere. The compulsive became extremely anxious. The phenomenon of group pressure to accept group standards was about to put him in the dilemma of joining in or leaving the group. Either solution would have been anti-therapeutic for all. The therapist had to relieve the pressure and change the standards. He had, on the one hand, to protect one patient from too much pressure until he was able to work through his defenses. On the other hand, he had to help the "freer" members to examine their own motivation in their consistent choice of flamboyant language. As therapy progressed, all members were able to see that neither had as free a choice as they had thought. Flexibility and real choice could now become the new standards, and the leader could leave these to the natural group processes with little further interference. In this typical case the leader had to wield the group forces in two directions. He had to help develop therapeutic group standards, but see to it that individual differences did not succumb to the natural force of group pressures.

Group-dynamics investigators have probably made more progress in measuring the dimensions of cohesiveness than in that of any other group force. The role of this phenomenon in therapy groups also illustrates the interrelationship of the therapeutic and the group processes. Experience with therapeutic groups has shown that cohesiveness plays an important role in these too. It has, like many other group factors, a certain therapeutic value, but at some points it interferes with the progress of the group. The therapist who wishes to understand the full implication for his goal of this natural group force will discover that the sources of cohesiveness are different in the therapeutic from those in the ordinary group. In most ordinary groups cohesiveness increases rapidly with the mutual identification among members, growing out of their activity in carrying out the work necessary for reaching the goal. Cohesiveness is also increased by the satisfaction of the members' unconscious needs. Playing and winning games, building a clubhouse or campaigning for a cause quite obviously satisfy certain aggressive or libidinal needs. In problem-solving groups certain unconscious satisfactions may also work toward cohesiveness, but on the whole artificial stimulation toward that end becomes necessary.

In the therapy group the situation is quite different. The natural forces tend, during the early sessions, to hinder rather than facilitate cohesiveness. The members are not aware at first of what satisfactions will come to them. They are anxious, and in their anxiety often wish for an exclusive relationship with the leader. Some would have preferred to avoid the group. These are usually more anxious about belonging than hopeful of gaining satisfaction from the group because their neurotic problems have so often interfered with their ability to achieve it. It is the leader who must use his therapeutic skill to develop the particular kind of cohesiveness that will best serve his aim.

This difference in the nature of cohesiveness leads us to another distinction between ordinary and therapeutic groups. Ordinary groups strive for an overt cohesiveness based on friendliness, mutual interests, and cooperation, which can usually be achieved through the channelling or repression of negative feelings. The goal of therapy requires that such negative feelings be brought out into the open, their sources understood, and worked through. For example, it is up to the leader to help the patients recognize and express their jealous need for exclusive possession of the leader in order that they may be enabled to form deeper relationships with the members. This makes for cohesiveness indirectly. He will also have to help them examine their suspicions of one another. If there are many paranoid trends in the group this will take rather a long time. Meanwhile if the leader has used his dynamic technique well, the members will begin to get satisfaction from mutual understanding. Due to these two therapeutic developments, a feeling of belonging begins to develop, leading to a very strong degree of cohesiveness. It will develop later than in normal groups but rest on a sounder substructure.

At a later stage when the forces making for cohesion in ordinary groups may well begin to flag, an extraordinarily strong cohesiveness takes place in the therapeutic group, and the leader may make full use of it. The safe family-like atmosphere of the group which derives from the developing transferences is a tremendous force for cohesion. Even the hostilities engendered by them do not interfere with it because they are accepted and dealt with therapeutically.

At some point in this process, however, the therapeutic goal demands a loosening of the forces of cohesiveness, as Papanek (7) has pointed out. The therapist must work toward the resolution of the transferences, for they are distortions. Moreover, he is interested in helping his patients develop good relationships in their total life situations. He has used the group relationship as a means to this end. Now he must prevent the means from becoming an end in itself. It can become so comfortable and easy for the members that they cling to their "family" group rather than venture forth into outside relationships. The therapeutic technique can in itself achieve this end, but the therapist who understands and can deal with the dynamic group processes will have better control than those who ignore them. In some therapeutic groups where there is a tendency to overstress the familial nature of the group and to use the group to provide a new and better family instead of analyzing the transference distortions, the continued satisfactions can lead to stickiness and overcohesiveness.

Many other group dynamics cut across the dynamics of the therapeutic process. We need only think of the way in which the development of an individual member's role playing is utilized for goal locomotion in ordinary groups, while it is broken down by analysis in therapeutic groups. For example, the "perfect lady" becomes a leader in a social group. In a therapeutic group it is often discovered that her perfect behavior forms a compulsive facade which binds her anxiety but leaves her empty and frightened underneath. The intellectual is a leader in a problem-solving group, but his reliance on ideas to the exclusion of feelings is treated as a defense in the therapeutic group. (I do not imply, of course, that the positive values of such character traits are broken down. The effort is only to remove the rigidity of the structure.) However, space permits us to examine only these few at present.

In retrospect we may, I think, conclude that the clinician who is skilled in the use of his therapeutic tools will not be unable to achieve his goals, even though he may not be cognizant of the full range of group-dynamics findings. He is bound to become acquainted with them in his own fashion in meeting with his therapeutic groups. However, knowledge of their viewpoint will assuredly broaden his foundations and provide him a fuller understanding of the nature of groups and provoke his interest in the dynamic basis of all kinds of groups. It may also add to his skill in using the therapeutic potentialities of the group processes themselves. He will therefore enrich his conception of his work and probably develop greater precision in executing it. The sociologist, on the other hand, who does not know the relationship of the therapeutic process to the group processes, will not be crippled in his research on the nature of other types of groups, but he may be misled, if he develops clinical interests, into confusing the therapeutic effect of group work with therapy as such.

In summary, we may say that, although we had to limit our discussion to a very few of the group-dynamic elements, these will serve to illustrate the following hypotheses: (1) that all types of group are comparable because they have a common dynamic basis in the psychology of ego interaction; (2) that findings derived from studies of other types of groups may be applied to therapy groups only if due account is taken of the differences in their situations and appropriate modifications are made; and (3) that group and therapeutic processes are on the whole mutually reinforcing but at times tend to work in opposite directions.

While the present attempt to establish these working hypotheses is based on clinical experience, my hope is that it will serve to stimulate experimental validation of them. Such scientific validation should shed further light on the relationship between the group processes and the therapeutic process; minimize errors in the application of results from one type of group to another; and, most important, increase the mutual understanding and eventual integration of the knowledge produced by these two main approaches to the understanding of the nature of groups.

Bibliography

1. Bach, G.: *Intensive Group Psychotherapy.* New York: Ronald Press, 1952.
2. Bales, R. F.:*Interaction Process Analysis—A Method of Study of Small Groups.* Boston, Mass.: Addison & Wesley Press, 1950.
3. Bavelas, A.: Communications Patterns in Task-Oriented Groups. *Acoustical Society of America,* 22:75, 1950.

4. Borgatta, E., Bales, R., Hare, P.: *Small Groups.* New York: A. Knopf, 1955.
5. Cartwright, C. and Zander, A., eds.: *Group Dynamics.* Evanston, Ill.: Row Peterson Co., 1953.
6. Freud, S. (1922): *Group Psychology and the Analysis of the Ego.* New York: Liveright, 1949.
7. Papanek, H.: Combined Group and Individual Therapy in Private Practice. *Am. J. Psychother., 8,* 1954.
8. Preston, M. and Heintz: Effects of Participatory and Supervisory Leadership. *J. Abn. & Soc. Psychol.,* 44:345–355,1949.
9. Redl, F.: The Phenomenon of Contagion and "Shock Effect" in Group Therapy. In: *Searchlights on Delinquency,* ed. K. R. Eissler. New York: International Universities Press, 1949.
10. Scheidlinger, S.: *Psychoanalysis and Group Behavior.* New York: Norton, 1952.
11. Wolf, A.: The Psychoanalysis of Groups. *Am. J. Pychother.,* 3, 4, 1949–50.

Transactional Analysis: A New and Effective Method of Group Therapy

ERIC BERNE, M.D.

Carmel, Cal.

Eric Berne (1910–1970) was an analytically trained psychiatrist who, after fifteen years in the psychoanalytic movement, in his own words "officially parted company (on the most friendly terms)." He developed a theory of structural analysis which he saw as a more comprehensive general theory of interaction than psychoanalysis. Berne was influenced by the work of Wilder Penfield when he was a medical student at McGill Medical School in Montreal. Penfield demonstrated how total experiences with the full attendant affect can be reexperienced under electrical stimulation of the brain, lending neurophysiological substance to the idea of a variety of ego states. Berne's ideas were refined over a number of years in the Group Therapy Seminars at Mount Zion Hospital and the Social Psychiatry Seminars, both in San Francisco. Berne's first major publication regarding transactional analysis (Transactional Analysis in Psychotherapy. New York: Grove Press, 1961), appeared just in time for the burgeoning encounter group movement, which promptly adopted many of its terms.

Berne specifically moved the focus of interest from intrapsychic phenomena to interpersonal transactions. Underneath the catchy phrases, this represented a major shift in keeping with Sullivan's interpersonal theory of development, a connection made quite explicit by Thomas A. Harris in "I'm OK — You're OK" (New York: Harper & Row, 1967). Most psychotherapy researchers have now moved to the same position. Berne saw group therapy as the logical modality for implementing his ideas (Principles of Group Treatment. New York: Oxford University Press, 1966). TA has a lower profile at present, perhaps because the idea of looking at the meaning of interpersonal transactions has become incorporated into most other therapeutic approaches. This article is an early paper presented at the Western Regional meeting of the American Group Psychotherapy Association in Los Angeles, November, 1957.   —Editor

Berne E: Transactional analysis: A new and effective method of group therapy. *American Journal of Psychotherapy* 12:735-743, 1958.

There is need for a new approach to psychodynamic group therapy specifically designed for the situation it has to meet. The usual practice is to bring into the group methods borrowed from individual therapy, hoping, as occasionally happens, to elicit a specific therapeutic response. I should like to present a different system, one which has been well-tested and is more adapted to its purpose, where group therapists can stand on their own ground rather than attempting a thinly-spread imitation of the sister discipline.

Generally speaking, individual analytic therapy is characterized by the production of and a search for material, with interpersonal transactions holding a special place, typically in the field of "transference resistance" or "transference reactions." In a group, the systematic search for material is hampered because from the beginning the multitude of transactions takes the center of the stage. Therefore it seems appropriate to concentrate deliberately and specifically on analyzing such transactions. Structural analysis, and its later development into transactional analysis, in my experience, offers the most productive framework for this undertaking. Experiments with both approaches demonstrate certain advantages of structural and transactional analysis over attempts at psychoanalysis in the group. Among them are increased patient interest as shown by attendance records; increased degree of therapeutic success as shown by reduction of gross failures; increased stability of results as shown by long-term adjustment; and wider applicability in difficult patients such as psychopaths, the mentally retarded, and pre- and post-psychotics. In addition, the intelligibility, precision, and goals of the therapeutic technique are more readily appreciated by the properly prepared therapist and patient alike.

This approach is based on the separation and investigation of exteropsychic, neopsychic, and archaeopsychic ego states. Structural analysis refers to the intrapsychic relationships of these three types of ego states: their mutual isolation, conflict, contamination, invasion, predominance, or cooperation within the personality. Transactional analysis refers to the diagnosis of which particular ego state is active in each individual during a given transaction or series of transactions, and of the understandings or misunderstandings which arise due to the perception or misperception of this factor by the individuals involved.

I have discussed in a previous publication (1) the nature of ego states in general, and of their classification according to whether they are exteropsychic, that is, borrowed from external sources; neopsychic, that is, oriented in accordance with current reality; or archaeopsychic, that is, relics fixated in childhood. These distinctions are easily understood by patients when they are demonstrated by clinical material, and when the three types are subsumed under the more personal terms Parent, Adult, and Child, respectively.

As this is a condensation in a very small space of a whole psychotherapeutic system, I can only offer a few illustrative situations, choosing them for their relative clarity and dramatic quality in the hope that they will draw attention to some of the basic principles of structural and transactional analysis.

Structural Analysis

The first concerns a patient named Matthew, whose manner, posture, gestures, tone of voice, purpose, and field of interest varied in a fashion which at first seemed erratic. Careful and sustained observation, however, revealed that these variables were organized into a limited number of coherent patterns. When he was discussing his wife, he spoke in loud, deep, dogmatic tones, leaning back in his chair with a stern gaze and counting off the accusations against her on his upraised fingers. At other times he talked with another patient about carpentry problems in a matter of fact tone, leaning forward in a companionable way. On still other occasions, he taunted the other group members with a scornful smile about their apparent loyalty to the therapist, his head slightly bowed and his back ostentatiously turned to the leader. The other patients soon became aware of these shifts in his ego state, correctly diagnosed them as Parent, Adult, and Child, respectively, and began to look for appropriate clues concerning Matthew's actual parents and his childhood experiences.

******

Several transactional diagrams have been omitted.

******

In the course of Matthew's therapy, he asked the physician to examine his father, who was on the verge of a paranoid psychosis. The therapist was astonished, in spite of his anticipations, to see how exactly Matthew's Parent reproduced the father's fixated paranoid ego state. During his interview, Matthew's father spoke in loud, deep, dogmatic tones, leaning back in his chair with a stern gaze, and counting off on his upraised fingers his accusations against the people around him.

It should be emphasized that Parent, Adult, and Child, are not synonymous with superego, ego, and id. The latter are "psychic agencies," (2) while the former are complete ego states, each in itself including influences from superego, ego, and id. For example, when Matthew reproduced the Parental ego state, he not only behaved like a stern father, but also distorted reality the way his father did, and vented his sadistic impulses. And as cathexis was transferred from the Parental ego state into that of the scornful Child, the planning of his attacks and the accompanying guilt feelings had a childlike quality.

In therapy, the first task was to clarify in Matthew's mind what was Parent, what was Adult, and what was Child in his feelings and behavior. The next phase was directed toward maintaining control through the Adult. The third phase was to analyze the current conflicts between the three ego states. Each of these phases brought its own kind of improvement, while the ultimate aim in this pre-psychotic case was to enable all three ego states to cooperate in an integrated fashion as a result of structural analysis.

There were two contra-indications in this case. The first was the universal indication against telling the Child to grow up. One does not tell a two-year-old child to grow up. In fact, from the beginning it is necessary in every case to emphasize that we are not trying to get rid of the Child. The Child is not to be regarded as "childish" in the derogatory sense, but childlike, with many socially valuable attributes which must be freed so that they can make their contribution to the total personality when the confusion in this archaic area has been straightened out. The child in the individual is potentially capable of contributing to his personality exactly what a happy actual child is capable of contributing to family life. The second contra-indication, which is specific to this type of case, was against investigating the history and mechanism of his identification with his father, which was a special aspect of his parental ego state.

Simple Transactional Analysis

A patient named Camellia, following a previous train of thought said that she had told her husband she wasn't going to have intercourse with him any more and that he could go and find himself some other woman. Another patient named Rosita asked curiously: "Why did you do that?" Whereupon Camellia, much to Rosita's discomfort, burst into tears and replied: "I try so hard, and then you criticize me."

This transaction was analyzed for the group as follows. The original *transactional stimulus* is Camellia's statement about what she told her husband. She related this in her Adult ego state, with which the group was familiar. It was received in turn by an Adult Rosita, who in her response exhibited a mature, reasonable interest in the story. The transactional stimulus was Adult to Adult, and so was the *transactional response*. If things had continued at this level, the conversation might have proceeded smoothly.

Rosita's question ("Why did you do that?") now constituted a new transactional stimulus, and was intended as one adult speaking to another. Camellia's weeping response, however, was not that of one adult to another, but that of a child to a critical parent. Camellia's misperception of Rosita's ego state, and the shift in her own ego state, resulted in a crossed transaction and broke up the conversation, which now had to take another turn.

This particular type of crossed transaction, in which the stimulus is Adult to Adult, and the response is Child to Parent, is probably the most frequent cause of misunderstandings in marriage and work situations, as well as in social life. Clinically, it is typified by the classical transference reaction, which is a special case of the crossed transaction. In fact this particular species of crossed transaction may be said to be the chief problem of psychoanalytic technique.

In Matthew's case, when he was talking about his wife, the crossing was reversed. If one of the other members, as an Adult, asked him a question, expecting an Adult response, Matthew instead usually answered like a supercilious parent talking to a backward child.

Therapeutically, this simple type of transactional analysis helped Camellia to become more objective about her Child. As the Adult gained control, and the Child's responses at home were suppressed for later discussion in the group, her marital and social life improved even before any of the Child's confusion was resolved.

The Analysis of Games

Short sets of ongoing transactions may be called operations. These constitute tactical maneuvers, in which it is the other members of the group who are maneuvered. Thus the conversation between Camellia and Rosita, taken as a whole, is an operation, and has to be analyzed again at a deeper level, when it soon appears that the need of Camellia's Child to feel criticized was one of the motives for telling this particular story to the group.

A series of operations constitutes a "game." A game may be defined as a recurring series of transactions, often repetitive, superficially rational, with a concealed motivation; or more colloquially, a series of operations with a "gimmick."

Hyacinth recounted her disappointment and resentment because a friend of hers had given a birthday party which she herself had planned to give. Camellia asked: "Why don't you give another party later?" To which Hyacinth responded: "Yes, but then it wouldn't be a birthday party." The other members of the group then began to give wise suggestions, each beginning with: "Why don't you . . ." and to each of these Hyacinth gave a response which began: "Yes, but . . . .."

Hyacinth had told her story for the purpose of setting in motion the commonest of all the games which can be observed in groups: the game of "Why don't you . . . Yes but . . . .." This is a game which can be played by any number. One player, who is "it," presents a problem. The others start to present solutions, to each of which the one who is "it" objects. A good player can stand off the rest of the group for a long period, until they all give up, whereupon "it" wins. Hyacinth, for example, successfully objected to more than a dozen solutions before the therapist broke up the game. The gimmick in "Why don't you . . . Yes but . . ." is that it is played not for its ostensible purpose (a quest for information or solutions), but for the sake of the fencing; and as a group phenomenon it corresponds to Bion's basic assumption "F" (3).

Other common games are "How am I Doing?" "Uproar," "Alcoholic," "P.T.A.," "Ain't it Awful?" and "Schlemiel." In "Schlemiel," the one who is "it" breaks things, spills things, and makes messes of various kinds, and each time says: "I'm sorry!" This leaves the inexperienced player in a helpless position. The skillful opponent, however, says: "You can break things and spill things all you like; but please don't say 'I'm sorry!' " This response usually causes the Schlemiel to collapse or explode, since it knocks out his gimmick, and the opponent wins. I imagine that at this point many of you are thinking of Stephen Potter, but I think the games I have in mind are more serious; and some of them, like "Alcoholic," with all its complex rules published by various rescue organizations, are played for keeps. "Alcoholic" is complicated because the official form requires at least four players: a persecutor, a rescuer, a dummy, and the one who is "it."

The transactional analysis of Hyacinth's game of "Why don't you . . . Yes but . . ." was drawn and analyzed for the group. In the guise of an Adult seeking information, Hyacinth "cons" the other members into responding like sage parents advising a helpless child. The object of Hyacinth's Child is to confound these parents one after the other. The game can proceed because at the superficial level, both stimulus and response are Adult to Adult, and at a deeper level they are also complementary, Parent to Child stimulus ("Why don't you . . . ? ") eliciting Child to Parent response ("Yes, but . . ."). The second level is unconscious on both sides.

The therapeutic effect of this analysis was to make Hyacinth aware of her defensive need to confound, and to make the others aware of how easily they could be conned into taking a parental role unawares. When a new patient tried to start a game of "Why don't you . . . Yes but . . ." in this group, they all played along with her in order not to make her too anxious, but after a few weeks they gently demonstrated to her what was happening. In other words, they now had the option of playing or not playing this game, as they saw fit, where formerly they had no choice but to be drawn in. This option was the net therapeutic gain, which they were able to apply profitably in their more intimate relationships.

The Analysis of Scripts

A script is an attempt to repeat in derivative form not a transference reaction or a transference situation, but a transference drama, often split up into acts, exactly like the theatrical scripts which are intuitive artistic derivatives of these primal dramas of childhood. Operationally, a script is a complex set of transactions, by nature recurrent, but not necessarily recurring, since a complete performance may require a whole lifetime. A common tragic script is that based on the rescue fantasy of a woman who marries one alcoholic after another. The disruption of such a script leads to despair. Since the magical cure of the alcoholic husband which the script calls for is not forthcoming, a divorce results and the woman tries again. A practical and constructive script, on the other hand, may lead to great happiness if the others in the cast are well chosen and play their parts satisfactorily. A game usually represents a segment of a script.

The ultimate goal of transactional analysis is the analysis of scripts, since the script determines the destiny and identity of the individual. Space, however, does not permit a discussion of the technique, aim, and therapeutic effect of script analysis, and this topic will have to be reserved for another communication.

Self-Analysis

Structural and transactional analysis lend themselves to self-examination more readily than orthodox psychoanalysis does, since they effectively bypass many of the difficulties inherent in self-psychoanalysis. The therapist who has some knowledge of his own personality structure has a distinct advantage in dealing with his countertransference problems: that is, the activity of his own Child or Parent with its own favorite games, its own script, and its own motives for becoming a group therapist. If he has a clear insight, without self-delusion, as to what is exteropsychic, what is neopsychic, and what is archaeopsychic in himself, then he can choose his responses so as to bring the maximum therapeutic benefit to his patients.

I have condensed into this brief communication material which would easily fill a book, and which is best made clear by six months or a year of clinical supervision. In its present form, however, it might stimulate some people to more careful observation of ego states in their patients, and to some serious and sustained experiments in structural interpretation.

Summary

(1) A new approach to group therapy is outlined, based on the distinction between exteropsychic, neopsychic, and archaeopsychic ego states. The study of the relationships within the individual of these three types of ego states, colloquially called Parent, Adult, and Child, respectively, is termed structural analysis, and has been discussed in a previous publication.

(2) Once each individual in the group has some understanding of his own personality in these terms, the group can proceed to simple transactional analysis, in which the ego state of the individual who gives the transactional stimulus is compared with the ego state of the one who gives the transactional response.

(3) In the next phase, short series of transactions, called operations,

are studied in the group. More complex series may constitute a "game," in which some element of double-dealing or insincerity is present. In the final phase, it is demonstrated that all transactions are influenced by complex attempts on the part of each member to manipulate the group in accordance with certain basic fantasies derived from early experiences. This unconscious plan, which is a strong determinant of the individual's destiny, is called a script.

(4) Clinical examples are given, and the therapeutic gain expected from each phase of structural and transactional analysis is indicated.

References

1. Berne, E.: "Ego States in Psychotherapy." *Am. J. Psychother.* XI: 293-309, 1957.
2. Freud, S: *An Outline of Psychoanalysis.* W. W. Norton, New York, 1949. 3. Bion, W. R.: "Group Dynamics: A Re-View." *Internat. J. Psycho-Anal.,* XXXIII: 235-247, 1952.

Psychoanalysis and Group Therapy:
A Developmental Point of View

FRITZ REDL, PH.D.

Distinguished Professor of the Behavioral Sciences,
Wayne State University, Detroit, Michigan

Fritz Redl (1902–1988) was Distinguished Professor of the Behavioral Sciences at Wayne State University, Detroit, Michigan, when he wrote this paper. Prior to that he had been Chief of the Child Research Branch at the National Institute of Health in Washington, DC. Redl was a student of August Aichhorn in Vienna, the first adolescent group psychotherapist. He was interested, like Slavson, in progressive education when he came to America in 1936. In Detroit he established a network of clubs for adolescents and participated in a residential program for delinquent youth (Pioneer House). A general introduction to the work of early adolescent group psychotherapists is available (Rachman AW, Raubolt RR: The pioneers of adolescent group psychotherapy. International Journal of Group Psychotherapy 34:387–413, 1984). Redl was an influential figure in promoting the application of Freudian ideas to the group format. He was active in the American Psychoanalytic Association and was President of the American Orthopsychiatric Association.

This paper was originally presented as a memorial lecture for the Boston training analyst, Dr. Leo Berman, who was particularly interested in how ego psychology and social psychology could be integrated through psychoanalytically oriented group psychotherapy.

Only the second half of the paper is presented here, that dealing with group phenomena. The first portion describes the gradual rapprochement of the psychoanalytic community to the idea of group psychotherapy. Redl describes four stages: (1) suspicion and contempt with no toleration of any validity for group approaches; (2) the acceptance of some facts as long as they were identified with a clearly separate tradition, for example phenomena found in non-clinical group settings; (3) extramarital slumming, whereby analytic candidates received passive permission to indulge in group work outside of their formal educational stream; and finally (4) official sanction of a few group specialists, especially if they represented marginal areas such as institutional hospital settings, were only said to be concerned with symptomatic relief, or were primarily researchers.

—Editor

Redl F: Psychoanalysis and group therapy: a developmental point of view. *American Journal of Orthopsychiatry* 33:135–147, 1963.

Besides his work on and his contribution to the question of just what psychoanalysis does to and with group therapy, Leo Berman was equally concerned with the supplementary question: What are the implications of some of the by now undeniable facts of group life—especially of life in therapy groups—for psychoanalytic theory? If even a few of the observations made by psychoanalysts who have exposed themselves to group therapy hold up, don't they constitute a challenge to our customary theoretical formulations, and especially to our model of personality, which has proved so adequate for our work in the individual therapy situation? Don't some of the data thus discovered constitute, if not a threat, then at least a demand for reformulation? Should we expect all the group psychological phenomena we run into to be explained with the same set of metapsychological assumptions used to explain the individual therapy process?

A challenge to our theory should be a wonderful and welcome event for anybody who follows in the footsteps of Sigmund Freud. For, you may remember, he operated on the very same principle. If, in the course of clinical work, phenomena appear to be undeniable— however crazy or amazing they may seem—for which our present theoretical constructs have no appropriate places, well then, let those theoretical formulations go. They had better be discarded, modified or supplemented to cope with the new facts. There is no need to remind this audience of what this basic principle of scientific thought did to Freud— and what he did with it. We ought to be proud that right now we are allowed to face a situation similar to those he faced several times. Coping with the impact of new group psychological data of clinical relevance to our theoretical constructs was another one of Leo's life ambitions. Within the limits of this occasion, of course, I must confine myself to just putting on the table, so to speak, a few of the items of concern. I will leave it to you to carry on from there.

In a nutshell, it seems to me that the following four phenomena constitute the "facts of group life" that emerge clearly in therapy groups, but which our present model of personality is not flexible enough to explain: (1) the phenomenon of "contagion and shock effect"; (2) the power of "group psychological role suction"; (3) the tax-imposition and tax exemption power of group structure and group code; and (4) the action-threshold impact of spatial designs and of things.

It will not be easy to present enough of a description of what I refer to as "group psychological facts" to convince you that I am not talking about what we already know anyway, that the phenomena I have in mind really contain some core as yet hard to explain. It fills me with horror that my short and colorful illustrations may be interpreted as if they were meant to be adequate evidence for what I am trying to prove. So, let me make sure it is understood that what I say from here on in only illustrates a special angle I am trying to convey. I think I have some proof for it, but I cannot, of course, unpack anything as complex as "evidence" in the fleeting moments that remain.

1. *The phenomenon of contagion and shock effect.* This poses the following challenge to our psychoanalytic theory: Freud rightly opposed Le Bon's explanation of some group phenomena on the basis of his concept of "imitation," and showed, as we all know, how much more complex what looks like simple imitation really is, when viewed in the light of such concepts as identification. On the other hand, Freud directed his remarks primarily at "imitation" events as they were expected to occur in specific types of leader-related groups. He left untouched a wide range of group situations we have since run into. I, too, am well aware that much "imitative" behavior in groups follows exactly Freud's formula. Yet, under certain circumstances, one individual may "pick up" behavioral cues from other individuals in the group in a situation lacking any of the conditions Freud postulates—where there is neither libidinous nor any other type of dependency of the acting individual on the one whose behavior he seems to "imitate," and where, nevertheless the impact of this other individual seems "coercive" to the "actor" in question. This goes beyond what we could easily explain.

> *Example*: Therapy group session, relatively new, most group members resisting therapist's frantic attempts to "pull them in," and reacting to everything that is said with nearly tangible emanations of a deeply hostile silence. Suddenly, one group member—and, in this case again, one without any traceable sign of status or role in the group—"warming up" naively and without being aware what chance he really takes, and starting to talk and to react cooperatively to the therapist's attempts at discussion. All of a sudden the "ice" seems to be broken, and the whole group is coming through with the goods. What gave this person the power to force them to drop their resistance and "do as he did?" Or, what made it possible for the others to drop their resistance just because they saw somebody else act that way?

> *Example*: Therapy group of adults well under way, pretty good over-all atmosphere developed by now, group well at work on whatever the theme of their major discussion happens to be. Suddenly, one group member, through undeniable evidence of her deep-seated resistance and defense against anything the group or the therapist may be doing, spreads such an aura of "hostile silence" around that everybody else dries up in the process. What is the source of the power of that person to reinforce the otherwise well-relating group member's defenses and resistances by her mere oozing of hostility and defense? She was not admired or loved, she had no other status or power weapons at her disposal. Why should the other group members freeze up just because of the hostility from that one unimportant corner of the room?

The phenomenon of "shock effect" is equally hard to explain. In this specific instance, I mean by it the impact of one member of a group that forces new intensities of defense on another group member, against the very impulsivity he allows himself to indulge in.

Example: Cabin of primarily delinquency-oriented thieves. Grouped with them, by mistake, is a child with a long history of stealing, which was more on a neurotic basis, and which this child, as a result of previous therapy, had already tried hard to conquer in himself. Is the delinquency of the rest going to make him steal again? Guaranteedly not. However, the contrary pathology is going to emerge: Our youngster will be severely threatened, his only partially overcome internal conflict will be revived and he will have to produce a double dose of "reaction formation" against his previous symptom trend. He will become a goody-goody or tattler, or he will be so plagued by newly evoked neurotic symptoms such as anxiety, sleep disturbances or what not, that his stay in the group will be inadvisable. How is it that the overtly visible behavior of the other kids, whom our youngster neither loved nor liked nor selected as "identification objects" could throw him into such an internal revival of his conflict, and that the *mere visualization of their behavior* started all this off in him?

In short, under certain conditions the very *visualization of behavior by others* is enough to start off either a chain of the same behavior or a heavy load of "defenses against it" in the individual who perceives it—and all without the specific libidinous and identification-related processes we would usually assume.

Question: How is it that others can have such influence on behavioral production in a child and, even worse, how does that child perceive the precise basis for the behavior of the others?

2. The power of "group psychological role suction." Here I limit the term "role" to those situations in which certain performances basic to the need gratification of a group are demanded by someone in it. Please let me get away with this heuristic oversimplification of the role concept, for it is all too obvious that any fertile discussion of a concept as involved as that of group roles cannot be attempted now.

Most teachers with some experience have observed that sometimes the nicest kids who are quite friendly and pleasant in individual interaction become a pain in the neck when they hit the group. They may turn into clowns, little rebels, rabble rousers or the ones who "tattle" on others' mischief. Sometimes, teachers remark that, in this special group, an otherwise wild and unruly kid seems to be eager for chores and jobs, accumulating with glee before they know it all the janitorial chores classroom life has to give away. Or, they may say that,whenever things get tight, you can "bet" on Johnny to come through with a good and appropriate joke that makes everybody laugh and relax, or express their relief that Mary invariably yells "shut up" to the rest of the noisy crowd just a moment before she, the teacher, would have had to do it. Group therapists, in recent years, have also produced ample evidence for the analogous trend among adults. Such as "therapist's little helper," "group scapegoat, self-appointed," "isolate," "underdog," "defender of the underdog," "group admonisher," and "umpire" have recently entered the standard vocabulary of this field.

Most of this poses no special problem. In fact, psychoanalysts, more than most other people, find it easy to discover just why such individuals play such roles in a group. I have no quarrel with this. My only request is, let's not stop there: It is not enough. Our usual explanation fits a large number of cases, but it does not hold true all along the line. We usually assume that the given individual had strong conscious or unconscious needs in that direction and has finally either forced them on this group, or used the group's inability to defend itself against him to allow himself behavior he otherwise might not have had enough opportunity for.

Two facts seem to puncture this otherwise quite plausible explanation: First, some people do not use groups indiscriminately to live out their individual pathology or personality needs. They seem to reserve some role-acting for some groups only, and do not show much of it in the rest of their lives. If that is so, I would like to know just what it is *in that group* that seems to bring out "the worst," or "the best," of them. Assuming the real cause is a basic need to act that way anyway, just what sets this off—or pushes it back—in specific group situations? Obviously, it must be a property of the group they are in, regardless of their own motivations. If so, what is it?

The second challenge is this: While many a clown or "therapist's little helper" may be sufficiently explained on the basis of his personal pathology, I don't think this is true for them all. Granted that nobody would do anything that he lacks the latent capacity to do, the push from within by no means always explains precisely what evokes the behavior. I think I have seen situations in which Johnny's need to tattle was among the least vehement forces in the child, when, in fact, it belonged to trends heavily opposed by his own superego. Only in certain group situations, for instance, when panicked by a too frightening lack of control within the group, would he assume the "tattler's role." Far from using the group to satisfy his tattling greed, he actually, with great disgust within himself, performed the salutary task for the sake of the group, for otherwise the group would soon have gone to pieces, or things would have gotten out of hand. And not every kid who yells "shut up" when the group gets too noisy is a conceited egotist or a namby-pamby teacher's pet. Some of them really yell "shut up" just in time and in just the right way, because their own perception of group drive processes shows them that the group is helpless, that some behavior needs to be terminated, that nobody else seems to be ready to do it, so maybe they had better, since somebody must.

In all those cases—and I wouldn't care if you could convince me that they are few compared with the other type for even one would be enough to get my theoretical visor up—it seems to me that something like a "role suction" emanating from something within the dynamic events of the group itself is just as relevant in explaining behavior as is whatever we know about inner needs. If so, what is it, how can I nail it down, and what theoretical constructs do I need to explain the fact that the *transition of a mild wish into open behavior can be influenced by something as "superficial" and intangible as a dimly perceived group need?* A tracing, no matter how thorough, of the history of the youngster's individual readiness for such action certainly would not suffice.

3. *The tax imposition and tax exemption power of group structure and group code.* We know what a superego is made of, and the source of its value content. We also know that, by the time kids reach their post-latency years or become adults, most of that process has long been under way and the basic structure of the various individual superegos must be well established, on whatever level.

If any changes are to be made, we know they will require new libidinous relationships toward important "parent surrogate" figures in a person's life, which he will then ward off because of his fear of re-sexualization of the original wishes, and so forth, and that, on the basis of such renunciation of original wishes, he will incorporate ego ideals or superego content into his own superego. It takes all that to bring about a modification in superego content.

How does it happen, then, that under certain circumstances a group of youngsters suddenly live way above or way below their usual level of operation? And I mean they do so without any of the basic, analytically assumed conditions, but by the sheer force of situations that are difficult to assume are powerful enough to account for all that.

> *Example*: Delinquent gang, moved into the camp setting, and kept together. No need to describe what it takes to survive with them and to make them survive with each other and with the rest of the camp. Suddenly somebody thought of some especially well advised "project" which happens to catch the fancy of the kids. For about a week, with no other personal changes having occurred in the individuals, this group abandons its collective warfare against society and operates on a high level of reliability and work orientation, and its members even develop temporary changes in their superego functions. Individuals feel guilty if they do anything that endangers their project, they feel ashamed if caught slacking behind the effort expected, they stop steeling, raiding, destroying —their normal side enterprises—they live as though they had changed. The termination of the project, of course, terminates this whole episode, and concomitant work with the individuals makes it clear that no lasting changes in their superegos have as yet occurred. Yet, what was source of the power of the group atmosphere created by that specific project to influence their superego even to the point of production of appropriate guilt feelings, and how is it that something like group organization around a program was able to produce such atmosphere changes to begin with?

Example: A group of otherwise respectable adults well oriented in their values find themselves at a convention, in a hotel in somebody else's town. How is it that a wide range of behavior suddenly becomes "tax exempt from guilt feelings" for the duration, while their individual superegos apparently emerge undamaged after their return home? How can solid agents such as superegos and basic processes be modified by changes as seemingly simple as geography and group organizational pattern?

By the way, the very power of therapy groups to bring about some changes in individuals at a time when their individual readiness for such changes was seriously in doubt has impressed us in many a case. Those of us with longer experience with many groups will also remember that we must keep in mind how many changes that turn up within the confines of a patient's group life maybe limited to the very condition of his being immersed in the overall value pattern of that specific group, and that we must question whether we have a group psychological process on our hands or a real personality change, before we let him out as cured. By the way, what constitutes a real change anyway, and, come to think of it, is some of this perhaps also at work when we predict what will happen when a patient leaves the two-person group of the individual therapy room?

4. The action threshold impact of spatial designs and things. This issue seems to be a new one, not faced either by psychoanalysis in general or by group therapy, although both have pointed to it with ample illustrations. After we have said all there is to say in our capacity of analytically oriented group therapists on the basis of such concepts as transference, counter-transference and libidinal cathexis, we are sometimes astounded by the incredible impact "simple facts" can have on the behavior of people in a group. We know now, for instance— what nursery school teachers have always known—that occasionally the simple geography of a seating order may make or break a group session, or may actually be a decisive factor in the formation of or failure to form a subgroup or in what shading the member-leader relationship will assume. We have also developed, without theoretical astonishment and sheerly for our survival as practitioners, a holy respect for issues as "superficial" as the size of the room in which we hold our sessions, the presence or absence of water faucets, the privacy or the heavy traffic of the terrain or whether a recorder—although visibly unused—stands around on the table. Anyone who tries group therapy with body-restless adolescents or children will willingly add to this inventory a variety of "gadgets" that better be left out, or else. That baseball bat, for instance, is O.K. when we take them out for a game; but leave it around on the table or a chair while the group is supposed to sit down for a serious discussion of an incident they are all really eager for, and you know what will happen in spite of their "readiness" for the discussion. In short, it seems that a variety of properties of space, timing and equipment, or anything that can be used as a prop for anything else, have a latent power over the behavior of people, which our psychoanalytic theory does not seem to me to explain sufficiently. Only those who deal with the borderline cases of psychotics and delinquent acter-outers have, even in their individual therapy, conceded that power, although conceding it is a far cry from being able to explain it. All of us seem to have forgotten what Freud had to say in his initial insistence on the conditions for analytic therapy. If the emotional interaction between therapist and patient by means of words, thoughts and emotions is the main current through which treatment takes place, why should such little issues as a prone or upright position, a couch versus a chair, an exit or an entrance or the soundproofness of a room be deemed so important? I think we were able to neglect all this for so long because we had learned how to control such factors efficiently in individual therapy with certain types of neuroses. In individual therapy with children, it was already harder and, the moment we invite other patients into the room—individuals who may become live props for each other—the impact of spatial arrangements, gadgets and props can no longer be ignored.

My question: How do we know just which spatial arrangements, time sequences and physical properties of the therapy environment will assume such dramatic importance, and why? How can a silly thing like a baseball bat lying in the wrong place elicit open behavior, which might otherwise have been fantasized, but not acted out?

This, by the way, seems to me to be the crucial challenge to our over-all theoretical design: we have paid ample respect to the ego's role as a watchdog on the threshold between the conscious and the unconscious. I don't think we have studied thoroughly enough another function that certainly belongs into the job description of a well-functioning ego, namely, its power to decide which fantasy, emotion, urge, should remain just that and which should be allowed access to the muscular machinery, and therefore find entrance into the realm of behavior that can be called "acted out".

I have no answer to all of this. Whatever thought crowds itself into my mind pretending to be an answer soon turns out to be premature and oversimplified. But I know that Leo Berman was concerned with issues like these as seriously as I am. I also know that we shared the conviction that an answer to all this is as important to psychoanalysis as it is to group therapy. Furthermore, it is obvious that the task of building some of the above-mentioned "facts of group life"—and many others—into our psychoanalytic model of the personality and of the world requires the most experienced and the sharpest theoretical minds. I, for one, do not feel well enough equipped for the task. One of those who would have been, we have lost. It may not be inappropriate to close this memorial assembly for a man of Leo Berman's stature with the hope that the psychoanalytic community may pick up and continue the task in which we were so rudely interrupted by his untimely death.

The Process of the
Basic Encounter Group

CARL R. ROGERS, PH. D.

Carl Rogers (1902–1987) received his early training at Columbia University Teachers College, New York, in a psychoanalytically oriented approach. Once in practice at the Rochester Guidance Center, New York, he found himself emphasizing the importance of focusing on the client's feelings, a direction reinforced through contact with Otto Rank. In a talk at the University of Minnesota in 1940, Rogers began his identification of the "necessary and sufficient conditions" required for effective psychotherapy, including nonpossessive warmth, accurate empathy, and genuineness in a noncontrolling atmosphere of unconditional positive regard. Perhaps his greatest productivity is associated with his tenure at the University of Chicago Department of Counseling Psychology (1945–1957), where his ideas were augmented by the work of a generation of graduate students including Robert R. Carkhuff, Charles B. Truax, and Godfrey T. Barrett-Lennard (Rogers CR: Client-Centered Therapy. Boston: Houghton Mifflin, 1951). Rogers was Vice-President of the American Orthopsychiatric Association (1941–1942), and President of the American Psychological Association (1946–1947).

Rogers' work marked a major breakthrough in the scientific study of psychotherapy. A large research output demonstrated that his critical dimensions were indeed correlated with better outcome. However, over time it has become clear that these factors play a definite but limited role. In their absence, helpful therapy is unlikely. But if they are present even to only a modest degree then it is patient variables that better predict outcome. The current "therapeutic alliance" literature provides some continuity with Rogers' work.

This article gives a good flavor of the passion and hope that infuse Rogers' work. It was written while he was a resident Fellow at the Western Behavioral Sciences Institute in La Jolla, California and was shifting his focus from individual to group methods. —Editor

Rogers CR: The process of the basic encounter group. In Bugental JFT, *Challenges of Humanistic Psychology.* New York: McGraw-Hill, 1967.

I would like to share with you some of my thinking and puzzlement regarding a potent new cultural development—the intensive group experience. It has, in my judgment, significant implications for our society. It has come very suddenly over our cultural horizon, since in anything like its present form it is less than two decades old.

I should like briefly to describe the many different forms and different labels under which the intensive group experience has become a part of our modern life. It has involved different kinds of individuals, and it has spawned various theories to account for its effects.

As to labels, the intensive group experience has at times been called the *T-group* or *lab group*, 'T' standing for training laboratory in group dynamics. It has been termed *sensitivity training* in human relationships. The experience has sometimes been called a *basic encounter group* or a workshop—a workshop in human relations, in leadership, in counselling, in education, in research, in psychotherapy. In dealing with one particular type of person—the drug addict—it has been called a synanon.

The intensive group experience has functioned in various settings. It has operated in industries, in universities, in church groups, and in resort settings which provide a retreat from everyday life. It has functioned in various educational institutions and in penitentiaries.

An astonishing range of individuals have been involved in these intensive group experiences. There have been groups for presidents of large corporations. There have been groups for delinquent and predelinquent adolescents. There have been groups composed of college students and faculty members, of counsellors and psychotherapists, of school dropouts, of married couples, of confirmed drug addicts, of criminals serving sentences, of nurses preparing for hospital service, and of educators, principals, and teachers.

The geographical spread attained by this rapidly expanding movement has reached in this country from Bethel, Maine (starting point of the National Training Laboratory movement), to Idyllwild, California. To my personal knowledge, such groups also exist in France, England, Holland, Japan, and Australia.

In their outward pattern these group experiences also show a great deal of diversity. There are T-groups and workshops which have extended over three to four weeks, meeting six to eight hours each day. There are some that have lasted only 2 1/2 days, crowding twenty or more hours of group sessions into this time. A recent innovation is the "marathon" weekend, which begins on Friday afternoon and ends on Sunday evening, with only a few hours out for sleep and snacks.

As to the conceptual underpinnings of this whole movement, one may almost select the theoretical flavor he prefers. Lewinian and client-centered theories have been most prominent, but gestalt therapy and various brands of psychoanalysis have all played contributing parts. The experience within the group may focus on specific training in human relations skills. It may be closely similar to group therapy, with much exploration of past experience and the dynamics of personal development. It may focus on creative expression through painting or expressive movement. It may be focused primarily upon a basic encounter and relationship between individuals.

Simply to describe the diversity which exists in this field raises very properly the question of why these various developments should be considered to belong together. Are there any threads of commonality which pervade all these widely divergent activities? To me it seems that they do belong together and can all be classed as focusing on the intensive group experience. They all have certain similar external characteristics. The group in almost every case is small (from eight to eighteen members), is relatively unstructured, and chooses its own goals and personal directions. The group experience usually, though not always, includes some cognitive input, some content material which is presented to the group. In almost all instances the leader's responsibility is primarily the facilitation of the expression of both feelings and thoughts on the part of the group members. Both in the leader and in the group members there is some focus on the process and the dynamics of the immediate personal interaction. These are, I think, some of the identifying characteristics which are rather easily recognized.

There are also certain practical hypotheses which tend to be held in common by all these groups. My own summary of these would be as follows: In an intensive group with much freedom and little structure, the individual will gradually feel safe enough to drop some of his defenses and facades; he will relate more directly on a feeling basis (come into a basic encounter) with other members of the group; he will come to understand himself and his relationship to others more accurately; he will change in his personal attitudes and behavior; and he will subsequently relate more effectively to others in his everyday life situation. There are other hypotheses related more to the group than to the individual. One is that in this situation of minimal structure, the group will move from confusions, fractionation, and discontinuity to a climate of greater trust and coherence. These are some of the characteristics and hypotheses which, in my judgment, bind together this enormous cluster of activities which I wish to talk about as constituting the intensive group experience.

As for myself, I have been gradually moving into this field for the last twenty years. In experimenting with what I call *student-centered* teaching, involving the free expression of personal feelings, I came to recognize not only the cognitive learnings but also some of the personal changes which occurred. In brief intensive training courses for counsellors for the Veterans Administration in 1946, during the postwar period, I and my staff focused more directly on providing an intensive group experience because of its impact in producing significant learning. In 1950, I served as leader of an intensive, full-time, one-week workshop, a postdoctoral training seminar in psychotherapy for the American Psychological Association. The impact of those six days was so great that for more than a dozen years afterward, I kept hearing from members of the group about the meaning it had for them. Since that time I have been involved in more than forty ventures of what I would like to term—using the label most congenial to me—*basic encounter groups*. Most of these have involved for many of the members experiences of great intensity and considerable personal change. With two individuals, however, in these many groups, the experience contributed, I believe, to a psychotic break. A few other individuals have found the experience more unhelpful than helpful. So I have come to have a profound respect for the constructive potency of such group experiences and also a real concern over the fact that sometimes and in some ways this experience may do damage to individuals.

The Group Process

It is a matter of great interest to me to try to understand what appear to be common elements in the group process as I have come dimly to sense these. I am using this opportunity to think about this problem, not because I feel I have any final theory to give, but because I would like to formulate, as clearly as I am able, the elements which I can perceive at the present time. In doing so I am drawing upon my own experience, upon the experiences of others with whom I have worked, upon the written material in this field, upon the written reactions of many individuals who have participated in such groups, and to some extent upon the recordings of such group sessions, which we are only beginning to tap and analyze. I am sure that (though I have tried to draw on the experience of others) any formulation I make at the present time is unduly influenced by my own experience in groups and thus is lacking in the generality I wish it might have.

As I consider the terribly complex interactions which arise during twenty, forty, sixty, or more hours of intensive sessions, I believe that I see some threads which weave in and out of the pattern. Some of these trends or tendencies are likely to appear early and some later in the group sessions, but there is no clear-cut sequence in which one ends and another begins. The interaction is best thought of, I believe, as a varied tapestry, differing from group to group, yet with certain kinds of trends evident in most of these intensive encounters and with certain patterns tending to precede and others to follow. Here are some of the process patterns which I see developing, briefly described in simple terms, illustrated from tape recordings and personal reports, and presented in roughly sequential order. I am not aiming at a high-level theory of group process but rather at a naturalistic observation out of which, I hope, true theory can be built.

Milling Around: As the leader or facilitator makes clear at the outset that this is a group with unusual freedom, that it is not one for which he will take directional responsibility, there tends to develop a period of initial confusion, awkward silence, polite surface interaction, "cocktailparty talk," frustration, and great lack of continuity. The individuals come face-to-face with the fact that "there is no structure here except what we provide. We do not know our purposes; we do not even know one another, and we are committed to remain together over a considerable period of time." In this situation, confusion and frustration are natural. Particularly striking to the observer is the lack of continuity between personal expressions. Individual A will present some proposal or concern, clearly looking for a response from the group. Individual B has obviously been waiting for his turn and starts off on some completely different tangent as though he had never heard A. One member makes a simple suggestion such as, "I think we should introduce ourselves," and this may lead to several hours of highly involved discussion in which the underlying issues appear to be, "Who is the leader?" "Who is responsible for us?" "Who is a member of the group?" "What is the purpose of the group?"

Resistance to Personal Expression or Exploration: During the milling period, some individuals are likely to reveal some rather personal attitudes. This tends to foster a very ambivalent reaction among other members of the group. It is the public self which members tend to reveal to one another, and only gradually, fearfully, and ambivalently do they take steps to reveal something of their inner world.

******

Here and throughout the paper, a number of verbatim examples
have been deleted.

******

Description of Past Feelings: In spite of ambivalence about the trustworthiness of the group and the risk of exposing oneself, expression of feelings does begin to assume a larger proportion of the discussion. The executive tells how frustrated he feels by certain situations in his industry, or the housewife relates problems she has experienced with her children.

Expression of Negative Feelings: Curiously enough, the first expression of genuinely significant "here-and-now" feeling is apt to come out in negative attitudes toward other group members or toward the group leader. In one group in which members introduced themselves at some length, one woman refused, saying that she preferred to be known for what she was in the group and not in terms of her status outside. Very shortly after this, one of the men in the group attacked her vigorously and angrily for this stand, accusing her of failing to cooperate, of keeping herself aloof from the group, and so forth. It was the first *personal current feeling* which had been brought into the open in the group. Frequently the leader is attacked for his failure to give proper guidance to the group.

Why are negatively toned expressions the first current feelings to be expressed? Some speculative answers might be the following: This is one of the best ways to test the freedom and trustworthiness of the group. "Is it really a place where I can be and express myself positively and negatively? Is this really a safe place, or will I be punished.?" Another quite different reason is that deeply positive feelings are much more difficult to express than negative ones. "If I say, 'I love you,' I am vulnerable and open to the most awful rejection. If I say, 'I hate you,' I am at best liable to attack, against which I can defend." Whatever the reasons, such negatively toned feelings tend to be the first here-and-now material to appear.

Expression and Exploration of Personally Meaningful Material: It may seem puzzling that following such negative experiences as the initial confusion, the resistance to personal expression, the focus on outside events, and the voicing of critical or angry feelings, the event most likely to occur next is for an individual to reveal himself to the group in a significant way. The reason for this no doubt is that the individual member has come to realize that this is in part his group. He can help to make of it what he wishes. He has also experienced the fact that negative feelings have been expressed and have usually been accepted or assimilated without any catastrophic results. He realizes there is freedom here, albeit a risky freedom. A climate of trust (Gibb, 1964, Ch. 10) is beginning to develop.

The Expression of Immediate Interpersonal Feelings in the Group: Entering into the process sometimes earlier, sometimes later, is the explicit bringing into the open of the feelings experienced in the immediate moment by one member about another. These are sometimes positive and sometimes negative. Examples would be: "I feel threatened by your silence." "You remind me of my mother, with whom I had a tough time." "I took an instant dislike to you the first moment I saw you." "To me you're like a breath of fresh air in the group." "I like your warmth and your smile." "I dislike you more every time you speak up." Each of these attitudes can be, and usually is, explored in the increasing climate of trust.

The Development of a Healing Capacity in the Group: One of the most fascinating aspects of any intensive group experience is the manner in which a number of the group members show a natural and spontaneous capacity for dealing in a helpful, facilitative, and therapeutic fashion with the pain and suffering of others. As one rather extreme example of this, I think of a man in charge of maintenance in a large plant who was one of the low-status members of an industrial executive group. As he informed us, he had not been "contaminated by education." In the initial phases the group tended to look down on him. As members delved more deeply into themselves and began to express their own attitudes more fully this man came forth as, without doubt, the most sensitive member of the group. He knew intuitively how to be understanding and acceptant. He was alert to things which had not yet been expressed but were just below the surface. When the rest of us were paying attention to a member who was speaking, he would frequently spot another individual who was suffering silently and in need of help. He had a deeply perceptive and facilitating attitude. This kind of ability shows up so commonly in groups that it has led me to feel that the ability to be healing or therapeutic is far more common in human life than we might suppose. Often it needs only the permission granted by a freely flowing group experience to become evident.

In a characteristic instance, the leader and several group members were trying to be of help to Joe, who was telling of the almost complete lack of communication between himself and his wife. In varied ways members endeavored to give help. John kept putting before Joe the feelings Joe's wife was almost certainly experiencing. The facilitator kept challenging Joe's facade of "carefulness." Marie tried to help him discover what he was feeling at the moment. Fred showed him the choice he had of alternative behaviors. All this was clearly done in a spirit of caring, as is even more evident in the recording itself. No miracles were achieved, but toward the end Joe did come to the realization that the only thing that might help would be to express his real feelings to his wife.

Self-acceptance and the Beginning of Change: Many people feel that self-acceptance must stand in the way of change. Actually, in these group experiences, as in psychotherapy, it is the *beginning* of change. Some examples of the kind of attitudes expressed would be these; "I *am* a dominating person who likes to control others. I do want to mold these individuals into the proper shape." Another person says, "I really have a hurt and overburdened little boy inside of me who feels very sorry for himself. I am that little boy, in addition to being a competent and responsible manager."

This feeling of greater realness and authenticity is a very common experience. It would appear that the individual is learning to accept and to be himself, and this is laying the foundation for change. He is closer to his own feelings, and hence they are no longer so rigidly organized and are more open to change.

The Cracking of Facades: As the sessions continue, so many things tend to occur together that it is difficult to know which to describe first. It should again be stressed that these different threads and stages interweave and overlap. One of these threads is the increasing impatience with defenses. As time goes on, the group finds it unbearable that any member should live behind a mask or a front. The polite words, the intellectual understanding of one another and of relationships, the smooth coin of tact and cover-up—amply satisfactory for interactions outside—are just not good enough. The expression of self by some members of the group has made it very clear that a deeper and more basic encounter is *possible*, and the group appears to strive, intuitively and unconsciously, toward this goal. Gently at times, almost savagely at others, the group demands that the individual be himself, that his current feelings not be hidden, that he remove the mask of ordinary social intercourse. In one group there was a highly intelligent and quite academic man who had been rather perceptive in his understanding of others but who had not revealed himself at all. The attitude of the group was finally expressed sharply by one member when he said, "Come out from behind that lectern, Doc. Stop giving us speeches. Take off your dark glasses. We want to know *you*."

If I am indicating that the group at times is quite violent in tearing down a facade or a defense, this would be accurate. On the other hand, it can also be sensitive and gentle. The man who was accused of hiding behind a lectern was deeply hurt by this attack, and over the lunch hour looked very troubled, as though he might break into tears at any moment. When the group reconvened, the members sensed this and treated him very gently, enabling him to tell us his own tragic personal story, which accounted for his aloofness and his intellectual and academic approach to life.

The Individual Receives Feedback: In the process of this freely expressive interaction, the individual rapidly acquires a great deal of data as to how he appears to others. The "hail-fellow-well-met" discovers that others resent his exaggerated friendliness. The executive who weighs his words carefully and speaks with heavy precision may find that others regard him as stuffy. A woman who shows a somewhat excessive desire to be of help to others is told in no uncertain terms that some group members do not want her for a mother. All this can be decidedly upsetting, but as long as these various bits of information are fed back in the context of caring which is developing in the group, they seem highly constructive.

Confrontation: There are times when the term "feedback" is far too mild to describe the interactions which take place, when it is better said that one individual *confronts* another, directly "leveling" with him. Such confrontations can be positive, but frequently they are decidedly negative, as the following example will make abundantly clear. In one of the last sessions of a group, Alice had made some quite vulgar and contemptuous remarks to John, who was entering religious work. The next morning, Norma, who had been a very quiet person in the group, took the floor:

NORMA (*loud sigh*): Well, I don't have any respect for you, Alice. *None!* (*Pause.*) There's about a hundred things going through my mind I want to say to you, and by God I hope I get through 'em all! First of all, if you wanted us to respect you, then why couldn't you respect *John's* feelings last night? Why have you been on him today? Hmm? Last night—couldn't you—couldn't you accept—*couldn't you* comprehend in any at all that—that he felt his unworthiness in the service of God? Couldn't you accept this, or did you have to dig into it today to find something *else there*? And his respect for womanhood—he *loves* women—yes, he does, because he's a real person, but you—you're not a real woman—to me—and thank God, you're not my mother!!! I want to come over and beat the hell out of you!!! I want to slap you across the mouth so hard and—oh, and you're so, you're many years above me and I respect age, and I respect people who are older than me, *but I don't respect you, Alice. At all!* And I was so *hurt* and *confused* because you were making someone else feel *hurt* and *confused*. . . .

It may relieve the reader to know that these two women came to accept each other, not completely, but much more understandingly, before the end of the session. But this was a confrontation!

The Helping Relationship outside the Group Sessions: No account of the group process would, in my experience, be adequate if it did not make mention of the many ways in which group members are of assistance to one another. Not infrequently, one member of a group will spend hours listening and talking to another member who is undergoing a painful new perception of himself. Sometimes it is merely the offering of help which is therapeutic. I think of one man who was going through a very depressed period after having told us of the many tragedies in his life. He seemed quite clearly, from his remarks, to be contemplating suicide. I jotted down my room number (we were staying at a hotel) and told him to put it in his pocket and to call me anytime of day or night if he felt that it would help. He never called, but six months after the workshop was over he wrote to me telling me how much that act had meant to him and that he still had the slip of paper to remind him of it.

The Basic Encounter: Running through some of the trends I have just been describing is the fact that individuals come into much closer and more direct contact with one another than is customary in ordinary life. This appears to be one of the most central, intense, and change-producing aspects of such a group experience. To illustrate what I mean, I would like to draw an example from a recent workshop group. A man tells, through his tears, of the very tragic loss of his child, a grief which he is experiencing *fully* for the first time, not holding back his feelings in any way. Another says to him, also with tears in his eyes, "I've never felt so close to another human being. I've never before felt a real physical hurt in me from the pain of another. I feel *completely* with you." This is a basic encounter.

Such I-Thou relationships (to use Buber's term) occur with some frequency in these group sessions and nearly always bring a moistness to the eyes of the participants.

One member, trying to sort out his experiences immediately after a workshop, speaks of the "commitment to relationship" which often developed on the part of two individuals, not necessarily individuals who had liked each other initially. He goes on to say:

"The incredible fact experienced over and over by members of the group was that when a negative feeling was fully expressed to another, the relationship grew and the negative feeling was replaced by a deep acceptance for the other....Thus real change seemed to occur when feelings were experienced and expressed in the context of the relationship. 'I can't *stand* the way you talk!' turned into a real understanding and affection for you the *way* you talk."

This statement seems to capture some of the more complex meanings of the term "basic encounter."

The Expression of Positive Feelings and Closeness: As indicated in the last section, an inevitable part of the group process seems to be that when feelings are expressed and can be accepted in a relationship, a great deal of closeness and positive feelings result. Thus as the sessions proceed, there is an increasing feeling of warmth and group spirit and trust built, not out of positive attitudes only, but out of a realness which includes both positive and negative feeling. One member tried to capture this in writing very shortly after the workshop by saying that if he were trying to sum it up, ". . . it would have to do with what I call confirmation—a kind of confirmation of myself, of the uniqueness and universal qualities of men, a confirmation that when we can be human together something positive can emerge."

Some may be very critical of a "leader" so involved and so sensitive that she weeps at the tensions in the group which she has taken into herself. For me, it is simply another evidence that when people are real with each other, they have an astonishing ability to heal a person with a real and understanding love, whether that person is "participant" or "leader."

Behavior Changes in the Group: It would seem from observation that many changes in behavior occur in the group itself. Gestures change. The tone of voice changes, becoming sometimes stronger, sometimes softer, usually more spontaneous, less artificial, more feelingful. Individuals show an astonishing amount of thoughtfulness and helpfulness toward one another.

Our major concern, however, is with the behavior changes which occur following the group experience. It is this which constitutes the most significant question and on which we need much more study and research.

Sometimes the changes which are described are very subtle. "The primary change is the more positive view of my ability to allow myself to *hear*, and to become involved with someone else's 'silent scream.'"

At the risk of making the outcomes sound too good, I will add one more statement written shortly after a workshop by a mother. She says:

> "The immediate impact on my children was of interest to both me and my husband. I feel that having been so accepted and loved by a group of strangers was so supportive that when I returned home my love for the people closest to me was much more spontaneous. Also, the practice I had in accepting and loving others during the workshop was evident in my relationships with my close friends."

Disadvantages and Risks

Thus far one might think that every aspect of the group process was positive. As far as the evidence at hand indicates, it appears that it nearly always is a positive process for a majority of the participants. There are, nevertheless, failures which result. Let me try to describe briefly some of the negative aspects of the group process as they sometimes occur.

The most obvious deficiency of the intensive group experience is that frequently the behavior changes, if any, which occur are not lasting. This is often recognized by the participants. One says, "I wish I had the ability to hold permanently the 'openness' I left the conference with." Another says 'I experienced a lot of acceptance, warmth, and love at the workshop. I find it hard to carry the ability to share this in the same way with people outside the workshop. I find it easier to slip back into my old unemotional role than to do the work necessary to open relationships."

Some Data on Outcomes: What is the extent of this "slippage"? In the past year, I have administered follow-up questionnaires to individuals who have been in groups I have organized or conducted. The information has been obtained from two to twelve months following the group experience, but the greatest number were followed up after a three- to six-month period. Of these individuals, two (i.e.; less than one-half of 1 percent) felt it had changed their behavior in ways they did not like. Fourteen percent felt the experience had made no perceptible change in their behavior. Another fourteen percent felt that it had changed their behavior but that this change had disappeared or left only a small residual positive effect. Fifty-seven percent felt it had made a continuing positive difference in their behavior, a few feeling that it had made some negative changes along with the positive.

A second potential risk involved in the intensive group experience and one which is often mentioned in public discussion is the risk that the individual may become deeply involved in revealing himself and then be left with problems which are not worked through. There have been a number of reports of people who have felt, following an intensive group experience, that they must go to a therapist to work through the feelings which were opened up in the intensive experience of the workshop and which were left unresolved. It is obvious that, without knowing more about each individual situation, it is difficult to say whether this was a negative outcome or a partially or entirely positive one. There are also very occasional accounts and I can testify to two in my own experience, where an individual has had a psychotic episode during or immediately following an intensive group experience. On the other side of the picture is the fact that individuals have also lived through what were clearly psychotic episodes, and lived through them very constructively, in the context of a basic encounter group. My own tentative clinical judgment would be that the more positively the group process has been proceeding, the less likely it is that any individual would be psychologically damaged through membership in the group. It is obvious, however, that this is a serious issue and that much more needs to be known.

Other Hazards of the Group Experience: There is another risk or deficiency in the basic encounter group. Until very recent years it has been unusual for a workshop to include both husband and wife. This can be a real problem if significant change has taken place in one spouse during or as a result of the workshop experience. One individual felt this risk clearly after attending a workshop. He said, "I think there is a great danger to a marriage when one spouse attends a group. It is too hard for the other spouse to compete with the group individually and collectively." One of the frequent after effects of the intensive group experience is that it brings out into the open for discussion marital tensions which have been kept under cover.

Another risk which has sometimes been a cause of real concern in mixed intensive workshops is that very positive, warm, and loving feelings can develop between members of the encounter group, as has been evident from some of the preceding examples. Inevitably some of these feelings have a sexual component, and this can be a matter of great concern to the participants and a profound threat to their spouses if these feelings are not worked through satisfactorily in the workshop. Also the close and loving feelings which develop may become a source of threat and marital difficulty when a wife, for example, has not been present, but projects many fears about the loss of her spouse—whether well founded or not—onto the workshop experience.

Still another negative potential growing out of these groups has become evident in recent years. Some individuals who have participated in previous encounter groups may exert a stultifying influence on new workshops which they attend. They sometimes exhibit what I think of as the "old pro" phenomenon. They feel they have learned the "rules of the game," and they subtly or openly try to impose these rules on newcomers. Thus, instead of promoting true expressiveness and spontaneity they endeavor to substitute new rules for old—to make members feel guilty if they are not expressing feelings, are reluctant to voice criticism or hostility, are talking about situations outside the group relationship, or are fearful of revealing themselves. These old pros seem to be attempting to substitute a new tyranny in interpersonal relationships in the place of older conventional restrictions. To me this is a perversion of the true group process. We need to ask ourselves how this travesty on spontaneity comes about.

Implications

I have tried to describe both the positive and the negative aspects of this burgeoning new cultural development. I would like now to touch on its implications for our society.

In the first place, it is a highly potent experience and hence clearly deserving of scientific study. As a phenomenon it has been both praised and criticized, but few people who have participated would doubt that *something* significant happens in these groups. People do not react in a neutral fashion toward the intensive group experience. They regard it as either strikingly worthwhile or deeply questionable. All would agree, however, that it is *potent*. This fact makes it of particular interest to the behavioral sciences since science is usually advanced by studying potent and dynamic phenomena. This is one of the reasons why I personally am devoting more and more of my time to this whole enterprise. I feel that we can learn much about the ways in which constructive personality change comes about as we study this group process more deeply.

In a different dimension, the intensive group experience appears to be one cultural attempt to meet the isolation of contemporary life. The person who has experienced an I-Thou relationship, who has entered into the basic encounter, is no longer an isolated individual. One workshop member stated this in a deeply expressive way:

"Workshops seem to be at least a partial answer to the loneliness of modern man and his search for new meanings for his life. In short, workshops seem very quickly to allow the individual to become that person he wants to be. The first few steps are taken there, in uncertainty, in fear, and in anxiety. We may or may not continue the journey. It is a gutsy way to live. You trade many, many loose ends for one big knot in the middle of your stomach."

Another implication which is partially expressed in the foregoing statement is that it is an avenue to fulfillment. In a day when more income, a larger car, and a better washing machine seem scarcely to be satisfying the deepest needs of man, individuals are turning to the psychological world, groping for a greater degree of authenticity and fulfillment. One workshop member expressed this extremely vividly:

"It has revealed a completely new dimension of life and has opened an infinite number of possibilities for me in my relationship to myself and to everyone dear to me. I feel truly alive and so grateful and joyful and hopeful and healthy and giddy and sparkly.... With persons everywhere, but especially my family, I have found a new freedom to explore and communicate. I know the change in me automatically brings a change in them. A whole new exciting relationship has started for me with my husband and with each of my children—a freedom to speak and to hear them speak."

Though one may wish to discount the enthusiasm of this statement, it describes an enrichment of life for which many are seeking.

Rehumanizing Human Relationships: This whole development seems to have special significance in a culture which appears to be bent upon dehumanizing the individual and dehumanizing our human relationships. Here is an important force in the opposite direction, working toward making relationships more meaningful and more personal in the family, in education, in government, in administrative agencies, in industry.

An intensive group experience has an even more general philosophical implication. It is one expression of the existential point of view which is making itself so pervasively evident in art and literature and modern life. The implicit goal of the group process seems to be to live life fully in the here and now of the relationship. The parallel with an existential point of view is clear cut. I believe this has been amply evident in the illustrative material.

There is one final issue which is raised by this whole phenomenon: What is our view of the optimal person? What is the goal of personality development? Different ages and different cultures have given different answers to this question. It seems evident from our review of the group process that in a climate of freedom, group members move toward becoming more spontaneous, flexible, closely related to their feelings, open to their experience, and closer and more expressively intimate in their interpersonal relationships. If we value this type of person and this type of behavior, then clearly the group process is a valuable process. If, on the other hand, we place a value on the individual who is effective in suppressing his feelings, who operates from a firm set of principles, who does not trust his own reactions and experience but relies on authority, and who remains aloof in his interpersonal relationships, then we would regard the group process, as I have tried to describe it, as a dangerous force. Clearly there is room for a difference of opinion on this value question and not everyone in our culture would give the same answer.

Conclusion

I have tried to give a naturalistic, observational picture of one of the most significant modern social inventions, the so-called intensive group experience, or basic encounter group. I have tried to indicate some of the common elements of the process which occur in the climate of freedom that is present in such a group. I have pointed out some of the risks and short- comings of the group experience. I have tried to indicate some of the reasons why it deserves serious consideration, not only from a personal point of view, but also from a scientific and philosophical point of view. I also hope I have made it clear that this is an area in which an enormous amount of deeply perceptive study and research is needed.

References

Bennis, W. G., Benne, K. D., Chin, R. (Eds.) *The planning of change.* New York: Holt, Rinehart and Winston, 1961.

Bennis, W. G., Schein, E. H., Berlew, D. E. & Steele, F. I. (Eds) *Interpersonal dynamics.* Homewood, Ill.: Dorsey, 1964.

Bradford, L., Gibb, J. B., & Benne, K. D. (Eds.) *T-group theory and laboratory method.* New York: Wiley, 1964.

Casriel: D. *So fair a house.* Englewood Cliffs, N.J.: Prentice-Hall, 1963.

Gibb, J. R. Climate for trust formation. In L. Bradford, J. R. Gibb, & K. D. Benne (Eds.), *T-group theory and laboratory method.* New York: Wiley, 1964.

Gordon, T. *Group-centered leadership.* Boston: Houghton Mifflin, 1955.

Hall, G. F. *A participant's experience in a basic encounter group.* (Mimeographed) Western Behavioral Sciences Institute, 1965.

YEARS OF CONSOLIDATION
1968–1981

Analytic Group Psychotherapy

MORRIS B. PARLOFF

Morris Parloff was, at the time this article appeared, Chief of the Section on Personality at the National Institute of Mental Health. He was later to serve as Chief of the Psychotherapy and Behavioral Intervention Section, where he made a major contribution to the promotion of clinical research into the psychotherapies. One of his final projects before retirement was the development of the large Multi-Center Collaborative Study of Depression which has recently reported its provocative findings.
  Dr. Parloff has been a regular contributor to the group literature and in years past presented at AGPA meetings. Parloff is noted for his marvelous dry sense of humor; for example, a scholarly discussion of outcome criteria is entitled "Assessing the effects of headshrinking and mind-expanding" (International Journal of Group Psychotherapy 20:14–24, 1970).
  The widely quoted article featured below appeared in a book sponsored by the American Academy of Psychoanalysis. The editor, Judd Marmor of UCLA, produced a volume that was quietly revolutionary. In his introductory chapter, Marmor espouses an "open system" approach of viewing the individual in the context of his group or "field situation." He suggests that the regression commonly found in intensive psychoanalytic treatment is an "iatrogenic artifact" of the highly structured and controlled situation, and that excessive reliance on cognitive understanding has been a failure. A decade later Marmor was to write the definitive early paper on the techniques of brief psychotherapy.
  Parloff takes a critical look at the state of psychoanalytically oriented group psychotherapy in the late 1960s. This had been a decade of exciting developments. The use of group modalities was expanding through large scale social changes and the funding of the community mental health centers in 1963, and the British group-as-a-whole theories were gaining recognition in North America. Parloff comes down firmly on the importance of integrating individual dynamics with group social system theory. This chapter has been considerably shortened to focus on the central issues of how theory is translated into clinical technique, reflecting Parloff's interest in the mechanisms of psychotherapeutic change. —Editor

Parloff MB: Analytic group psychotherapy. In J. Marmor (Ed.), *Modern Psychoanalysis* (pp. 492–531). New York: Basic Books, 1968.

That groups appear to have powerful emotional effects on their members, effects which may be utilized in the furtherance of the psychotherapeutic process, is now widely accepted. Group psychotherapy has moved out of its earlier defensive position and no longer appears to be preoccupied with establishing its effectiveness as a treatment modality. It has been accepted as one of the appropriate and respectable forms of psychotherapy and the prospects for its even wider adoption as a treatment form are excellent.

Increasingly, group therapy is viewed as the treatment of choice with some patients and no less effective than most other treatment forms with other patients. Therapists such as Ziferstein and Grotjahn (1956) are so convinced of the efficacy of group analytic treatment that they predict that it will become the primary therapeutic tool and that individual analysis will be used primarily as a research tool and a training device. We are not prepared, at this point, to assign to this view the status of a "significant trend," but forces other than clinical experience support the prediction that the number of group psychotherapists may soon exceed the number of individual therapists. The normal increase in the demand for psychiatric service will soon be augmented, for psychiatric treatment will be available to a broad segment of the population through the expanding, federally supported, community mental health programs. If serious effort is to be made to provide psychiatric services to those in need of such treatment, the current method of dealing with psychiatric cases will be inadequate and group psychotherapy will be called on even more.

In my view, the field is moving toward the treatment of groups as entities; rather than tending in the direction of psychoanalytic orthodoxy, it seems to be heading toward the broader reaches of general psychology and group psychology. Regardless of which of these positions more closely approximates the truth, neither commits the offense that Moreno decries, namely, that of implying that group therapy is merely an elaboration of psychoanalysis (Moreno, 1962). That the group has gained widespread acceptance among analytically trained therapists is not disputed, but whether this indicates a trend toward the adaptation of psychoanalytic practice to group psychotherapy is very doubtful. I believe that one can make at least as good a case for a position that group therapy as practiced by analytically trained therapists represents a progressive dilution of psychoanalytic concepts of practice.

The present state of the field of analytic group psychotherapy reflects the dynamic interaction between two contrasting beliefs concerning the role of the group in the treatment of the individual: (1) adaptation of the principles and techniques of individual analytic treatment to the group; and (2) the identification, development, and utilization of forces and processes indigenous to groups to facilitate treatment. The resolution which is sought by many is the development of a genuinely distinct form of psychotherapy which utilizes group phenomena as an integral part of the treatment, yet retains the insights and powers of analytic theory and practice.

Three major approaches to group psychotherapy will be described here, as illustrative of the major positions and directions of the field of analytic group psychotherapy.

1. *Intrapersonalist.* This designation is applied to those therapists who appear to have transposed their views regarding individual treatment proc-

esses to the group setting. They maintain their focus on the individual and seek to effect changes in intrapsychic structures and in their internal balance. Proponents of this approach to treatment insist that since intrapsychic change may best be affected by analytic methods, then analytic theory and practice should be adopted insofar as possible in the group treatment setting. Such theorists appear to acknowledge that the group setting represents a challenge to the application of such formal techniques of the analytic method as free association, genetic review, dream interpretation, and the establishment of a transference neurosis. They respond to this challenge in two contrasting ways: by conceding that the aims and patients appropriate for analytic group therapy are restricted (Slavson, 1952); or by admitting no important differences yet reinterpreting the meaning of various psychoanalytic concepts to fit group treatment practices (Wolf and Schwartz, 1962; and Locke, 1961).

2. Transactionalist (Interpersonalist). This category encompasses those who attempt to focus on the dyad or subgroup. They deal primarily with interpersonal relationships and "transactional" units.

It is difficult to designate the theorists who best represent the Transactional position since there is no single individual or group that is acknowledged as a spokesman for this wide-ranging "school." The Transactionalists include such divergent views as those held by Frank (1957a), Bach (1954), Berne (1966), and Mullan and Rosenbaum (1962). All these perceive the group as providing stimuli which permit the individual member to demonstrate his idiosyncratic modes of relating and responding to a broad range of individuals. Psychotherapy depends in part on the therapeutic potential of the interrelationships among patients and between therapist and patients. Therapists of this persuasion recognize to a far greater degree than Intrapersonalists that there are properties of groups which facilitate a productive therapeutic experience.

Although the Transactionalists believe that patients' behavior in groups may be understood in part as a manifestation of properties of the group, they are much more concerned with the personality characteristics of the patients than with the dynamics of the total group. Intrapersonalists and Interpersonalists both appear to assume that the major advantage of the group is that it permits the study of the individual as he responds to a number of other individuals and provides the opportunity for therapeutic change by means of the relationships effected.

3. Integralist. This term is applied to those who place major emphasis on group processes. They believe that study of the group as an entity reveals the functioning of the individual member in his full complexity, since all group activity reflects overt or covert aspects of the behavior of the individuals composing it. The group as a unit engages in activities which provide the individual with experiences and responses which are different in degree and perhaps in kind from those found in the dyad. The Integralist believes that a major aspect of the patient's problem is his inability to be an effective member of a task-oriented group.

These three classifications do not represent equally popular approaches. On the basis of publications and an informal evaluation of the views expressed at professional meetings, we believe that the Transactionalists have the largest number of adherents and the Integralists the smallest number. Since we are concerned here with trends and directions, the criterion of popularity need not be invoked. As in all fields, relatively few therapists possess the necessary fortitude and acrobatic skill to assume and maintain extreme positions. Yet, by attention to the extremes represented by these few, we can more clearly discern direction. For purposes of this review, which concerns theory of group psychotherapy rather than technique, we will limit ourselves to an examination of some acknowledged leaders in this area.

Consistent with the purpose of this chapter, we intend to place major emphasis on the Integralist's position since it represents a relatively new direction in analytic group psychotherapy. This emphasis stems from the view, which we share with many, that advances in the field require self-conscious efforts to incorporate elements of group process in analytic group psychotherapy. The Integralists have made such efforts, and these we believe are finding growing interest and acceptance. Our emphasis represents neither a conviction that important therapeutic advances have been demonstrated by the Integralists nor that the theoretical positions advanced are compelling. They deserve detailed study, however, because they represent directions which are necessary ones for group psychotherapy to explore. The changes which are represented by the Integralists may best be highlighted by first reviewing briefly the major tenets of the Intrapersonal and Interpersonal positions. The latter two will be presented here as a single unit.

The Positions of the
Intrapersonalist and Transactionalist

The analytic group therapist who seeks to base his treatment on the authoritative statements of Freud finds surprisingly little that is supporting. He may be encouraged by the fact that Freud believed that individual psychology was a derivative of the more fundamental group psychology: "We must conclude that the psychology of groups is the oldest human psychology, what we have isolated as individual psychology, by neglecting all traces of the group, has only since come into prominence out of the old group psychology, by a gradual process which may still, perhaps, be described as incomplete" (Freud, 1921). However, Freud's further observation that members of groups appear to show heightened suggestibility, mutual identification, and repression of aggression is far less encouraging to the analytic group therapist. Such effects might indeed be interpreted as evidence of inherent limitations of the group as a setting for analytic treatment, since analytic therapy abjures conformity and repression and seeks to promote insight, freedom, and conscious choice. Freud may also be interpreted as implying that the patient's wish to be accepted by members of his group and to be in harmony with them may produce an antitherapeutic pressure, for he stated, ". . . experience has shown that in cases of collaboration, libidinal ties are regularly formed between the fellow workers which prolong and solidify the relation between them to a point beyond what is merely profitable" (Freud, 1921).

The "new integration" for the Intrapersonalists appears to refer mainly to adaptation of psychoanalytic principles to the group rather than the integration of "group dynamic" principles to group psychotherapy. The reports based on investigations of small group dynamics have received a very cool reception from the Intrapersonalists, but have achieved more acceptance from Transactionalists. The usual objection is that the group phenomena described by the students of small groups are, at best, irrelevant for the therapy group and, at worst, antitherapeutic. Moreover, the dimensions which have been studied by the social scientists have been deemed to be superficial, for they have not dealt with the unconscious.

To facilitate presentation and comparison of the major positions taken by analytic group therapists, we shall pay particular attention to each school's conception of the role of the group in three phases of the therapeutic process: (1) stimulation of the patient's typical "pathology" and defenses; (2) enhancement of the patient's accessibility to new experience, and (3) introduction of specific procedures believed by the therapist to have the potential of effecting desired change.

It is generally recognized that in order for attitudes and behaviors to be changed in psychotherapy they must first be given expression in the treatment setting. The effectiveness of the patient's characteristic defenses must be thwarted. It is necessary, however, that therapy provide conditions under which the patient can tolerate the anxiety consequent to the frustration of his usual behaviors and defenses, without resorting to even stronger defensive behavior and without experiencing a disruptive dissolution of his defenses. The patient's accessibility to new experience in therapy requires a commitment to treatment which may be assisted initially by the patient's identification with the therapist. The patient must also have some confidence in the power of the therapeutic agent. Depending on the particular theoretical orientation of the therapist a variety of procedures, techniques, and aims will be introduced as the prerequisite procedures and norms of the group.

Stimulation

Wolf and Schwartz (1962) insist that they engage in formal psychoanalysis in the group setting and that the stimuli provided by the group facilitate the accomplishment of psychoanalytic aims. They believe that the usual analytic procedures are fully available in the group.

That the concepts underlying the procedures must undergo considerable revision does not dismay these writers. The distinction between transference and transference neurosis is lost. Free association is redefined so that it no longer refers to the uninterrupted free flow of associations of a single individual, but includes all content and interventions of members of the group during a specified time sequence. Similarly, association to dreams is not restricted to the dreamer, but may include the fantasies and thoughts of fellow group members who free associate to one another's dreams. Such free associations to another's dream are believed to provide additional material which may bear on the latent meaning of the dream. The associations of others are viewed as an extension of the associations of the dreamer, and in this sense the associative process is not interrupted.

Slavson, considerably less sanguine about the effectiveness of these modifications, concludes that patients suffering from massive psycho-neuroses, requiring the establishment of a transference neurosis as part of treatment, are poor candidates for analytic group psychotherapy (Slavson, 1964). Slavson reasons that the presence of individuals other than the therapist may diminish the intensity of the transference which can be established with any one person, even though the total "quantum" of affect may be multiplied many times, and that therefore the intensity of the therapy is reduced. As a consequence the group may not be conducive to deep regression and may hamper the emergence of fantasies.

The Transactional therapists are less concerned with establishing the pristine orthodoxy of analytic procedures, but utilize the group setting to further the analysis of observable interpersonal relationships and transactions. They share with the Intrapersonalists the view that the group offers a unique opportunity for stimulating relevant affects, thoughts, resistances, and defenses. This category of therapist includes the full range of neo-Freudian theorists and encompasses the vast majority of all analytically oriented group therapists.

Within the limits of such variables as composition, orientation, leadership, and the like, the group is viewed as providing a setting in which individuals are confronted with: (1) conflicting values of other members; (2) a wide range of life experiences; and (3) an intensified rivalry for the doctor's attention. All three factors stimulate the individuals to respond verbally and nonverbally with typical sensitivities, anxieties, defenses, and resistances. Members of the group may be provoked into expressing their agreement or disagreement with the ideas of others. The group provides an opportunity for the patient to become aware not only of his own reactions to others, but also of the reactions of others to him. In addition to recognizing such stimulating effects of groups, the Transactional theorists point out that all individuals by virtue of membership in the group must cope with the problems of (1) inclusion, (2) control, and (3) intimacy. Inclusion involves the patient's fear of being left out or not being accepted, but can also refer to his fear of becoming overly involved with the group. The patient must deal with the attractive and repellent features of the opportunity to control others and of the possibility of being controlled. He must also cope with the threat and the potential satisfactions of experiencing his own and others' personal emotional feelings, such as resentment, hostility, warmth, and sympathy (Schutz, 1958; Bennis and Shepard, 1956). These three concepts appear to be extensions of the group phenomena described by Bion (1959) as the Basic Assumptions of Dependency, Fight-Flight and Pairing.

The Transactional therapists may or may not speak directly in terms of transference, free association, regression, and projection, but the transition from the extreme psychoanalytic position to their own has been made much easier by virtue of the modifications of analytic theory accepted by even the most orthodox group therapist.

Accessibility

Stimulation of characteristic patterns of ego functioning and defenses would be of little value if the therapy setting did not provide conditions which permit the patient to utilize the new experiences. The patient's accessibility to therapeutic influence is initially attributed by all Intrapersonalists to his identification with the therapist. This is consistent with Freud's belief that the essence of group formation consists of the libidinal tie which the group member experiences with the leader. With the development of the group, fellow patients as well as the therapist provide multiple models and objects of identification. The behavior attitudes and values of others who are cathected may be imitated and ultimately internalized.

Among other therapeutic assets of the group cited by both categories of therapists is the fact that the self-esteem of members may be increased by the experience of mutual acceptance. The group also helps to reduce the patient's self-alienation, self-criticism, and self-depreciation by revealing that others have the same or similar problems and are victims of similar impulses and feelings (Frank, 1957b; Durkin, 1964).

While acknowledging the fact that positive transference to the therapist increases the patient's amenability to the treatment process,

Intrapersonal therapists believe that the therapist's enhanced power for influencing the patient is not to be utilized to persuade or directly to influence the patient to conform to or adopt certain standards or modes of conduct. Intrapersonal therapists place great emphasis on the principle that patient change should not be effected as a consequence of conformity either to the therapist or to fellow patients, but should be the result of the patient's increased freedom to exercise conscious control over those behaviors and feelings which had previously been out of his awareness.

One of the areas of disagreement between the Intrapersonalists and Interpersonalists is the role each assigns to the group phenomenon of cohesiveness for aiding the patient to become more accessible to therapeutic influence. The Intrapersonalists believe that cohesiveness implies both an antitherapeutic collusion of mutual good fellowship and a pressure to accept group norms which may be antagonistic to analytic psychotherapy. Although such theorists may admire the elegance of the research performed by social scientists in the area of cohesiveness, they question its relevance. The Transactionalists tend to interpret the term cohesiveness in a manner consistent with its usage by social scientists to refer to the degree of attractiveness which membership in a particular group has for its members (Cartwright and Zander, 1960; Borgatta, Bales, and Hare, 1955). Such attractiveness not only may be based on mutual liking, but also may evolve from the experience of considerable conflict and antagonism in the group (Frank, 1957a).

A further danger to the individual's autonomy, according to Intrapersonalists, is implicit in what Redl (1942) has called "group emotional contagion." This refers to the communication of emotional feelings from one individual to another even when the content or the cause of the group feeling is contrary to the individual's apparent intellectual convictions and standards. In effect, the group, by common consent or approval, reduces the ego and superego restraints of its members and therefore may make the patient more accessible to experiencing and expressing hostility and aggression. The motivation for such loss of self is further enhanced by the desire for social acceptance. From this point of view, the more an individual becomes a part of the group, the less he can retain his autonomy, his individuality, and his responsibility for self-determination. This view is not shared by Existentialists and Transactionalists such as Mullan and Rosenbaum (1962), who believe that the group represents a lifelike setting in which the patient can aim at becoming more and more "human" without concern as to whether he becomes more and more individualistic. They state further that they have not found the group process to be a conforming force, but rather an "impelling" force that exposes the person to his responsibility as a member of the human society. The definition and role of group dynamics in analytic group therapy, as performed by Intrapersonalists and Transactionalists, remain ambiguous and confused.

Mechanisms of Therapeutic Change

Intrapersonalists place great emphasis on the analysis of resistance and defenses by means of interpretation. While therapists of this school recognize the value of catharsis as "a way of purging one's self of noxious states of the psyche" (Slavson, 1964, p.142), the experience is not valued if it is unaccompanied by insight. This is in sharp contrast to the recent well-publicized formulations of Mowrer (1964), a nonanalytically oriented therapist, who believes that one of the principal values of the group is that it provides an opportunity for "confession" and atonement.

These therapists also believe that the group is particularly effective in analyzing resistances. Group members frequently make frontal assaults on other patients' resistances, and challenge such behaviors as silence, withdrawal, lateness, absence, monopoly, autism, or pseudo-relating. Some therapists believe that this role of the group in treatment derives from the fact that members are particularly sensitive to behavior in others which they tend to reject in themselves. In addition, it is acknowledged that group analysis of resistances represents the acceptance and implementation of therapeutic models and mores introduced by the therapist.

Intrapersonal theorists acknowledge the value of the group for testing reality, yet decry exclusive emphasis on this aspect. They do not believe that any technique which addresses itself predominantly to reality or the analysis of group tensions, or limits itself to the immediate here-and-now situation, can be viewed as effective analytic group psychotherapy. This belief is based on the assumption that neuroses are essentially autonomous and that effective therapy requires that the basic sources of neuroses be worked through by dealing with memories, early relationships, anxieties, and guilt. Intrapersonal therapists believe that efforts to effect changes in interpersonal relationships by means of interpersonal techniques alone can be successful only with those patients whose disturbances are of a surface nature. Since the intrapsychic conflict underlies the manifest interpersonal problem, it must be resolved. Treatment of the interpersonal or transactional relationships is secondary to this aim. Only after the expression and clarification of the dynamics underlying pathology can the patient benefit from confrontation with realistic alternatives in behavior. Following insight into conflicts the process of working through may be effected.

In contrast, the Transactional therapist concentrates on the immediate observable interaction of group members. Eliciting personal history material is neither consistently encouraged nor discouraged, but such material is sometimes effectively used to document and underscore a behavior pattern which has been highlighted in the immediate group situation. The reality-testing aspect of the group is emphasized. The group, in effect, provides a laboratory in which each member has an opportunity to learn how he affects others and how they stimulate him.

Depending on the therapist's orientation, the treatment may stress conscious awareness of one's behavior and feelings or emphasize the understanding of the motivation behind the behavior. The level of interpretation frequently aims at uncovering the immediate gains served by the patient's behavior in the group, rather than at attempting to identify his underlying conflicts or "basic motivations" (Berne, 1961).

Another approach to Transactionalist therapy is represented by Frank. He states that as the patient experiences successes due to his more effective way of handling his interpersonal and internal conflicts, his new ways of behaving are reinforced. As a consequence of such repeated experiences, the maladaptive patterns are extinguished and the successful interactions are strengthened. This theory of psychotherapy suggests that the dynamic of treatment is the self-reinforcement value of new behavior which more adequately deals with conflicts. He does not assume that such specific behavioral change is the end point of therapy, but hypothesizes that these changes will enable the patient to experience further emotional growth (Frank, 1961).

The Positions of the Integralists

Integralists hold the view that membership in a therapy group evokes shared unconscious or preconscious conflicts and motivations. The therapist, by attending to such shared group concerns, may effectively treat each patient in his group. This conception of the group as guided by common unconscious forces is consistent with Freud's observation that to the degree that a group lacks formal organization, its members are stimulated to display basic similarities in their unconscious drives. Such groups encourage members to throw off, albeit temporarily, the repressions which constrain the expression of their instinctual impulses (Freud, 1921).

In attempting to treat the group as a unit, the Integralists tend to ascribe to it characteristics of an individual. As a consequence, psychotherapy of the group concerns the analysis of interaction and transactions between the group as an entity and the therapist, or between the group and one of its members. Since the group is treated as if it were an individual, the familiar conflict and tension-reduction models of individual psychotherapy are applied to the group as a whole. Among the clinicians and theorists who attempt to treat the group as a unit, Bion (1959) is preeminent.

Bion's formulations are concerned primarily with the description and specification of the common motivational elements of all groups. In his efforts to develop a framework for describing and conceptualizing dimensions which organize the seemingly discrete behaviors of each of the patients, he has carefully avoided the imposition of psychoanalytic concepts. As a consequence, unlike such students of group psychotherapy as Mann (1955) and Semrad and Arsenian (1951), Bion does not utilize concepts like "group ego" or "group superego." Although Bion has applied his theories to the treatment of patients, the major focus of his interest and his writings is in the identification and description of group phenomena relevant to all groups. Bion is far more concerned with explicating group phenomena than with presenting any compelling evidence concerning the therapeutic consequences which follow the application of his theory or techniques of analytic group psychotherapy.

The implementation of Bion's views by clinicians was facilitated greatly by the work of Ezriel and of Sutherland, who in effect bridged the gap between Bion's group dynamics and the group therapist's views of the analytic group psychotherapy treatment process. Perhaps the fullest theoretical statement concerning the role of the group in the treatment process is that presented by Whitaker and Lieberman (1964). Although they were initially greatly influenced by the thinking of both Bion and Ezriel, Whitaker and Lieberman have developed an original and effective theoretical position which integrates their own clinical and research experience with groups.

Bion's work answers the serious objection which group therapists have long expressed regarding the work of "group dynamicists"—namely, their failure to deal with psychotherapy groups or to represent group phenomena in terns of unconscious motivational states. Despite this, Bion's work has not been widely accepted by clinicians in the United States. Perhaps one of the factors which has acted to dampen the enthusiasm in this country is Bion's use of Kleinian rather than Freudian concepts to expound his theory. In addition, the sociological notion that groups are organized around a shared task—rather than by libidinal ties to a central person as postulated by Freud and amplified by Redl (1942)—is not accepted as tolerantly in the United States as it is in England.

The popular belief that group psychotherapy requires an integration of group processes with individual psychodynamics in their genetic complexity is not shared by Bion or his closest followers. They believe instead that group psychotherapy is best focused on the group processes per se, since these will more effectively reveal the pertinent aspects of the individual. Bion does not accept the distinction between individual and group dynamics and rejects the position that "group psychology" comes into being only when a number of people are collected together in one place at one time. He believes that group phenomena exist in individuals, since no individual, however isolated in time and space, can be regarded as outside of a group or lacking in active manifestations of group psychology. "The apparent difference between group psychology and individual psychology is an illusion produced by the fact that the group brings into prominence phenomena that appear alien to the observer unaccustomed to using the group" (Bion, 1959, p.169).

Stimulation

The Integralists who have been influenced by Bion assume that a primary source of stimulation inheres in the fact that therapy groups, like individuals, are motivated not only by manifest overt aims, but also by latent covert purposes which may conflict with the accomplishment of the overt purposes. Such covert motivations appear to be shared unwittingly by the group membership. Bion, in contrast to other Integralists, postulates but does not emphasize or utilize in his theory individual predispositions to behave in idiosyncratic fashion; instead Bion attempts only to describe characteristic group phenomena. On the basis of his observations, Bion concluded that each group appears to behave as if it were in fact two groups—or, more precisely, as if it had developed two quite different cultures. The aims of the covert culture, although apparently inconsistent with the stated purposes of the group, might coincide, on occasion, with the primary task. The two cultures are identified as the work group and the basic assumption (Ba) group. The term "work group" is used to describe the facet of a group's functioning that seems to be purposeful and effective in achieving the primary task. Members cooperate with one another in formulating and implementing a program for realistically achieving the group's aims. Participation in such a group requires effort and utilization of relevant experiences and learned skills.

The Ba group appears to be less reality-oriented, seeks instantaneous satisfaction, and is characterized by the impulsive expression of uncritical fantasy. Participation in such a group requires no special training, skills, or self-conscious effort. Such group behavior may be understood as a reflection of a shared, unverbalized, yet tacitly accepted assumption which motivates the group. Bion has identified three such assumptions or emotional states, all three of which are oriented around the issue of leadership. Leadership is a salient issue in Bion's groups and in all other Integralist groups since the therapist usually appears to the patients to have abdicated his leadership role. This leaves the group members to deal with an apparent leadership vacuum.

Bion's three basic assumptions are dependency, fight-flight, and pairing. Bion insists that his descriptions of the motivations underlying each Ba group are to be taken quite literally rather than metaphorically. The dependency group behaves as if the group's purpose is to obtain protection, comfort, and nurturance from a leader whom it has endowed with godlike qualities of wisdom, knowledge and power. The group members act stupidly and helplessly, as if to underscore their desperate need for an omniscient and omnipotent leader. In the group treatment setting the group turns first to the therapist for such assistance. The leader cannot fulfill this assignment, and, in the view of Bion, should not attempt to undertake it. As a consequence the group's wish for a dependency leader will be frustrated. When the group has exhausted its repertoire of techniques for inducing the leader to fill its dependency needs, it will attempt to seek out an alternate leader from among the membership. He, too, will inevitably fail to live up to the group's expectations. When the emotional state of dependency prevails, the group experiences a sense of closeness and "groupiness" which it attempts to maintain.

With regard to the second basic assumption, fight-flight, the group acts as if its aim is to preserve itself. It seems to see its alternatives as either attack or flight from someone or something. Unlike the Ba dependency group, the fight-flight group appears relatively unconcerned with the welfare of the individual and shows little if any tolerance for "sickness." Such groups appear to be pointedly unconcerned with self-study or rational thought. They are preoccupied with action. The group seeks out a leader who can mobilize it for attack or for flight. Candidates for leadership who do not lead in these directions are disavowed or ignored.

The third Ba group, which uses the assumption of pairing, behaves as if its purpose is to produce a new leader and savior. The relationship between members, regardless of sex, is treated with an air of hopeful expectation that this "sexual" union will produce a new leader or a new concept which will bring about the desired ideal state. When this Ba is operative, the group does not actively seek a leader but appears to wait for one to emerge. The group is characterized by optimism, but Bion emphasizes that the state of hopeful anticipation can be sustained only as long as the group does not in fact produce either a leader or an idea. Reality, apparently, cannot sustain imagination's promises.

Bion's concept of valency suggests that the very fact that some members move into a basic assumption attitude might be sufficient to induce other members to follow. However, Bion is also careful to note, as are his followers, that although the individual may experience a strong inclination to merge with the group, he sharply confronts his counterwish to maintain his own individuality. Part of the anxiety which group members experience in a relatively unstructured group is attributable to their conflict regarding being drawn into a Ba culture. The patient experiences an intensification of emotions, which are associated with his unconscious anxiety that the basic assumptions will become dominant and his intellectual capacity will be reduced. The individual is impelled to seek satisfaction of his needs in the group "by total submergence in the group," yet is simultaneously inhibited by the fears that such activity will sacrifice his sense of "individual independence."

A second source of conflict inheres in the clash between the individual's need to maintain his view of the group as a source of security and his recognition that the group also produces anxiety and frustrations within him. To reconcile the apparent discrepancy between the "good" and the "bad" groups, the group member may, according to Bion, invoke massive denial and projection. The members may split off the negative aspects of the group. The source of frustration may be attributed not to the group but to members, the therapist, subgroups, or events and individuals outside of the group. Projection permits group members to identify rejected aspects of themselves in other individuals. Members may also split off their own competence and invest it in another, such as a leader.

A third source of conflict, which acts to stimulate group members to manifest their predispositions, distortions, and defenses, derives from the hypothesized opposition between the cognitive and affective states represented by the two major group cultures: work and basic assumptions. These two group states appear to be expressions of the conflict represented in an individual patient between his conscious wish to learn about the source of his personal difficulties and to alter his behavior, and his preconscious and unconscious resistances against any such efforts which threaten to heighten anxiety. The work group is concerned with reality, exposing inappropriate ego-functioning and attempting to uncover the source of such disturbances. The Ba represents an attempt to escape from reality into group-shared assumptions and regressive affective states.

Whitaker and Lieberman, with some modifications, subscribe to Ezriel's view that each patient, on entering the group, projects his own unconscious fantasy-objects onto other group members as he attempts to manipulate the group members into assuming assigned roles. In effect, each member attempts to influence the group in order to make it correspond to his fantasy group. To the degree that the individual's internalized objects do not coincide with reality, or the assigned roles are not accepted by members of the group, the underlying unconscious dynamics of the patient are stimulated and his particular defense mechanisms for coping with such tensions are manifested. Although each individual plays a "private game," the impact of these separate acts on each other provides the basis of common group tensions which reflect the unconscious fantasies of all of the group members. The unconscious group tension produces interactions which are aimed at resolving or diminishing some aspect of the individual's unconscious tension. The group thus stimulates each member to adopt a particular role which corresponds to his own way of defending himself against unconscious fears. The intrapersonal conflicts or relations with internalized objects express themselves in interpersonal relations as the internalized objects are projected onto group members.

Whitaker and Lieberman accept Bion's and Ezriel's view that the wishes and fears of group members evolve into a group-shared unconscious conflict. Increasingly direct analysis of the nature of the impulses and of the defenses against their expression is facilitated by "enabling solutions" achieved by the group. The contrary is true of groups that have a history of accepting defensive or restrictive solutions. An enabling solution is one that is directed at alleviating fears and at the same time allows for some expression of the disturbing motive; a restrictive solution aims primarily at alleviating fears, and does so at the expense of satisfying or expressing the disturbing motive. Whitaker and Lieberman identify group themes as a sense of focal conflicts centered around a single disturbing motive. These themes are reminiscent of Bion's basic assumptions in that they are described as dealing with sex, aggression, and dependency. Whitaker and Lieberman also use the term "group culture" in a manner analogous to the way in which Bion uses it, but they refine it. They define culture as the collective effect of group-accepted solutions (whether enabling or restrictive) on group focal conflicts. Group culture concerns the character of the relationship among patients and between patients and therapists, the freedom with which affect is expressed, the acceptability to patients of a wide range of content, and so forth.

Foulkes and Anthony (1957) represent yet another approach to the group as a unit. Although they share the view of the other Integralists that the group responds to the unconscious needs and motivations of the individual members, they believe that this kind of response develops slowly, rather than precipitously and spontaneously. The sharing of unconscious motivations, according to Foulkes, occurs only in the advanced stages of group formation. Anthony does not accept the fact that group members may appear to be dependent on the therapist during the early phases of the group as evidence of shared unconscious group motivation. He believes instead that such leader-centered activity occurs during the phase when the group members are acting more like a collection of individuals than a group. If groups are permitted to remain at this level of development, then, according to Anthony, the relevant group phenomena will not be manifested (1966). It is for this reason, he believes, that many group therapists are unaware of the unique potential of the group therapy setting and persist in dealing with individuals. The evidence accepted by Anthony that the group is guided by the members' sensitivity to or understanding of one another's needs is somewhat different from that proposed by the previously mentioned Integralists. He believes that the shared group unconscious is demonstrated principally in the fact that some patient behavior and needs appear to represent the complement or the supplement of the behavior and needs of other patients. Thus, dominance of one is supported by the submissiveness of the other, activity in some is enhanced by the passivity of others, and so forth (Anthony, 1966).

The development of this alleged unconscious symbiotic relationship is facilitated by confrontation, growing imitation, and identification.

Accessibility

The Integralists have added very little to the material presented by the Intrapersonalists and Interpersonalists regarding the conditions which make the individual more accessible to change. The circumstances which enable patients to tolerate their anxieties and permit them to respond with reduced defensiveness are not adequately developed by the Integralists. It may be inferred that membership in the basic assumption groups provides cohesiveness and a sense of belonging which facilitates the patients' accessibility as described previously. However, although these feelings of closeness may provide support for the patients, they may also strengthen resistances. The major therapeutic benefit, according to Bion, lies not in such cohesiveness, but in the conscious experiencing of a high order of work group activity—that is, learning to cooperate in a work group.

Mechanisms of Change

The principal technique for effecting change, according to Bion, is the therapist's confrontation of the group with the basic assumption it appears to have accepted. The therapist in effect interprets the group's transference toward him and toward others in the group. Interpretations are made primarily by the therapist. They are used when the therapist is reasonably clear about the group's attitude toward him or toward a patient. Interpretations are also made when a patient acts as if he believed the group had a definite and specific attitude toward him. The focus of interpretations is on the here-and-now, highlighting group-shared behavior concerning the issue of securing leadership that will provide fulfillment of primitive wishes.

A serious limitation of Bion's presentation of his theories, to date, is his incomplete account of therapeutic movement. This aspect of the theory has been dealt with more fully by Ezriel and Whitaker and Lieberman. These writers view the therapist's role as principally that of influencing the processes whereby group solutions may be established, maintained, or modified.

They believe that the occurrence of a given group conflict may permit the achievement of more useful solutions provided that the culture of the group has shifted appropriately. This view of group-functioning represents a considerable deviation from Bion's, since he believes that the same Ba issue, no matter how often repeated, leads to inevitable frustration unless the therapist's interpretations are accepted.

An assumption underlying their view of the treatment process, based on the thinking of the psychoanalyst French, is that the group focal conflict is a derivative of each individual's nuclear conflict (1952). Although they accept Bion's conviction that attention to the shared group conflicts will usefully influence the individual, they believe it is appropriate to deal also with the individual psychodynamics and with observed interpersonal relationships.

Among the Integralists we include Foulkes, who represents an approach to groups derived from Freudian theory. The mechanisms of change stressed by Foulkes concern the interpretation of the group's contributions as equivalents of free association. When all conversations in the group are presumed to be equivalent to free associations in their unconscious aspects, interpretations of such group free associations are believed to give access to the repressed unconscious of the members. The interpretations are aimed at enlarging the group's area of awareness by bringing unconscious components into consciousness.

Although Foulkes recognizes that group therapy can be used to communicate insights regarding unconscious problems of each individual, he is diffident about assuming this as the relevant mechanism for analytic group psychotherapy. He insists that interpretations are to be group-oriented and hypothesizes that even interpretations addressed specifically to an individual may be interpreted as directed toward the group, since, like any other communication, interpretations are of a multidimensional and multipersonal consequence. Thus, Foulkes sees interpretations directed to the individual as relating also to the group, while Bion sees interpretations directed to the group as relating to the individual.

Foulkes and Anthony believe that analytic group therapy does not compete with psychoanalysis in the area of analysis of transference neurosis: "It is not that group-analysis does less; it does something different . . ." (Foulkes and Anthony, 1957, p.22). Foulkes places emphasis on the analysis of transference in the sense of distortions. Like most group therapists he is concerned with the relationship between the therapist and the patient in the present rather than with uncovering the psychogenesis of illness. Anthony appears to have moved toward a model approaching that of "discrimination-learning." He suggests that an essential dynamic of therapeutic value may derive from the fact that the individual in the group is confronted with the discrepancy between his expectations regarding the group behavior or the leader's behavior and his actual experience with the group and the leader. From such a discrepancy the patient may learn that his expectations are inappropriate and that other more relevant attitudes and behaviors can be utilized (Anthony, 1966).

Discussion and Conclusions

Integralists appear to have extended the Intrapersonalists' and Interpersonalists' observation that the verbal and nonverbal participation of group members may be interpreted as free associations around a common theme, conflict and basic motivation. The Integralists believe that the contributions of the group members deal not only with the analysis of the idiosyncratic conflicts of the individual, as believed by the Intrapersonalists and Interpersonalists, but with the shared conflicts. The value of the group is based on the assumption that the group shares the same conflicts and irrational aims and can, therefore, be treated as a unit rather than as a set of individuals. Interpretations and confrontations with reality are believed to be effective for each member to the degree that he participates in the group-stimulated and -shared problem. The Integralist places more emphasis on the immediate conditions which stimulate and maintain the conflicts than on their genetic origins for each individual.

It is clear that the therapist who attempts to deal with the individual patient has no shortage of stimuli to occupy him in his treatment efforts. When the therapist is confronted with a number of patients in a group, the stimuli that are presented to him are multiplied not arithmetically but geometrically by reason of the multiplicity of interactions. As a consequence, the group therapist has a great need to adopt a simplifying principle that will permit him to treat the patients with economy of effort and no loss of effectiveness. That the solution is simply the recognition that a group of diverse individuals represent a composite "single patient" is, at the very least, one of the most fortunate therapeutic coincidences yet discovered. The need for such a solution has been more adequately demonstrated than has the effectiveness of the solution.

Integralists other than Bion do not appear to assume that all group behaviors reflect shared conflicts, but believe that it is more useful to deal only with those aspects of group behavior which can convincingly be interpreted as shared. A problem which is shared by all group-oriented therapists is that of deciding when they have identified a common unconscious group tension. The process is essentially a deductive one based on the behavior of each individual. There is the "clear and present danger" that the greater the therapist's conviction regarding the nature of the conflicts which may be found in the group, the less evidence he requires for confirmation of his expectations. It is therefore possible that the behavior of an individual may be interpreted as evidence for a group conflict or of a "basic assumption."

One of the more dubious conventions adopted by Bion and other Integralists is that silence and nonparticipation of group members may be interpreted as agreement and consent to the group activity. As a consequence two people who are interacting in an otherwise silent group provide the therapist with the basis for an interpretation of a group-shared conflict. The silent members, by not actively opposing or commenting on the activity, share responsibility for it. The danger of generalizing to the group from the behavior of one or even a few group members is somewhat reduced, however, by the procedure introduced by Ezriel. He requires that group interpretations be documented by explicit reference to the individual ways in which patients respond to the group shared conflict.

A related problem is that the Integralist, by offering interpretations of presumably unconscious group-shared phenomena, is by definition the only uninvolved member of the group. He is, therefore, the only one capable of making and judging the accuracy of the interpretation. This is a problem which is not unfamiliar to the individual treatment setting. One of the frequently cited advantages of the group therapy treatment form is that the group provides the opportunity for a more objective analysis of transference and countertransference. Among Intrapersonalists and Transactionalists, particularly the latter, it is assumed that patients and therapist all share the opportunity to observe and to evaluate the interpersonal interactions and transactions of others in the group. A consensus thus achieved regarding the behavior and the "meaning" of such behavior carries considerable weight. The likelihood that a therapist's countertransference would go undetected is lessened in Transactional groups.

It must also be recognized that the group-therapy setting provides a uniquely powerful social influence situation. It combines the conditions of ambiguity of treatment process, authority of the therapist, and the suggestibility of patients. The group rarely is able to achieve complete agreement on any issue, even on the rejection of an interpretation offered to the group as an entity. One of the important pressures operating to produce acceptance of a group interpretation is the fact that the group presents a seemingly diffuse set of data and stimulation; the interpretation offers to bring order out of this chaos. This is a very attractive offer. However, when a member seems to offer documentation of an interpretation (post hoc), it must be remembered that this "confirmation" can also be a function of suggestion.

The theoretical advances in analytic group psychotherapy represented by the Integralists appear to be: (1) the formulation by Bion that the seemingly divergent and individualistic concerns of the group members represent a fairly narrow range of shared issues; (2) the modification by Ezriel and Whitaker and Lieberman that behavior of the group (like that of the individual) may be conceptualized as centering around motivational conflicts and their attempted resolutions; and (3) the idea that group-centered interpretations of shared unconscious and preconscious motivations can be made with no loss of power and with considerable gain in efficiency. What now remains is the demonstration that this theoretical "advance" has been accompanied by therapeutic advance.

Although Integralists have relatively little to add to what Intrapersonalists and Interpersonalists have previously stated regarding the utility of the group in facilitating the patient's accessibility to new experience, Bion's descriptions of group phenomena which he regularly encounters raise some serious questions. Most theorists believe that the treatment situation must develop and maintain an optimal level of anxiety in patients. The extremes of panic or apathy are to be avoided as they are not conducive to the development of either curiosity or insight about one's self. The Ba groups are described, however, as evoking a high degree of anxiety, sufficient in some cases to precipitate a psychotic-like regression. It is not clear, therefore, why such states are considered as conducive to analytic work. According to Bion's own descriptions of the Ba groups, the patients in such affective states become less accessible to verbal communications and to rational thought and, indeed, may actively resist any efforts at rational thought.

Bion's unique emphasis on maintaining all therapist interventions at the group level rather than the individual has been tempered by his followers to a point which may be more acceptable to Intrapersonalists and Interpersonalists. The problem remains, however, whether interpretations of generalized motivations and conflicts can be effective in producing individual change independent of explicit efforts to specify their unique relevance to each member of the group. We do not quarrel with the view that the concepts of pairing (sex), fight-flight (aggression), and dependency may adequately classify the motivational states of patients in a group. Psychoanalysts have long contented themselves with only the concepts of sex and aggression, and the addition of dependency may be useful. The problem, however, lies in the implication that these three concepts adequately represent the basic dynamics of groups.

Bion has in effect undertaken to describe characteristic group processes which are independent of group composition, stated goals, size, leadership, etc. This approach to groups appears to be analogous to that of the "trait" theorist and suffers from all the limitations that have been experienced by such personality theorists.

The value of group dynamics for the advancement of the field must lie in the further specification of the variables which influence the development of such group phenomena. One of the least developed aspects of the theory is the description of the conditions which permit the individual and the group to move from one group culture to another or from one basic assumption to another. The concept of valency and the assumption that exposure to reality has a compelling effect have no more explanatory power than coincidence or a deus ex machina. What is lacking is a detailed theory regarding therapeutic change.

The three types of therapists appear to encompass two distinct, yet quite familiar, traditional approaches to the conception of mental health and well-being. The Intrapersonalists and Interpersonalists believe that mental health is represented by man's expression of his unique individuality and by his ability to free himself from the constraints of his environment, the group, the culture, and the like. The Integralists take the diametrically opposed position that man's well-being depends on his full participation and integration in the group, the culture, and society. An additional, overlapping view is represented by Existentialists, who are concerned with preserving and enhancing man's ineffable humanness and are less concerned with the aims of individuality or "finding oneself by losing oneself" in the group.

At the present state of the art of psychotherapy, the practitioner's use of what may be therapeutic is based more on the congeniality of the philosophy he adopts than the empirical evidence of its therapeutic consequences. It may be dreary and possibly mischievous to recapitulate the now familiar exhortation that the field cannot resolve its theoretical differences until it undertakes to specify what it will accept as evidence of meaningful outcome. Such a complaint is frequently interpreted as an invitation to specify the aims of therapy, which becomes yet another exercise in rhetoric without referent and grammar without syntax. The fact remains that the therapist cannot defer treatment pending receipt of the ultimate answers from the ultimate researcher.

Group therapy's widespread popularity is further evidence of the therapist's courage, which permits him to "bash on regardless." After some thirty years of claiming success, group therapists find themselves in the rather anomalous position of only now becoming preoccupied with understanding in what ways—if any—the group contributes to the therapeutic process. The need to cope with the multiplicity and complexity of group phenomena requires that the therapist adopt some simplifying principles. Some have found it convenient to maintain their gaze fixedly on the individual; others, on the interaction, the transactional unit, or, more recently, the group as an entity. To treat the group as a unit requires the assumption either that the group members share, albeit unconsciously, the same motivations or that the leader will deal only with those issues which can be identified as shared, and will ignore all others. In the face of complexity, the clinician, like the scientist, tends to invoke Occam's razor, but in group therapy, as in any other enterprise, the principle of adopting the most parsimonious explanation may not lead to clarity but only to simplicity.

In our view, the fundamental task for group therapists and individual therapists alike is increased understanding of the treatment process as it relates to the particular patients and particular problems that are to be treated. The premise has direct implications for the therapist's growing interest in group dynamics and group processes, which is based on the seemingly plausible assumption that students of small groups have accumulated information that, if made available to the group therapist, would make treatment in the group setting more effective. The group therapist who immerses himself in the vast literature of group dynamics may be rewarded by recognizing phenomena and principles which can be utilized to facilitate the therapeutic process. The probability of making such discoveries would be significantly enhanced, however, if the therapist's approach to the literature and to his social science colleagues were more focused. The question is not simply what has the researcher learned about groups, but rather what has the researcher learned about groups that would facilitate the achievement of specific events that the therapist believes appropriate and necessary for treatment. The therapist must be quite explicit regarding his hypotheses, not only about the ultimate aims of therapy, but also about the mediating goals—that is, the clinician's assumptions about the steps and stages which must be achieved if treatment is to be effective.

The group therapist, like all therapists, is interested in advances in basic research; however, he cannot expect that the researcher, by sheer serendipity, will stumble on principles which will make the therapist's job easier. The therapist must himself be in a position to recognize and to utilize such basic contributions. Such recognition depends on the "prepared" mind.

The fundamental problem which confronts the group psychotherapist is not the process of group psychotherapy, but the process of any and all psychotherapy. The aim of the psychotherapist, independent of the setting, remains the same—namely, to increase the patient's social effectiveness and personal comfort. When a general theory of change is achieved, it will be necessary only to devise adaptations of the general theory to the group setting. The special conditions to be developed or the unique attributes which inhere in a particular setting could then be identified. This step is contingent on the development of clear criteria of therapeutic change. It is unlikely that we shall recognize answers if we do not recognize the questions.

Note: I am deeply grateful to Mr. Barry Wolfe and to Drs. Merton Gill, David Shakow, Margaret Rioch, and Pierre Turquet for their generous assistance in the preparation of this chapter. They do not, however, assume any responsibility for the accuracy of the reporting, nor may it be assumed that they share the author's formulations and interpretations.

References

Ackerman, N. W. "Symptom, Defense and Growth in Group Process." *International Journal of Group Psychotherapy, 2* (1961), 131–142.

Anthony, E. J. "The Generic Elements in Dyadic and in Group Psychotherapy." Presented at the American Group Psychotherapy Association Meeting, January 28, 1966.

Asch, S. E. *Social Psychology.* New York: Prentice-Hall, 1952.

Bach, G. *Intensive Group Psychotherapy.* New York: Ronald Press, 1954.

Bennis, W. G., and Shepard, H. A. "A Theory of Group Development." *Human Relations, 9* (1956), 415–437

Berger, M. "An Overview of Group Psychotherapy: Its Past, Present, and Future Development." *International Journal of Group Psychotherapy, 12,* No. 3 (1962), 287–294

Berne, E. "'Psychoanalytic' versus 'Dynamic' Group Therapy." *International Journal of Group Psychotherapy, 10* (1960), 98–103.

Berne, E. *Transactional Analysis in Psychotherapy.* New York: Grove Press, 1961.

Berne, E. *Principles of Group Treatment.* New York: Oxford University Press, 1966.

Bion, W. R. *Experiences in Groups.* New York: Basic Books, 1959.

Borgatta, E. F., Bales, R. F., and Hare, A. P. *Small Groups*. New York: Knopf, 1955.
Cartwright, D., and Zander, A. (eds.) . *Group Dynamics: Research and Theory*, 2nd ed.; Evanston, Ill.: Row, Peterson, 1960.
Crutchfield, R. S. "Personal and Situational Factors in Conformity to Group Pressure." *Acta Psychologica et Pharmacologica Neerlandica (Amsterdam)*, 15 (1959), 386–388
Cushing, J. G. N. "Report of the Committee on the Evaluation of Psychoanalytic Therapy." *Bulletin of the American Psychoanalytic Association*, 8 (1950), 44–50.
Durkin, Helen E. "Toward a Common Basis for Group Dynamics." *International Journal of Group Psychotherapy*, 1 (1957), 115–130.
Durkin, Helen E. *The Group in Depth*. New York: International Universities Press, 1964.
Ezriel, H. "A Psychoanalytic Approach to Group Treatment." *British Journal of Medical Psychology*, 23 (1950), 59–74.
Ezriel, H. "Notes on Psychoanalytic Group Therapy. II. Interpretation and Research ." *Psychiatry*, 15 (1952), 119–126.
Ezriel, H. "Experimentation within the Psychoanalytic Session." *British Journal of Philosophical Sciences*, 7 (1956), 29–48.
Ezriel, H. "The Role of Transference in Psychoanalytic and Other Approaches to Group Treatment." *Acta Psychotherapeutica*, 7 (1959), 101–116.
Foulkes, S. H. *Introduction to Group-Analytic Psychotherapy*. London: Heinemann, 1948.
Foulkes, S. H. "Group Analytic Dynamics with Specific Reference to Psychoanalytic Concepts." *International Journal of Group Psychotherapy*, 7 (1957), 40–52.
Foulkes, S. H. "Group Process and the Individual in the Therapeutic Group." *British Journal of Medical Psychology*, 34 (1961), 23–31.
Foulkes, S. H. *Therapeutic Group Analysis*. New York: International Universities Press, 1964.
Foulkes, S. H., and Anthony, E. J. *Group Psychotherapy: The Psychoanalytic Approach*. Baltimore: Penguin, 1957.
Frank, J. D. "Some Aspects of Cohesiveness and Conflict in Psychiatric Out-patient Groups." *Bulletin of the Johns Hopkins Hospital*, 101 (1957), 224–231.(a)
Frank, J. D. "Some Determinants, Manifestations, and Effects of Cohesiveness in Therapy Groups." *International Journal of Group Psychotherapy*, 7 (1957), 53–63. (b)
Frank, J. D. "Therapy in a Group Setting." In M. I. Stein (ed.), *Contemporary Psychotherapies*. New York: The Free Press of Glencoe, 1961. Pp. 42–59.
French, T. M. *The Integration of Behavior*. Chicago: University of Chicago Press, 1952. Vols. I, II.
Freud, S. "On the History of the Psycho-analytic Movement" (1914). *The Standard Edition of the Complete Psychological Works of...*. London: Hogarth Press. Vol. 14, pp. 7–66. (Also in *Collected Papers of...*. New York: Basic Books, 1959. Vol 1 , pp. 287–359.)
Freud, S. "Group Psychology and the Analysis of the Ego" (1921) . *The Standard Edition of the Complete Psychological Works of...*. London: Hogarth Press. Vol. 18, pp. 69–143.
Freud, S. "An Outline of Psychoanalysis" (1938). *The Standard Edition of the Complete Psychological Works of...*. London: Hogarth Press. Vol. 23.
Fromm-Reichmann, Frieda. *Principles of Intensive Psychotherapy*. Chicago: University of Chicago Press, 1950.

Gill, M. M. "Ego Psychology and Psychotherapy." *Psychoanalytic Quarterly, 20* (1951), 62–71 .

Gill, M. M. "Psychoanalysis and Exploratory Psychotherapy." *Journal of the American Psychoanalytic Association, 2* (1954), 771–797.

Harvey, O. J, and Consalvi, C. "Status and Conformity to Pressures in Informal Groups." *Journal of Abnormal Social Psychology, 60,* No. 2 (1960), 182–187.

Hill, W. F. "Therapeutic Mechanisms." In W. F. Hill (ed.), *Collected Papers on Group Psychotherapy.* Provo: Utah State Hospital, 1961.

Illing, H. A. "On the Present Trends in Group Psychotherapy." *Human Relations, 10* (1957), 77–84.

Kelman, H. C. "The Role of the Group in the Induction of Therapeutic Change." *International Journal of Group Psychotherapy, 13,* No. 4 (1963), 399–432.

Kubie, L. S. "Some Theoretical Concepts Underlying the Relationship between Individual and Group Therapy." *International Journal of Group Psychotherapy, 8* (1958), 3–19.

Lewin, K. "Frontiers in Group Dynamics: Concept, Method, and Reality in Social Sciences: Social Equilibria and Social Change." *Human Relations, 1* (1947), 5–41.

Lewin, K. *Field Theory in Social Science.* New York: Harper, 1951.

Locke, N. *Group Psychoanalysis: Theory and Technique.* New York: New York University Press, 1961.

Locke, N. "Group Psychotherapy, Group Psychoanalysis, and Scientific Method." In J. L. Moreno (ed.), *The International Handbook of Group Psychotherapy.* New York: Philosophical Library, 1966. Pp. 294–298.

Mann, J. "Some Theoretic Concepts of the Group Process." *International Journal of Group Psychotherapy, 5* (1955), 235–241.

Moreno, J. L. "The Group Psychotherapy Movement, Past, Present and Future." *International Journal of Group Psychotherapy, 15,* No. 1 (1962), 21–23.

Mowrer, O. H. *The New Group Therapy.* Princeton, N. J.: Van Nostrand, 1964.

Mullan, H., and Rosenbaum, M. *Group Psychotherapy.* New York: The Free Press of Glencoe, 1962.

Osborn, A. F. *Applied Imagination.* New York: Scribner's, 1953.

Parloff, M. B. "Group Dynamics and Group Psychotherapy: The State of the Union." *International Journal of Group Psychotherapy, 13* (1963), 393–398.

Parnes, S. J., and Meadows, A. "Effects of Brainstorming Instructions on Creative Problem-solving by Trained and Untrained Subjects." *Journal of Educational Psychology, 50* (1959), 171–176.

Redl, F. "Group Emotion and Leadership." *Psychiatry, 5* (1942), 573–596.

Scheidlinger, S. *Psychoanalysis and Group Behavior.* New York: Norton, 1952.

Scheidlinger, S. "Group Process in Group Psychotherapy. Part I." *American Journal of Psychotherapy, 14* (1960), 104–120. (a)

Scheidlinger, S. "Group Process in Group Psychotherapy. Part II." *American Journal of Psychotherapy, 14* (1960), 346–363. (b)

Schutz, W. C. *FIRO: A Three Dimensional Theory of Interpersonal Behavior.* New York: Rinehart, 1958.

Schwartz, E. K., and Wolf, A. "Psychoanalysis in Groups: The Mystique of Group Dynamics." In *Topical Problems of Psychotherapy.* New York: Karger, 1960. Vol. 2, pp. 119–154.

Semrad, E., and Arsenian, J. "The Use of Group Process Group Dynamics." *American Journal of Psychiatry*, *108* (1951), 358–363.

Sherif, M. "A Study of Some Special Factors in Perception." *Archives of Psychology*, No. 187 (1935).

Slavson, S. R. *Analytic Group Psychotherapy*. New York: Columbia University Press, 1952.

Slavson, S. R. "A Critique of the Group Therapy Literature." *Acta Psychotherapeutica*, *10* (1962), 62–73.

Slavson, S. R. *A Textbook in Analytic Group Psychotherapy*. New York: International Universities Press, 1964.

Stock, Dorothy, and Thelen, H. A. *Emotional Dynamics and Group Culture*. New York: International Universities Press, 1958.

Stock, Dorothy, and Lieberman, M. A. "Methodological Issues in the Assessment of Total Group Phenomena in Group Therapy." *International Journal of Group Psychotherapy*, *12*, No. 3 (1962), 312–325.

Sutherland, J. D. "Notes on Psychoanalytic Group Psychotherapy." *Psychiatry*, *15* (1952), 111–117.

Trist, E. L., and Sofer, C. *Explorations in Group Relations*. Leicester, Eng.: Leicester University Press, 1959.

Wassell, B. B. *Group Psychoanalysis*. New York: Philosophical Library, 1959.

Whitaker, D. S., and Lieberman, M. A. *Psychotherapy Through the Group Process*. New York: Atherton Press, 1964. P. 305.

Whitman, R. M., and Stock, Dorothy "The Group Focal Conflict". *Psychiatry*, *21*, No. 3 (1958), 269–276.

Wolf, A., and Schwartz, E. K. *Psychoanalysis in Groups*. New York: Grune & Stratton, 1962.

Ziferstein, I., and Grotjahn, M. "Psychoanalysis and Group Psychotherapy." In Frieda Fromm-Reichmann and J. L. Moreno (eds.), *Progress in Psychotherapy*. New York: Grune & Stratton, 1956. VoL 1, pp. 248–255.

Group Relations:
Rationale and Technique

MARGARET J. RIOCH, PH. D.

Dr. Rioch is currently Professor Emeritus, The American University, Washington, DC, where she has been a highly esteemed teacher and supervisor. She was Chairman of the Group Relations Conference Committee of the Washington School of Psychiatry in Washington, DC, when this paper was written. Rioch has been a major contributor to Group Relations training in the USA and has written a definitive paper on the concepts of Bion (Rioch MJ: The work of Wilfred Bion. Psychiatry 33:56–66, 1970).

This paper was chosen because it describes the origins and basic principles of Group Relations, or Tavistock, training experiences. These have continued to flourish in the USA under the sponsorship of the AK Rice Institute. This format extends the group-as-a-whole approach to its extreme. Issues related to authority and responsibility are primary, and the supportive or containing use of the group environment is purposefully avoided. As the author points out, this can be a stressful experience, and is designed as a method to understand group dynamics. Its direct translation into therapy groups is not recommended.

This paper is directly related to the others in this book concerned with group dynamics, namely, those by Bion and Rickman, Lewin, Durkin, Ezriel, Foulkes, and Stock, Whitman, and Lieberman. —Editor

Rioch MJ: Group relations: rationale and technique. *International Journal of Group Psychotherapy* 20:340–355, 1970.

In June 1965, The Washington School of Psychiatry, the Yale University Department of Psychiatry, and the Centre for Applied Social Research of the Tavistock Institute of London held their first Group Relations Conference in the United States at Mount Holyoke College. With this event began the transplantation of educational methods that had developed within the Tavistock Institute of Human Relations of London to American soil.

These methods of Group Relations Training go back to a two-week residential conference organized by the Tavistock Institute and the University of Leicester in September 1957, which has been described by Trist and Sofer (1959). In the introduction to their book, *Explorations in Group Relations*, these authors speak of the contribution of social psychology especially the work of Kurt Lewin; of the contribution of group psychotherapy, especially the work of W. R. Bion; and of the influence of Bethel, on the thinking which went into the arrangement of this conference. The primary emphasis at that time was on the study of small groups, with secondary emphasis on the application of this study to the problems that members encountered in their own work. The membership was drawn from a variety of organizations, over half of the participants being from industry or allied fields. The staff were all professional psychologists or members of allied social science disciplines who had psychological training. The small groups, called Study Groups, were conducted only by those who had experience in psychoanalysis. The aim of the training offered by this conference was "to encourage in those who participate a constructively analytical and critical approach to the way they perform their roles in the groups to which they belong" (Trist and Sofer, 1959). This conference seems to have been very similar to those being run in the 1950's in the United States by the National Training Laboratories. In fact, during the planning stages, a member of the Planning and Policy Committee of the National Training Laboratories consulted with the Executive Committee.

In the twelve years following the conference described by Trist and Sofer (1959), major changes took place in the theory and practice of the British conferences, which are now under the sponsorship of the Centre for Applied Social Research of the Tavistock Institute, so that when they were transplanted to the United States in 1965 they were no longer very similar to the comparable events of the National Training Laboratories. The British and the American institutions had gone separate ways. The changes in the British conferences will be described in the next sections of this paper. They have been in large part due to the work of A. Kenneth Rice, who directed all of the Tavistock-Leicester Conferences from 1962 through 1968. Until 1968 Rice was Chairman of the Centre for Applied Social Research in which he acted as senior staff member until his untimely death on November 15, 1969. This Centre is one of the divisions of the Tavistock Institute.

******

Factual information regarding administrative structures and implementation details has been omitted in this section.

******

In 1963, two members of the Washington School of Psychiatry faculty (Morris Parloff and Margaret Rioch) attended the Tavistock-Leicester Conference. They formed the opinion that the introduction of this kind of conference into the United States would mean a valuable addition to the methods of group relations training in this country.

The Tavistock Institute had no formal responsibility for financing and administering the conference, but as the institution supplying the Director (A. K. Rice) and two other senior staff members (P. Turquet and J. Sutherland) and representing the tradition that was being built upon, it was actually the center of the conference.

The Executive Committee of the Conference consisted of the Director and two American members, F.C. Redlich, then Chairman of the Yale Department of Psychiatry, now Dean of its Medical School, and M. J. Rioch, member of the Executive Council of the Washington School of Psychiatry. The Conference was held at Mount Holyoke College. This location has now become part of the tradition of the two-week conferences that have been held there every year since 1965 in June.

In September 1966, the first one-week American conference was held at Connecticut College in New London. Since then a one-week conference has been held every year in late August at Amherst College. There has been a special effort in these conferences to build an American staff which can function independently. Since 1967, the Director has been an American, and the intention is to maintain and develop American leadership in these conferences.

Rationale

In order to understand man in society, it is necessary to shift one's view from the individual and the pair to a larger whole. The thrust of the Washington School of Psychiatry-Tavistock Conferences is the attempt to make this shift.

Nineteenth-century science tended to break things down into smaller and smaller pieces, and great progress was made in this way, but the task now is one of integration and organization of the small pieces into intelligibly patterned wholes. This is true in biology and medicine as well as in the social sciences. One investigator, in the field of medicine, Dr. Thomas McP. Brown of George Washington University, likens the task to that of a person sitting on a merry-go-round in which the horse is not only going around and up and down but also sideways, while the whole thing, mounted on a huge truck, is racing along at 100 miles per hour. In this position the investigator is supposed to describe and understand phenomena which are on a similar merry-go-round proceeding down the road alongside him (Brown, 1969). The usual approach to a situation like this is to try to limit attention to one small aspect which can be encompassed and kept in view all the time, like the one horse in front of us on our own merry-go-round. But this will not yield a solution to complex problems in medicine and biology, and still less so in the social sciences. In order to see the total pattern, attention must shift from the single horse, or, in other words, from the single individual, and we must take in a larger view. This is very easy to say, but in actual practice it is very difficult to do, especially for those who were trained in individual psychology or in looking through a microscope at the individual cell in biology. Even the social psychologist who by definition is interested in something quantitatively larger than the individual, often finds his task so exceedingly difficult that he opts for something like a study of how individuals differ in their behavior in groups.

The two major changes which have taken place in the Tavistock-Leicester conference model in the years of A. K. Rice's directorship are both related to this shift in perspective. The first has to do with leadership and authority. In Rice's (1965) *Learning for Leadership*, he stated, "I am now working on the assumption that the primary task of the residential conferences with which my colleagues and I are concerned is to provide those who attend with opportunities to learn about leadership." His concept of leadership is a complex one which carries with it all of his very rich thinking about organizational structure and the life of institutions. More recently the conferences have been described as being about authority, and in 1969, the aim of the conference was defined in its brochure as being "to provide members with opportunities to learn about the nature of authority and the interpersonal and intergroup problems encountered in its exercise."

There is no attempt on the part of the conference staff to prescribe how members shall define or use the words authority and leadership. In considering the various meanings of these terms as they are experienced in concrete situations, members sometimes acquire greater clarity in their own thinking about these important topics. In using the word authority the conference staff indicates its concern with this significant issue in present-day society.

By focusing on problems of leadership and authority, it is possible to see the patterns of the group emerging with regard to these concepts. The leader or leadership in a group can be thought of as representing or embodying the function of the group, especially its major function or primary task. "Primary task" is one of Rice's central concepts, and it has been defined and explained in several of his works (Rice, 1963, 1965; Miller and Rice, 1967). Briefly, he means by this term that task which an organization or institution must perform in order to survive. The organization may, and usually does, also perform secondary tasks. An important question then becomes, how do the members of the group relate to the primary task as represented by the leader? Do they accomplish the parts of it that, when put together, complete the total task? Do they fight to destroy it, betray it, sabotage it, work toward redefining or changing it? Do they compete for the position of leader? How do they conceive of authority in the group? Looking at these and other attitudes toward leader, leadership, and authority are ways of understanding the functioning of the group as a whole.

The second major change that has taken place under Rice's directorship is a shift in emphasis away from the small group to the institution as a whole. The total conference is conceived as an interplay of the various groups of which it is constituted. Further, the institution as a whole includes the relationship with groups outside, such as the college in which the conference is located, the institutions that provide staff, members, and sponsorship; and the national and international environment that impinges upon the life of the conference. This means, of course, that the conferences deal with a much larger order of complexity than was the case in 1957. Anyone who has worked with a small group knows of the enormous number of factors operating in it and feels the need both to organize these factors into some kind of pattern and/or to exclude some of the data impinging upon his nervous system in order to make any kind of meaningful statement about the group. If one is focusing upon an institution of 50 to 70 members, its constituent parts, and its relationship to institutions outside itself, the situation is obviously even more difficult. In order to manage it at all, it is necessary, first, to have some experience and practice in taking this overall view, and, second, to have some concepts and guidelines that help to make sense out of the overwhelming mass of data. Thus, the sharp focus upon a particular aim, such as the study of the nature of authority and leadership, is the other side of the coin which necessarily accompanies the wider view of the institution as a whole, including its external relationships.

It is quite possible, of course, to design a conference with another primary task than that of the study of leadership and the nature of authority. It is one essential characteristic of these conferences that they attempt to state their aim clearly and to focus upon it, whatever that aim may be. The staff of each conference at the present time tries to make a clear statement about its own purpose and position and to adhere to this purpose and position no matter how difficult it may become. At the same time the staff invites and encourages questioning of its task, purpose and position, on the part of the members, and is constantly engaged in self-questioning of its own activities. A major value to which the leadership is committed is ruthless honesty in thinking about oneself and one's group without any assumption that such honesty will necessarily lead to resolution of conflict. Thought, intellect, and rationality are highly valued, as are clear and firm decisions made in the service of a stated goal.

There is recognition on the part of the leadership of the conferences that human beings readily—all too readily—form groups, that they form mobs that lynch, groups that glorify fanatical leaders, groups that easily slip into orgiastic experiences or into the warm glow of togetherness. On the other hand, the formation of a human group seriously and consistently dedicated to a serious task, without fanaticism or illusion, is an extremely difficult process and a relatively rare occurrence. Human beings have the potentiality for this kind of group formation, however, and when it occurs, even briefly and imperfectly, it is one of the most valuable human phenomena, as well as one of the most individually satisfying experiences. Without some element of this, groups, both large and small, tend to remain childishly dependent upon a leader or a set of slogans, to seek an enemy against whom to unite, or to disintegrate in one way or another.

One of the major aims of the conferences is to contribute to people's ability to form serious work groups committed to the performance of clearly defined tasks. Whether or not members of such groups feel friendliness, warmth, closeness, competitiveness, or hostility to each other is of secondary importance. It is assumed that these and other feelings will occur from time to time, but this is not the issue. The issue is the common goal to which each individual makes his own differentiated contribution. A second major aim, closely related to the first, is the development of more responsible leadership and followership in group life.

Methods

The conferences have been set up as residential events in order to create an optimal situation in which people can concentrate their full energies and attention on the undertaking. In ordinary life the exigencies of daily work are so pressing that it is difficult to free time and energy for a profound involvement in the learning experience. In a residential conference there is no need to interrupt the learning process by fulfilling the usual demands of job, family and social life. Nonresidential workshops and courses do not have this advantage but they may, nevertheless, call forth sufficient involvement on the part of participants to permit a significant learning experience to take place.

There are four events which constitute the main work of the conference. In the first three of these the staff members, who function as consultants, call attention to the processes as they see them which are occurring in the group there and then. The usual session lasts one and one-half hours. The number of sessions varies with the event and the duration of the conference. In addition to the separate events, the conference as a whole is the subject for discussion in one or two plenary sessions toward the end and is the main object of concern to the conference leadership throughout the one or two weeks of its duration. Concepts about groups and organizations which have proved useful to the staff are introduced through lectures or in the fourth event, i.e., the Application Groups. The four major events are:

1. *Small Groups.* These consist of from eight to twelve members. The task of each group is to study its own behavior in the "here and now." Each

group has the services of a consultant whose task is to help the group examine its own behavior.

2. The Large Group. This consists of all the conference members together with consultants. The task of the large group is to study behavior in meetings that consist of more people than can form a face-to-face group. Members have the opportunity to experience, and to learn to deal with, situations in which sides are taken spontaneously, existing subgroups adhere and split, other factions are formed for apparently irrational reasons, and the individual can feel bereft of support.

This exercise was introduced by A. K. Rice. It is one aspect of the shift in emphasis in the Conference from the intimacy of small groups to the difficult problems of anonymity and of mob phenomena in large groups.

3. The Intergroup Event. This provides opportunities for all members to study the relationships between and among groups as they happen. Members form groups among themselves for this purpose. Consultants are available to groups so formed and to any intergroup activities that occur.

This exercise is also one of the innovations of A. K. Rice. While the whole conference institution is thought of as the interplay of groups, in this exercise there is special opportunity for the formal study of this kind of interrelationship. Consultants in this exercise try to make clear that effective intergroup relations require the exercise of authority of some people on behalf of others, and, as the other side of the coin, they require the delegation of authority by some people to others. Problems of representation become paramount if one group is to communicate clearly with another. Who speaks for whom and with what authority are major questions. If they are not solved, chaos results.

4. Application Groups. These consist of from five to ten members drawn from those in similar or complementary roles in their ordinary work. These groups meet toward the end of the conference, each one with a staff member. They serve a threefold purpose. They attempt to examine and articulate some of the unresolved conference problems. They attempt to deal with problems of leaving the conference and of returning to the world outside. They consider the relevance of the conference to members' own work.

In all of these events the consultants maintain a highly disciplined style. The message that this style is intended to convey is the seriousness of the task and the commitment of each staff member to the role that he has taken upon himself. The consultants must try constantly to do two things at once: to experience in themselves what the group is doing to them and to think about this interpretively. They hope that the members will gradually share their leadership in this.

Rules are never made for members except for those imposed by the community in which the events are taking place. But very firm rules are made for staff. It is ordinarily a matter of pride on the part of staff members to abide by these since it is well known to anyone who joins the staff group that this is an essential part of the method. Time boundaries, for example, are strictly kept. Consultants always begin and end the various events promptly, whereas members are, of course, free to come and go at any time.

The teaching of responsible leadership and followership is not done by teaching any techniques of leadership or of how to become more accepted or better liked or of how to manipulate people. It is done partly by setting a model within the staff. It is also done by the staff members keeping their attention fixed upon the group as a whole and holding consistently to their job of studying and interpreting as best they can the way the groups are relating to them as the leaders who represent the task of the group. The members recognize the consultants as the authorities in the conference. They also tend to ascribe to them power which they do not actually possess. In the process of consistently and persistently interpreting the way in which the group members tend to divest themselves of authority and responsibility but also to undercut the authority of anyone else who tries to assume leadership, the consultants are sometimes able to help the group members become aware of the many self-defeating manoeuvres in which they engage. Staff members try to make clear how the total group is actually responsible for what is going on in its midst, for how it eggs on its leaders or refuses to let them function, and also for how it sometimes actively and constructively supports its leaders in their jobs so that they can accomplish their purpose. When the purpose of the conference is accomplished, members are able to see that their group, like others in the "real world," got the leaders that they deserved.

In studying the processes that go on in groups, consultants try to stress the covert processes that are, to some extent at least, outside people's awareness, so that participants may become increasingly aware of the complex and often irrational factors that influence the behavior of groups. The conferences provide opportunities to observe how the emotional and irrational elements of group life further or hinder task performance. However, confessionals about people's private lives and early childhoods are never encouraged. If anyone starts to engage in the kind of self-revelation that would be appropriate in psychotherapy, it is interpreted by the consultant as a group phenomenon and the group is asked to think about how it is using the member who is engaging in this kind of activity. In order to understand the irrational and emotional elements that are present in any group, it is of course necessary for the group members to feel the emotions and the anxiety that are part of the conflicts of group life. The consultant's task is to try to see to it that the group does not get lost either in an orgy of feeling or in sterile intellectualization. The ideal is that of bringing together emotion and intellect, study and experience.

Selection of Staff

As in any organization, staff selection poses a chronically knotty problem. Whereas in the 1957 British conference the requirement was that staff members, particularly small-group consultants, should have psychoanalytic experience, the present policy does not make this a requirement. In fact, the tendency is to try to find people who do not take a "clinical" approach. Since the institution is educational and since it wishes to educate with regard to institutions and the leadership thereof, the idea is that those who competently maintain reasonable leadership provide the best models from whom members can learn. Reasonable leadership, especially in an educational institution of this kind, includes at its best the ability to understand and articulate the processes occurring in the institution.

Membership in at least two conferences held in the Tavistock tradition is a prerequisite for a staff position. New staff members usually begin by taking small groups and are given some supervision in this by an experienced staff person. The usual policy is not to appoint a new staff member to a very short conference or workshop in which the time available for staff training is minimal. Although these policies have worked reasonably well, the need has often been felt for better and longer staff training. Limitations on this have been set by lack of time and money to develop an appropriate program.

Selection of Members

The membership of the British conferences has from the beginning been drawn from various types of organizations, including commercial, industrial, educational, medical, social service, and religious ones. This heterogeneity has been felt to be a source of strength in that no particular kind of jargon or set of assumptions held by one profession can go unchallenged by another group. In the United States the fact that the original sponsoring institutions were identified with psychiatry led inevitably to a heavy weighting of the membership in the field of mental health. The people recruited by the Washington School of Psychiatry and the Yale Department of Psychiatry were very largely psychiatrists, psychologists, and people in related professions. In the first two-week conference, only 24 per cent of the members were from fields outside mental health. In the 1968 conference, 39 per cent came from fields outside mental health. This is considered a desirable trend by those responsible for the conferences, and efforts are consistently made to prevent membership from being concentrated too heavily in any one group.

By and large, participants are accepted if they apply early. But preference is given to those in leadership positions because of the greater likelihood of their ability to wield important influence.

Each applicant is asked, on his application blank, to give the name of an officer of his organization or institution who can speak for his integrity and good standing. It is obvious that there is no way in which membership of such conferences can be screened in an adequate way, but the request for such a statement is, in effect, an indication that the conferences are appropriate only for those people who will take some responsibility for their institutions and who are considered responsible by their institutions. Obviously, no statement in writing beforehand can actually insure this, but it is the best that can be done.

Relationship to T-Groups, Encounter, and Therapy Groups

Differences between the methods and philosophy developed by the Tavistock-Washington School of Psychiatry Conferences and those used in T-groups and encounter groups have probably emerged in the fore-going account. Perhaps the major difference is the consistent emphasis on the group as a whole rather than on individuals within it. There is no doubt some overlap in this with other organizations, especially with the more conservative elements in the National Training Laboratories.

One of the major characteristics of the Tavistock style is that it is imperative to define and articulate as clearly as possible the primary task of the conference or workshop and to try to have all staff decisions insofar as possible flow from this task definition. There will, of course, always be constraints upon this, but they will be recognized as constraints rather than as implementary functions.

Another major characteristic, closely related to the foregoing, is the emphasis on task and work. The concept of work as understood in these conferences was developed by W. R. Bion (1959). Rice's concept of primary task is related to it in the sense that when a group is "working" in Bion's sense, it is accomplishing its "primary task" in Rice's sense. Both of these concepts require the elaboration given them by their authors, and a brief explanation cannot do them justice. But in both there is implicit a dedication to something larger than, though not inimical to, one's personal growth and interest. In both the thought is implicit that something is possible which is not just a compromise between individual and group needs, but is more like a synthesis in which important needs of the individual are, at least for a short time, fulfilled by his immersion in the work of the group. The strong emphasis upon learning and work, rather than upon personal growth or self-expression, differentiates the Tavistock style from that of many other group experiences.

Astrachan and Klein (unpublished) have addressed themselves to the differences in approach between the Tavistock and the T-group model and have made some interesting comparisons. The present author takes issue with their view that the Tavistock "Study Group" consultant remains detached and remote but finds other aspects of their comparisons accurate.

With regard to the relationship of the Tavistock-Washington School of Psychiatry Conferences to group therapy, it is easy to state that the Group Relations Conferences are educational, not therapeutic in intention. The differences and similarities between education and therapy constitute an interesting and difficult subject of discussion which is not appropriate in this paper. The statement that the conferences are educational means that people who are in distress about their personal problems and who are finding it difficult to manage their ordinary lives without some therapeutic help should not come to them. The conferences can be, and really should be, stressful if they are to have their optimal effect. If this stress is added to an adjustment that is already precarious, it may be too much for a person to handle. It is devoutly to be wished that there might be a way of screening out those in whom the conference will arouse more anxiety than can be usefully worked through, but the best that can be done at present is to try to give fair warning and to suggest to people who are finding the conference very threatening that they would do better to leave. It requires a certain toughness on the part of the staff to refuse to turn the institution or any part of it into a "hospital" when an individual seems to need care. But the institution cannot carry on its task for the rest of its members if it turns aside from it for the sake of one individual.

The fact that the conferences are educational not therapeutic in intent does not mean, of course, that what is learned in them is inapplicable to group therapy. A greater understanding of the processes, especially the covert processes, which go on in groups should be of the utmost importance to group therapists. How they should use this understanding is a matter for discussion in terms of therapeutic methods, goals and constraints, and is not a part of the subject of this paper.

A Look at the Future

The various people connected with the American Tavistock Conferences probably have quite different views of what the future will and should hold. The following is the personal view of the present author and may or may not be shared by others of the conference staffs. I should like to see the following developments:

1) A slow growth in numbers and size of the Tavistock Conferences and related events, slow enough to allow for real integration and assimilation of the people involved.

2) An American staff that will operate with increasing competence and sureness independently of the strong British tradition.

3) Conferences, workshops, and other events that will not turn aside from facing the important social issues of the day, such as black-white problems and student unrest.

4) Responsible American leadership that will stand for rational, flexible, clear, and dedicated authority.

5) New developments along a number of different lines to fill the needs of a number of different segments of our society.

References

Astrachan BM and Klein FB: (Unpublished manuscript). Copies may be obtained from the authors, Department of Psychiatry, Yale University School of Medicine, New Haven, Conn.

Bion WR (1959) Experiences in groups. New York: Basic Books.

Brown T McP (1969) Personal communication.

Miller EG and Rice AK (1967) Systems of Organization London: Tavistock Publications.

Rice AK (1963) The Enterprise and its environment London: Tavistock Publications.

Rice AK (1965) Learning for Leadership London: Tavistock Publications.

Trist EL and Sofer C (1959) Explorations in Group Relations Leicester, England: Leicester University Press.

A Study of Encounter Group Casualties

IRVIN D. YALOM, M.D.
Stanford, Calif
MORTON A. LIEBERMAN, PH.D.
Chicago

No collection of group psychotherapy papers would be complete without a selection by Irv Yalom. Since "The Theory and Practice of Group Psychotherapy" was first published (New York: Basic Books, 1970), Yalom has dominated the field, with appeal to clinicians of all professional persuasions. His book placed great importance on the idea of group cohesion and group therapeutic factors. This focus provided for group psychotherapy what the concept of common factors did for individual therapy. Yalom has also written eloquently about existential factors in psychotherapy (Existential Psychotherapy. New York: Basic Books, 1980), and reached the New York Times Best Seller list with "Love's Executioner" (New York: Basic Books, 1989).

Yalom, Professor of Psychiatry at Stanford University, has also been a major contributor to the empirical research literature, a legacy of his early group training with Jerome Frank. It is one of these papers that has been chosen for this volume, a study funded primarily by the National Institute of Mental Health and the Ford Foundation. The sensitive issue of negative therapeutic effects is widely documented but often ignored in clinical practice. This paper is based on the Stanford Encounter Group Study, a research undertaking that remains as perhaps the largest in-depth study of small group behavior (Lieberman MA, Yalom ID, Miles MB. Encounter Groups: First Facts. New York: Basic Books, 1973). In addition to the question of casualties, the study was notable for its rich descriptions of therapist styles, which are discussed in this paper. The study also found that theoretical label has almost no correlation with what a leader actually does in a clinical situation. —(Editor)

Yalom ID, Lieberman MA: A study of encounter group casualties. *Archives of General Psychiatry* 25:16-30, 1971.

How psychologically dangerous are encounter groups? For several years mental health professionals have been in the uncomfortable position of having to answer this question without the necessary information. Despite the lack of systematic information, however, there has been no dearth of polemics.

On the one hand, many, alarmed by case reports of severe psychological decompensation following an encounter group experience (so-called "encounter group casualties"), have branded the whole encounter group field as dangerous. Some medical societies have proposed that state governments legislate regulations for encounter group practice. Clinicians' views towards encounter groups are based on heavily skewed information: they often see casualties or read about them in their professional journals, but they rarely have contact with encounter group members who have had satisfying experiences. Some psychiatric associations have attempted to garner relevant evidence by polling members for a list of all the casualties they have seen. Such an approach can demonstrate the existence but not the frequency of danger. Knowing the number of casualties without knowing the total number of participants from which the casualties issue offers useful but severely limited information. Anecdotal case reporting has another intrinsic flaw: multiple reporting may spuriously inflate casualty rates. An untoward outcome in a group member is generally a striking event not easily forgotten by the other group members; if the other 20 members (or, in a residential laboratory, 100 members) all describe this event to colleagues or friends, the single casualty soon assumes alarming proportions.

Encounter group leaders, enthusiastic members, and administrative staff of growth centers often take an opposite position. They report few casualties and generally do not view the encounter group as a hazardous venture—a not unexpected viewpoint. Most encounter group leaders and growth centers are limited in their source of information. Their groups are generally brief; once ended, the members scatter and the leaders have little opportunity, even were they so inclined, to gather follow-up data. A psychological decompensation occurring after the end of the group would be unlikely to come to their attention.

There are in addition to actual limitations of information, ideological sources of bias. Many encounter group leaders reject psychiatric definitions of "adverse effect"; they feel that extreme psychological discomfort, even to the degree that professional aid is required, may be not a failure but an accomplishment of the group. They view psychological decompensation, like the legendary "night journey" as a stage, even a desideratum, of personal growth. Other leaders express a lack of interest in adverse effects since their ideological base stresses the necessity and ability of each individual to assume responsibility for himself. They believe that the leader who takes responsibility for the welfare of others thus infantilizes them and impedes their growth.

The American Psychiatric Association was sufficiently concerned with these issues to commission in 1969 a task force (chaired by one of us, I.Y.) to survey the current state of knowledge. The Task Force report[1] reviewed the literature and noted that there was "distressingly little data": the available evidence consisted entirely of anecdotal reports or loosely designed studies which lacked a post-group follow-up.

With this background in mind when designing a systematic research project on encounter groups, we attempted to pay careful attention to the negative as well as to the positive outcomes of encounter groups.

Methodology

In the spring of 1969 we conducted an intensive study of a large number of encounter groups led by leaders from different ideological schools. The group members, all Stanford University undergraduates, were studied in a variety of ways. They completed a large battery of self-report questionnaires before beginning the groups, after each meeting, at the end of the group experience, and again, for a final follow-up, six months later. The groups each met for a total of 30 hours: some had spaced (ten three-hour) meetings, others a massed format in which the groups met for only a few time-extended "marathon" meetings.

The encounter group participants received three academic credits; no preparation paper or examination was required; the only requirements (though not enforced) were attendance and cooperation in the research endeavor. The groups, with a few exceptions, met on or near the Stanford campus, each meeting was tape-recorded and rated by two trained observers.

Eighteen groups were conducted. We deliberately selected leaders from a wide variety of ideological schools. Our 18 groups thus had these labels:

Group Labels

1. N.T.L. sensitivity groups (T-groups)	2 groups
2. Gestalt therapy (Esalen—Fritz Perls derivative)	2 groups
3. Psychodrama orientation	2 groups
4. Psychoanalytic	1 group
5. Transactional analysis	2 groups
6. Sensory awareness focus (Esalen derivative)	1 group
7. Marathon (rogerian; eclectic personal growth)	2 groups
8. Synanon	2 groups
9. N.T.L. West—"personal growth", black-white encounter focus	2 groups
10. Tape groups (leaderless; Bell & Howell Peer Program)[2]	2 groups

******

Here and in the following Methodology and Results sections some research details and clinical vignettes have been omitted.

******

Once we selected the "types" of groups, we then attempted to identify the most competent, senior leaders of each ideological school in Northern California. The leaders were well paid ($750 for the 30-hour groups, plus two to three hours of research interviews and questionnaires). We were fortunate enough to recruit highly experienced, well-recommended leaders. Indeed, several of the leaders have national reputations. The instructions to the leader were minimal: they were asked to lead the encounter groups in their usual manner—to "do their thing."

When students registered for the course they were randomly assigned (stratified by sex, race, and previous encounter group experience) to one of the 18 groups. A total of 209 students began the groups, 39 dropped out (ie, missed at least the last two meetings), and 170 completed the group.

The goals of the project were ambitious. We attempted a thorough study of the process and outcome of experiential groups—in short "everything you ever wanted to know about groups." This article describes only that part of the project pertaining to negative outcome. The reader is referred elsewhere[4] for a complete description of the experimental methodology and the measurement of process and of positive outcome.

Identification of Casualties

Since it was not possible to interview in depth all 209 subjects who began the groups, we used eight criteria to identify a potential high-risk subsample who could then be studied more intensively.

(1) *Request for psychiatric aid*: The most obvious mode of identifying a casualty, and the one used in most previous research, is the request for emergency aid during the course of the group.

(2) *Dropouts from groups*: We expected that those who dropped out of groups might have done so because of a noxious group experience.

(3) *Peer evaluation*: At the end of the group, all members were asked, "Did anyone get hurt in your group? Who? How?"

(4) *Self-esteem drop*: The Rosenberg Self-Esteem measure[5] was used as one measure of outcome. We calculated the pre-post change in self-esteem and studied the lowest ten percentiles (the 17 subjects who decreased the most in self-esteem) of the subjects.

(5) *Subjects' testimony*: At the end of the group the subjects were asked to rate their group on a number of seven-point differential scales (eg, constructive-destructive, low learning-high learning, pleasant-unpleasant, turned off-turned on). Again, the lowest 10% were included in our high risk sample.

(6) *Psychotherapy*: At the six-month follow-up subjects were asked whether they had started psychotherapy since the beginning of the group. All subjects answering positively were studied.

(7) *Leaders' ratings*: The leaders were asked at the end of the group to rate each student on the amount of progress he had made on a number of dimensions (eg, self-understanding, positive self-image, happiness, openness, sensitivity, ability to collaborate with others). The subjects (lowest 10%) who had the lowest leader ratings were included in the high-risk population.

(8) Several miscellaneous sources of information were available to us. For example, the observers occasionally reported concern about some member of a group which they observed, or subjects during an interview expressed concern about another member.

Our definition of casualty was fairly stringent: not only must the student have undergone some psychological decompensation but it must have been persistent and there must have been evidence that the group experience was the responsible agent. We did not consider as casualties several subjects who were shaken up and severely distressed by the group but who, a few days later, had recovered their equilibrium. Nor did we include several subjects who during the group or in the six months following had had some psychological decompensation that was due not to the encounter group but to other circumstances in the life of the individual.

Results

A total of 104 casualty suspects were identified. Of these 79 were contacted by telephone and 25 could not be located. Sixteen casualties were identified: this represents 7.5% of the 209 subjects who began the groups, or 9.4% of the 170 subjects who completed the groups.

The severity and type of psychological injury varied considerably. Three students during or immediately following the group had psychotic decompositions—one a manic psychosis, one an acute paranoid schizophrenic episode, and the third an acute undifferentiated schizophrenic-lysergic acid diethylamide episode. Several students had depressive or anxiety symptoms, or both, ranging from low grade tension or discouragement to severe crippling anxiety attacks to a major six-month depression with a 40-lb weight loss and suicidal ideation. Others suffered some disruption of their self-system: they felt empty, self-negating, inadequate, shameful, unacceptable, more discouraged about ever growing or changing. Several subjects noted a deterioration of their interpersonal life; they withdrew or avoided others, experienced more distrust, were less willing to reach out or to take risks with others.

The comparative efficiency of the various modes of identifying casualties showed that the most effective method is peer evaluation. A total of 30 subjects were listed by their comembers as having been hurt by the group and of these 30, 12 were casualties. There were 11 subjects who were multiply chosen (ie, more than one member of their group listed them); of these 11, eight were casualties (and a ninth was the subject who committed suicide). There were four casualties with only a single nomination, but three of these four were self-selected. *Therefore, if a group member is cited by more than one member of his group, or cites himself as having been hurt by the experience, it is highly probable that he represents a casualty of the group.* (In our sample, the probability is 73%.) Furthermore, all of the more severe casualties were identified by this method.

The leaders' ratings were a highly inaccurate mode of identifying casualties. Of the 20 subjects with the lowest leader ratings, only three were casualties. Moreover, some of the severe casualties were missed by this mode.

It is three times more likely that a subject who is in an encounter group will seek psychotherapy during the time he is in the group, or in the eight-month follow-up period, than a control subject.

Why does he enter psychotherapy? Information from interviews with the 14 subjects suggested several reasons: (1) Five sought psychotherapy for repair. They were all casualties and were so upset by the group experiences that they needed help in order to regain their equilibrium. (2) Six (including two casualties) entered psychotherapy for the same reasons they had entered the encounter group. Psychotherapy and the encounter group experiences were not causally related; both were manifestations of the individual's search for help. (3) Two had a very constructive encounter group experience and entered therapy to continue work started in the group. They credited the group with helping them to identify their problems and showing them that it was possible to obtain help by talking about them and working on them. (4) One entered therapy for reasons entirely unrelated to the encounter group, a crisis in his life which arose months after the end of the group.

Relationship Between the Type of Encounter Group and the Casualty Rate

Casualties were not evenly distributed amongst the 18 groups. Six groups had no casualties, while three had two casualties and one group had three casualties. To understand this skewed distribution of casualties we attempted to cluster together leaders with similar style. As we have previously indicated, the ideological school of the leader and his actual behavior were largely unrelated so that, for example, the two transactional analysis leaders were no more likely to resemble one another than they were to resemble leaders of any of the other schools. A new taxonomy of leadership style was, therefore, required—a task of no little complexity.

The entire methodology of the derivation of this taxonomy is described elsewhere[3] but, in brief, leader behavior was examined through two lenses—participant questionnaires, designed to tap the symbolic value of the leader to each member, and observer schedules. Observers rated, exhaustively, the leaders' behavior, their global style, and their primary focus in the group (group, individual, or interpersonal issues). Observers also recorded their personal reactions to the leaders. In all 48 scales of leader behavior were rated by observers and participants. By means of factor analyses, these 48 categories were reduced to four basic dimensions of leader behavior—emotional stimulation, caring, meaning attribution, and executive functions. These four dimensions accounted for 70% of the variance of total leader behavior. By means of statistical clustering, all the leaders in the study could be subsumed under seven types of leaders.

Type A Leaders: "Aggressive Stimulators." These five leaders (the two gestalt leaders, one psychodrama leader, and the two Synanon leaders) were characterized by their extremely high stimulus input. They were intrusive, confrontive, challenging, while at the same time demonstrating high positive caring; they revealed a great deal of themselves. They were the most charismatic of the leaders. They were authoritarian and often structured the events in the group. They focused upon the individual in the group rather than upon the group, and they often provided the individual with some cognitive framework with which to understand himself and the world. They asserted firm control and took over for the participants. They seemed ready, willing, and able to guide participants forward on the road to enlightenment.

Type B Leaders: "Love Leaders." These three leaders (NTL T-group leader. a marathon eclectic leader, and a transactional analytic leader) were caring, individually focused leaders, who gave love as well as information and ideas about how to change. They exuded a quality of enlightened paternalism; they were "good daddies"; they had an established frame of reference about how individuals learn which they used in the group but which they do not press.

Type C Leaders: "Social Engineers." These three leaders (NTL, rogerian, and psychodrama) focused on steering the work of the group as a whole rather than on the individual or interpersonal relationships. They offered relatively low levels of stimulus input and rarely confronted or challenged individuals. They were perceived by participants as being low on authoritarianism and were not perceived as charismatic. The distance between them and the participants was psychologically felt to be small compared to, for example, the type A leaders.

Type D Leaders: "Laissez-faire." These two leaders (psychoanalytic and transactional analytic) offered very little stimulation input, no challenging, no confrontation, and made very little use of themselves as an issue in the group; they offered little support and generally remained distant and cool; they were experienced by the participants as technicians and their major input to the group was the occasional communication of ideas about how people learn. They offered very little structure to the members.

Type E Leaders: "Cool, Aggressive Stimulators." These leaders (two personal growth leaders) were aggressive stimulators, but not to the extent of the type A leaders. They offered little positive support and were nonauthoritarian in that they rarely structured the meeting; they tended to focus more on the group ("social engineering") than did most of the other leaders except, of course, the type C leaders.

Type F Leaders: "High Structure." One leader (sensory awareness—Esalen) was so different from all others that he must be classified separately. He used a large number (an average of 8 per meeting) of structured exercises—group "games." He was exceedingly controlling and authoritarian.

Type G Leaders: The Tape Leaders. These are two groups which had as their leader the Bell & Howell encounter tape (Peer Program). At the start of each meeting the members turned on a tape-recorder which gave the group instructions for the conduct of that meeting. The tape programs focused upon learning how to give and receive feedback, how to make emotional contact with others, how to self-disclose. They fostered a warm, supportive climate and deemphasized interpersonal conflict.

The probable mode of injury also differed considerably amongst the 18 groups. Our interviews with the subjects uncovered several types of prototypical group events to which they attributed their negative outcome.

Attack by leader is cited only in type A groups, and is associated with some of the more severe casualties. We should note that the categories of injury mode were developed before and independently of the taxonomy of leader styles.

Attack by the group was a mode of injury that occurred either in the type A groups, in conjunction with attack by the leader, or in groups led by leaders who were distant and modelled little or no positive supportive behavior. These occurred in groups led by a "laissez-faire" leader (D), by the least caring of the "social engineers" (C), and by one of the "impersonal" leaders (E).

Rejection played a role for six casualties. For some the experience of rejection overlapped so heavily with the experience of attack that the distinction was but a semantic subtlety; others, however, explicitly emphasized being rejected by the leader or group, or both.

Failure to achieve unrealistic goals was reported by four of the casualties who entered the group with unrealistically high expectations given their existing defenses. Their needs were extreme and would have been an appropriate ticket of admission to any psychotherapy group.

Group pressure effects were reported by two casualties who experienced unusual reactions to the group. Both, unable to accommodate to the group pressure to experience and express feelings, ended the group with a sense of hollowness. They could not keep up with the others in a pell-mell charge to levels of deep intimacy. They grew alarmed at their failure and defined themselves as deficient or empty. If they acceded to the group pressure by feigning intimacy, they privately felt duplicitous as well.

Input overload was experienced by several casualties who seemed to have suffered from "overstimulation"—a mode of injury as vague as it is inferential. Three of the five subjects involved had psychotic episodes beginning during or shortly after the end of the group.

Prevention of Casualties

In studying the casualty suspects we interviewed many individuals who resembled the casualties in some manner (character structure, goals, type of group, experience in the group, etc) but who did not have a negative experience. What accounted for these different outcomes? Our interviews suggested several *post hoc* explanations which were, for the most part, untestable in the present study.

Many of the subjects interviewed appeared to have taken a more casual stance toward the group than did the casualties. They had neither a pressing need nor great expectations for the group. Intellectual curiosity or the three easy academic credits loomed a bit larger; loneliness, depression, or other psychological hang-ups were more rarely mentioned. "Uninvolvement" was often mentioned. They stayed out of the vortex of the group, they "did not take it seriously," the group was "artificial," "not meaningful," "boring," or "plodding." One subject in Synanon stated, "It's unreal, you know, for a group of strangers to meet once a week and scream at one another. How can you really take it seriously?" They detoxified the group by maintaining their objectivity, by forming alliance with an observing ego which kept before them the fact that the group was an artificial, time-limited aggregation in which deliberate magnification of emotions occurred. Others disengaged themselves physically and dropped out of the group.

There were several subjects who, in our view, might well have become casualties were it not for skillful management on the part of the leader. It appeared to us that some subjects started the group in highly vulnerable states, yet benefited considerably from their group experience. Several were not active central members of their groups but seemed to profit both from a sense of belongingness and vicariously from observing others work through problems. Some explicitly expressed gratitude towards their leaders who invited, encouraged, but did not demand participation and who always permitted them to select their own pace.

Predicting and Screening Out Casualties

A wide variety of tests and questionnaire information was available on all our participants prior to the group experience. From the pre-group data, 71 scales or indices were selected to test out whether casualties could be predicted (and these were reduced to 20 dimensions). Six of the 20 dimensions were particularly sensitive in discriminating between the casualties and non-casualties. Those who became casualties showed, before beginning the group, significantly lower levels of self-esteem and a lower level of positive self-concept than did those who did not become casualties.

Furthermore the casualties had a higher growth orientation and a greater anticipation that the encounter group would provide opportunities for fulfillment of their needs. Perhaps they overinvested in the possibility, perhaps they were more needy individuals who saw in the encounter group the unrealistic possibility of personal salvation. Whatever the origin of the more intense need—or the more "unrealistic" expectation—those individuals who came believing in miracles were more likely to reap pain.

The last area of specific prediction was in the coping-ego-defense scales, which indicate that individuals who are *less* likely to use direct interpersonal modes and *more* likely to use escape modes had a greater probability of becoming casualties.

The entire picture is a consistent one: individuals with generally less favorable mental health with greater growth needs and higher anticipations for their group experience and yet who lacked self-esteem and the interpersonal skills to operate effectively in the group situation were more likely to become casualties.

Comment

Eighteen encounter groups led by leaders with diverse styles were offered as university undergraduate courses. The process and outcome of these groups were intensively researched. We developed several criteria to identify potential casualties of the groups. We defined a casualty as an individual who, as a result of his encounter group experience, suffered considerable and persistent psychological distress. The most effective method of identifying casualties was to ask the group members at the end of the group whether anyone had been harmed by the experience. One of the least effective methods was a rating of negative change by the leaders; indeed many of the leaders were completely unaware that there had been casualties in their groups. This finding has some obvious and significant implications. Group leaders who do not provide themselves with the opportunity for follow-up interviews with their group members simply do not have the necessary information to make a statement about the hazards of their groups. That the members themselves were more accurate in identifying casualties is not surprising. There are a number of studies which attest to the evaluative sensitivity of peers; for example, the Peace Corps candidates were able to predict which of their number would eventually fail in their duties more frequently than were the instructors.[10]

A total of 209 subjects began the encounter groups. There were 16 casualties. This represents a very appreciable casualty rate. Although one aspect of our design—the random assignment of the subjects to one of the 18 groups—may have increased the risk, it was our impression that our casualties rate may, in fact, be a conservative estimate. The overall design of the project, in our opinion, decreased the risk of the groups. The research conditions imposed some restraints on the groups: all groups were observed and tape-recorded and the leaders were cognizant that they were being evaluated. Furthermore, we defined "casualty" in a rigorous manner and, finally, some "high risk" suspects could not be located for study.

A major finding of the study is that the number and severity of casualties and the manner in which the casualties sustained injury are all highly dependent upon the particular type of encounter group. Some leadership styles result in a high-risk group.

Particularly stressful is a leader style (type A) which is characterized by intrusive, aggressive stimulation, by high charisma, by high challenging and confrontation of each of the members, and by authoritarian control. We shall focus on the A style of leadership since groups led in this manner accounted for far more than their share of the total number of casualties: the five type A leaders accounted for seven (44%) of the 16 casualties. It was our impression, too, that these groups generated more severe casualties and, furthermore, that they bore more responsibility for the casualty. (The casualty seemed truly *caused*, not merely hastened or facilitated, by the leader style, and is thereby preventable by a change in leader style.) The type A leaders were forceful and impatient. If some significant sign of growth or change (crying, testimonial, breakdown, or breakthrough) was not given to them in the group, they increased the pressure on the participants. The "A" leaders appeared to operate on an immediate gratification system; they paid little heed to the concept of "working through" and demanded that their members change and change "now."

Another important characteristic of the type A leaders was their lack of differentiation of the individuals in their groups. It appeared as though these leaders felt that everyone in the group had the same needs and had to accomplish the same thing in the group. There is a curious paradox here. The type A leaders appeared highly unorthodox and innovative; they displayed at the same time the widest and yet the narrowest range of techniques—narrow because of a lack of discernment of the scope of intrapersonal and interpersonal problems. After all, not *everyone* needs to express himself more vigorously and spontaneously, to shuck his societal restrictions, to achieve a greater degree of freedom, to abandon all success-oriented goals. Some individuals may need quite the opposite: they already express themselves with far too much lability; they need more, not fewer controls, they need more, not less of an ego boundary; they need, perhaps, a more structured, more traditionally based hierarchy of values.

One other observation of interest concerning the type A leaders was their religious aura. These charismatic leaders had their own internalized charismatic leader. Synanon is still guided by the hand of Dietrich, its founding father, and many of the Synanon activities have distinct ceremonial, ritualized overtones. The gestalt leaders, too, have a highly revered, idealized leader in the person of the late Fredrick "Fritz" Perls; in fact there is a published gestalt therapy prayer with which some leaders begin their meetings. The fifth type A leader was heavily invested in a Far Eastern religious order, and at the time of this writing he had been persuaded by his religious Elder to abandon his career as a group leader. Perhaps the religious element helps us to understand these leaders' failure to discriminate between individuals since they may tend to imbue the individual with a system of beliefs and values (a single and final common pathway to salvation) rather than to encourage the individual to change according to his own needs and potential. (During the meetings, the type A leaders all revealed, to a greater extent than other leaders, their own personal belief systems.)

Whereas four of the type A groups had a total of seven casualties, one "A" group had no casualties, and although this leader resembled in many ways an "A" leader who had three casualties, he differed from him in a significant fashion. He stated that he realized immediately that there were several restricted, fragile individuals in his group and therefore he deviated from his usual style: "I pulled my punches, I didn't get into the heavy intrapersonal material I usually focus on, I did more interpersonal work, more classroom work, I gave them a type of tasting session so that they could see what groups could be like . . . I was constantly aware of keeping the lid on my group." The "A" leader whose group had three casualties, on the other hand, commented that it was a stubborn group, full of people "too infantile to take responsibility for themselves and to form an adult contract" with him. "I saw that most of the group didn't want to do anything so what I did was to just go ahead and have a good time for myself."

Occasionally a casualty from attack by the members, not leaders, occurred in groups led by laissez-faire or leaders who modeled little positive, caring behavior. (Laissez-faire leaders paid another type of penalty for their lack of involvement or low stimulus input—large numbers of their groups dropped out because they found the pace slow and plodding.)

Other mechanisms of injury included rejection by the leader or by the other members. That a member may have a truly destructive experience because of rejection is a function of several factors: the norms of the group which mediated the existence and degree of rejection, the consistency of self-image of the subject, the presence of internalized anchor groups, and the presence of other interpersonal resources to which the subject could turn for support.

Other casualties were caused (or perhaps, more accurately, hastened) by "input overload"; they were so challenged and overstimulated that rather than assimilate new perspectives on themselves and their world they were instead sucked into a maelstrom of confusion and uncertainty. The "unfreezing" process that occurs in almost any encounter group may produce this type of casualty. Clearly, we found that these subjects had some preexisting significant disturbance which met the process half-way.

A final mode of injury occurred in a curious manner. The subject observed other members quickly experiencing and expressing high intensity affect. Noting the apparent discrepancy between the others' productions and his own comparatively pallid affect, he judged himself as emotionally deficient and thenceforth identified himself as one of the hollow men.

The low-risk groups were those led by type B leaders and the two tape groups. The subjects in the tape groups had a positive, though not deeply intensive, experience. The Peer Program tapes promoted supportive, low-conflict groups. On the few occasions that negative interaction occurred, it was dealt with by flight: with no leader to help the group understand and resolve conflict, the members generally avoided unpleasant issues. The type B leaders offered considerable positive support for members. They helped create an accepting, trusting climate in the group which permitted members to participate at their own pace.

Although this paper is concerned only with the hazards of encounter groups, we wish to remind the reader that the positive gains from the experience were far-reaching for many subjects. There was, as we describe elsewhere[11], even more variation amongst the 18 groups in positive outcome than there was in casualty rates.

Although there were pre-group differences apparent between those subjects who went on subsequently to have a destructive experience and those who did not, these differences are not likely to provide us with powerful predictors at the present state of development. Our best means of prediction remains the type of group the subject enters and our best mean for prevention is *self-selection*. If responsible public education can teach prospective encounter group members about what they can with reasonable accuracy, expect in terms of process, risks, and profit from a certain type of group then, and only then, can they make an informed decision about membership. Individuals who are psychologically vulnerable and who overinvest their hopes in the magic of salvation through encounter groups are particularly vulnerable when they interact with leaders who believe that they can offer deliverance. Such an interaction is a potent synergistic force for destructive outcome.

References

1. *Encounter Groups and Psychiatry*, Task Force Report No. 1. Washington, DC, American Psychiatric Association, 1970
2. Berzon B, Solomon LN: The self-directed therapeutic group: Three studies. *J Couns Psychol* 13:491-497, 1966.
3. Lieberman MA, Yalom I: Dimensions of leader behavior, in Berzon B, Solomon LN (eds): *The Encounter Group: Issues and Applications*. San Francisco, Jossey-Bass, 1971.
4. Lieberman M, Yalom I, Miles M, et al: The group experience: A comparison of ten encounter technologies, in Blank L, Gottsegen G, Gottsegen M (eds): *Encounter Confrontation in Self and Interpersonal Awareness*. New York, Macmillan Co Publishers, 1971.
5. Rosenberg M: *Society and the Adolescent Self-Image*. Princeton, NJ, Princeton University Press, 1965.
6. Asch SE: Interpersonal influence: Effects of group pressure upon the modification and distortions of judgment, in Maccoby EE, Newcomb TM, Hartley EL (eds): *Readings in Social Psychology*. New York, Holt, Rinehart & Winston Inc, 1958, pp. 174-183.
7. Sherif M: Group influences upon the formation of norms and attitudes, in Maccoby EE, Newcomb TM, Hartley EL (eds): *Readings in Social Psychology*. New York, Holt, Rinehart & Winston Inc, 1958, pp. 219-232.
8. Schutz W: FIRO: A Three Dimensional Theory of Interpersonal Behavior. New York, Rinehart & Co. Inc, 1958.
9. Childs KE: *Prediction of Encounter Group Outcome as a Function of Selected Personality Variables*, thesis. Committee on Human Development, University of Chicago, 1971.
10. Boulger J, Coleman J: *Research Findings with Peer Ratings*, research note No. 8. Washington, DC, Division of Research, Peace Corps.
11. Lieberman M, Yalom I, Miles M: The impact of encounter groups on participants. *J Appl Behav Sci*, to be published.

On the Concept of the "Mother-Group"

SAUL SCHEIDLINGER, PH.D.

Saul Scheidlinger immigrated to America from Poland in 1938 at the age of 20 with no knowledge of the English language and no money. Four years later, while working part-time to survive, he graduated with four distinguished academic awards. He became associated with group psychotherapy at the Jewish Board of Guardians under the direction of Slavson. His extensive bibliography dates back to 1947 with a paper on group psychotherapy for children, his area of special interest. His Ph.D. dissertation formed the basis of his first book (Psychoanalysis and Group Behavior: A Study in Freudian Group Psychology. New York: Norton, 1952). His book of basic readings is a rich resource of material (Psychoanalytic Group Dynamics: Basic Readings. New York: International Universities Press, 1980).

Scheidlinger has provided both intellectual and political leadership for the field for over four decades. He served as Editor of the International Journal of Group Psychotherapy from 1970 to 1980, where his scholarly approach was evident. He was President of AGPA 1982-1984. He is Professor of Psychiatry (Psychology) at Albert Einstein College of Medicine in New York City. An edited volume has recently been published in his honor (Tuttman S (Ed.), Psychoanalytic Group Theory and Therapy: Essays in Honor of Saul Scheidlinger. New York: International Universities Press, 1991).

This paper is perhaps Scheidlinger's best known, although there was solid minority support from the Editorial Advisory Group for his earlier paper on regression (The concept of regression in group psychotherapy. International Journal of Group Psychotherapy 18:3–20, 1968). Scheidlinger here continues the theme of how best to understand the regressive pull in groups that activates early childhood patterns.
—Editor

Scheidlinger S: On the concept of "mother-group." *International Journal of Group Psychotherapy* 24:417–428, 1974.

There have been increasing references in the group process and group psychotherapy literature to observations that on the deepest levels group members perceive the group-as a-whole as a maternal image. This paper scrutinizes the historical roots of what one might term the concept of a "mother-group" and the varied usages of the term by students of group behavior. An attempt is made to relate this concept to the better-known concepts of group identification and of transferences.

The earliest reference to the group entity as a parental symbol appeared in a paper by R. Money-Kyrle (1950) in which he postulated three kinds of unconscious perceptions by members of groups:

(1) The "good parents," *particularly the mother*, representing the norms and ideals of the group; (2) the "bad parents" in the role of persecutors against whom the group values have to be defended; and (3) the "good parents," especially the father, who in his role as the mother's defender reappears as the group leader. While Money-Kyrle referred to larger societal groupings, Schindler (1951, 1952, and 1966) was the first group therapist to speak of the group as a mother symbol. He differentiated between transferences to the therapist as a father, to the group members as siblings, to the group entity as mother, on the one hand, and the "group personality" on the tripartite model of id, ego, and superego, on the other hand. W. R. Bion (1960) made repeated brief references in his writings to the group's being perceived unconsciously at times as a "part-object," such as the mother's breast or other body parts, in line with Melanie Klein's conceptualizations. Scheidlinger (1955 and 1964) hypothesized that the group members' identification with the group-as-a-whole represented a covert wish to restore an earlier state of unconflicted well-being inherent in the child's exclusive union with the mother.

Interestingly, S. R. Slavson's first and single mention of this theme occurred only 10 years ago, in 1964, when he briefly stated: "It has been shown that the group serves *in loco maternis*. The leader usually represents symbolically, the father figure, while the group represents the complementary figure of the mother" (p 27). Similarly, Foulkes (1964) asserted at that same time that ". . . on different levels the group can symbolize a variety of objects or persons, e.g., the body . . . the inside of the mother, the womb. It frequently, possibly universally, represents the 'Image of the Mother' hence the term 'matrix' " (p. 115). In the same year, Durkin (1964) postulated two separate transference manifestations in therapy groups: "(1) The idea of a group—i.e., a large totality of unknown power—conjures up the harsh, pre-oedipal mother image reactivating the individual's narcissistic fear of her; and (2) the individual perceives the group accordingly in distorted fashion, and behaves toward it in a way that resembles his mode of reacting to his mother. While the group member thus is afraid of the group as a whole, the therapist, in turn, is perceived in the image of the good all-giving omnipotent mother" (p. 329). Basing his observations on T-groups and on self-analytic classroom groups, Slater (1966) discussed at some length the group members' perceptions of the group-as-a-whole in a maternal vein. According to him, this "mother-group" was at times perceived as ". . . a source of succorance and comfort, even a refuge." At other times, this mother image was a frightening one involving primitive fantasies ". . . of being swallowed and enveloped." The "group revolt" against the leader which was depicted as occurring in the early phase of T-groups Slater tied up, on the one hand, with the members' trying to get the loving indulgent "mother-group" away from the depriving paternal figure; on the other hand, this dethroning of the leader he also associated with a ". . . dramatic heightening of sexual interest" among the group members. Still more recently, Grotjahn (1972) asserted that "as a general rule, the group is a truly good and strong mother, not only in fantasies of transference but also in the reality of the group process (p. 318). Ruiz (1972) described the early phase of a T-group in which the anxiety experienced by the participants appeared to be perceived as a threat to the idealized image of an unconflicted, nurturing "mother-group."

The most comprehensive discussion in the literature to date on this theme of the "mother-group" was that by Gibbard and Hartman (1973) who, following Slater (1966), asserted that the group members' ". . . affective response to the unconscious perception of the group-as-mother is profoundly ambivalent. The positive side of the ambivalence is the well-spring for what we [the authors] have called the utopian fantasy" (p. 127). This fantasy "offers some assurance that the more frightening, enveloping or destructive aspects of the group-as-mother will be held in check and that a host of oedipal feelings, libidinal and aggressive, will not become fully conscious and gain direct expression in the group. The essence of the utopian fantasy is that the good can be split off from the bad and that this separation can be maintained" (p. 126). (I shall return to some of the significant theoretical issues posed by Gibbard and Hartman at a later point in this paper.)

One might note here that, from the viewpoint of group therapy's history, the "mother-group" concept has begun to be discussed in the literature relatively late. The reasons for this are probably twofold: (1) the early psychoanalytic models of group formation, such as those postulated by Freud (1921) and Redl (1942), placed emphasis on the major role of a paternal "central person" in group psychology; and, (2) the recently growing stress on early object relations in psychoanalytic theory has affirmed the great significance of early mothering in personality development and in psychopathology. This stress has tended to focus the attention of individual and group therapists on the reactivation of early object relations in relation to the mother in the therapeutic process as well. An illustration of this trend is Stone's (1961) depiction of the classical psychoanalytic situation as representing on the unconscious level ". . . the superimposed series of basic separation experiences in the child's relation to his mother" (p. 35). More specifically, Stone viewed the analyst as representing what he termed "the mother of separation" as contrasted with the mother image associated with intimate bodily care.

In a previous publication of a decade ago (Scheidlinger, 1964) which dealt with the individual group members' identification with the group-as-a-whole, I defined identification (as distinct from transference and real object relations) as an endopsychic process calling for a degree of individual involvement with a perceived object or its symbolic representation. I hypothesized further that identification with the group entity entailed the following two related elements: (1) ascribing to the group an emotional meaning, i.e., as an instrument for need satisfaction or, on a genetically "deeper" level, as a mother symbol; (2) a self-involvement in the group, a "giving up" of an aspect of personal identity—from the *I* to the *We*—which can serve irrational purposes as well as those of adaptation or growth. I finally wondered whether, in a broader sense, the universal human need to belong, to establish a state of psychological unity with others, did not represent a covert wish to restore an earlier state of unconflicted well-being inherent in the infant's exclusive union with the mother to counteract a fundamental fear of abandonment and of aloneness in all of us. Continued observations of relevant aspects of group behavior since that time have strengthened my belief in the basic plausibility of the above hypotheses and have also led me to a search for additional data from current object-relations theory for their further elaboration.

Perhaps because of the impetus from the so-called "British School," recent psychoanalytic writings in America about early object relations have multiplied and have dwelled in considerably greater detail than did Freud on aspects of this crucial phase of development. Although Melanie Klein asserted that the infant's ego is capable in the first three months of life of perceiving and integrating parts of the first object, i.e., the mother's breast, serious questions have been raised by others whether an infant could conceivably be assumed to possess the perceptual capacity to accomplish this. Jacobson (1964) insists that for the baby to be able to relate psychologically to something external to himself which satisfies his bodily needs, he would have had to have passed through at least a rudimentary phase of ego development. This involves ". . . the laying down of memory traces, the organization of experiential states and the beginning ability perceptually to differentiate between the self and the object" (p. 34). Using Freud's better known terminology, the infant's transition from primary narcissism to secondary narcissism calls for some degree of reality-geared representations of self and of the maternal object and the perception of the latter as the source of tension relief and of need gratification. Only with this rudimentary recognition is the infant believed to experience anxiety in the absence of the mothering figure (Edgecumbe and Burgner, 1973). In this connection, Anna Freud (1965) postulated a separate stage of a *need-satisfying relationship* which falls developmentally between the phase of *primary narcissism* and that of *object-constancy*. This stage of a *need-satisfying relationship*, while still characterized by the baby's unique egocentricity, coupled with a symbiotic perception of the mother as a gratifier of needs, nevertheless represents an advance from primary narcissism in which a primitive state of experiential pleasure is assumed to prevail, devoid of any differentiation whatsoever between self and object-representations. According to Jacobson (1964), there is an ongoing conflict in the child between the wish to maintain this dependent, need-satisfying style of relating and opposing forces striving for independent ego-functioning. This conflict is believed to continue till the onset of the oedipal period.

In general, then, the term *need-satisfying relationship* refers to a specific mode of relating wherein the maternal object's need-satisfying functions are paramount. Furthermore, the maternal object is perceived as separate from the self only at moments of need; at other times, from the infant's subjective point of view, the object is believed to cease to exist as "somewhere out there." There is broad consensus in the literature that this phase of the need-satisfying relationship lasts from three months until the age of about 18 months. Gradually, this stage is believed to be supplanted by the psychologically more advanced stage of *object constancy*, in which concern for the mothering figure as an object takes precedence over her mere need-gratifying functions.

In returning to the earlier noted hypothesis regarding an aspect of identification with the group entity connoting a covert wish of group members to restore a state of unconflicted well-being characteristic of an earlier tie to the mother, I would like to be more specific. The group members' covert wish refers very likely to a yearning for a return to the need-gratifying relationship which I have just outlined. In this context I want to emphasize that the symbolic "mother-group" is accordingly perceived in purely positive, nonconflictual terms.

Guntrip (1961) related this phase of the child's positive early relationship to the mystic's experience of unity with the Deity, to Plato's "Idea of the Good," as well as to Freud's notion of an oceanic feeling, ". . . an indissoluble connection, of belonging inseparably to the external world as a whole" (p. 361). Guntrip felt, as I do, that this ". . . sense of identity or unity must be the basis of all kinds of feelings of oneness in both personal and communal living" (p. 362).

As I have noted elsewhere, the regressive emotional pulls which characterize the early group formative stages in unstructured groups tend to loosen the individual's self boundaries and to reactivate primitive wishes and modes of early object relations, including identifications. Such regressive patterns are not necessarily pathological insofar as even in the most mature personalities the infantile, need-satisfying modes of relating persist and are subject to reactivation at moments of threat and of anxiety. Greenacre (1972) asserted in this connection that ". . . the introjective-projective reaction leading ultimately to individuation, characteristic of the early stages of life, is never lost and may be revived with special strength in any situation of stress sufficient to cause a feeling of helplessness" (p. 147).

Similarly, Schafer (1968) stated that in the realm of primary process emotionality (which, as I have noted, characterizes the anxiety-laden period of group formation) ". . . the 'lost' object is not someone who will, it is hoped, return in the future: he is someone who still exists, though he is out of sight, touch, hearing, behind a wall, shattered, and so forth" (p. 222).

As mentioned, the most extensive discussion in the literature to date of the concept of the "mother-group" appeared in a recent paper by Gibbard and Hartman (1973) which is based on observations drawn from "self-analytic" classroom groups of college students. These authors not only found that the group entity was perceived by its members in a maternal vein but also that this shared unconscious fantasy comprised a splitting of the "good" mother image from the "bad." The "good" mother entailed nurturant and protective aspects; the "bad" mother, abandoning and destructive ones. The group members employed splitting ". . . to avoid both a state in which 'good' and 'bad' cannot be differentiated and a state in which both are experienced at the same time (genuine ambivalence)" (p. 127). These authors stressed, furthermore, that the utopian perception of the group as a benevolent maternal figure was a manifestation of defensiveness against dealing with painful intragroup conflicts. More specifically, according to Gibbard and Hartman ". . . the 'good' group functions as a defense both against the primitive, 'bad' engulfing and/or sadistic group (mother) and the fully heterosexual, oedipal group (which is no longer so clearly equated with the mother)" (p. 129).

I welcome Gibbard and Hartman's (1973) path of inquiry into the broader realm of group psychological regression and specifically into that of the relatively neglected concept of the "mother-group." While, as they have noted, there is much congruence between my earlier hypotheses regarding identification with the group-as-a-whole (1964) and their recent observations, I nevertheless would like to raise some questions here from the framework of group psychotherapy. To begin with, apart from Durkin's (1964) hypothesized split transference in which the group is perceived by the patients as a threatening pre-oedipal mother figure, with the therapist becoming the "good, all-giving omnipotent mother," I could find no reference in the group therapy literature to the kind of "bad" mother perception of the group entity which is stressed by Gibbard and Hartman (1973). Most other group therapists, as is evident from my earlier review of the relevant literature, refer to the group entity as being perceived in a benign maternal vein, on the one hand, with the *therapist* becoming the feared parental transference figure, on the other. Similarly, fears of abandonment by and of fusion with the group collectivity have been touched on only in rare instances in the American literature in connection with individual patients characterized by ego pathology in whom concern with self-object boundaries is marked. It should be noted in contrast that W. R. Bion (1960) and other British followers of Melanie Klein, such as Jaques (1970), have repeatedly written regarding group members' fears of engulfment by the group to the point of claiming that individual group belonging always entails a defense against loss of identity stemming from primitive, "psychotic" anxieties. (Jaques, to my knowledge, however, never referred to the group as a maternal image, while Bion made occasional references to the group entity's being perceived only as parts of the mother's body, in line with Kleinian postulates of part-objects.)

A number of possibilities suggest themselves as explanations here. It could be that the phenomena described by Gibbard and Hartman (1973) are in some way unique to short-term analytic classroom groups with their "normal" constituency, with assigned readings, an examination, and final grades. These groups are undoubtedly different in character from long-term psychotherapy groups with their composition of designated patients and their explicit goals of "repairing" identified personality pathology. (I was, in this connection, puzzled by the authors' occasional references in their paper to working through of conflicts or to "exploring in depth" the defensive nature of fantasies, which suggests, to me at least, a blurring of the aims of education and of therapy.)

There is also a question whether the verbal and nonverbal behavior noted in these classroom groups during their early periods of "manifest utopianism" might be subject to different theoretical explanations by others. Conversely, it is of course possible, too, that therapy groups would abound in the very same manifestations described by Gibbard and Hartman were it not for conscious or unconscious interferences with their open expression. For instance, in their understandable desire to prevent an unduly high anxiety level, especially in the groups' initial phase, group therapists might well be unwittingly discouraging the emergence of negative feelings toward the group entity. This would serve to reinforce the very mechanisms of repression and denial which Gibbard and Hartman postulated.

To answer such questions we obviously need carefully controlled observations of the relevant phases of group processes in therapy and other small groups, preferably by trained observers other than the therapists. These would not only serve to test the different hypotheses regarding the nature of the related individual and collective perceptions of the group entity in a maternal or perhaps other vein, but would also help to differentiate between the nature of these group manifestations in self-analytic and T-groups, on the one hand, and "true" therapy groups, on the other.

Pending such observations, I prefer to maintain the earlier stated, more parsimonious hypotheses regarding the perception of the group entity. In brief, according to these, the initial phase of unstructured therapy groups is characterized by nonpathological, regressive perceptions and relationships of all aspects of the group situation: of the leader, of the other group members, and of the group-as-a-whole. From a genetic, developmental viewpoint, these perceptions and relationships represent a reactivation, in the face of the individual and collective stresses and anxieties induced by group formation, of early patterns and especially of primitive identifications, including the search for the kind of nonconflictual, need-gratifying relationship to the mother which I discussed earlier in this paper. While the group entity is accordingly perceived in a positive and benign image, the group leader and the other members become almost immediately the objects of a gamut of partially ambivalent but largely hostile and fearful attitudes. As noted by Ruiz (1972) with reference to T-groups, and by Arsenian, Semrad, and Shapiro (1962) to therapy groups, when negative feelings thus aroused threaten the group's cohesiveness and basically positive climate, there is a tendency to displace negative feelings onto the leader, thus preserving the groups supportive character. While any perception or behavioral item can admittedly serve defensive purposes, I would like to await further evidence before accepting Gibbard and Hartman's conclusions regarding the regularity with which the members' perceptions of the benign "mother-group" represent an unwillingness "to come to grips with intragroup conflicts and other painful realities of group life." For it is also possible that this very perception is progressively utilized by both the members and by the therapist in the service of the "therapeutic alliance" or of group maintenance and cohesiveness so that the intragroup conflicts and personal problems can be subjected to analytic scrutiny in the context of an anxiety level which is not too threatening to the equilibrium of individual patients and of the group entity.

The complex theoretical issues posed by any attempt to scrutinize the conscious and unconscious aspects of concepts such as that of the "mother-group" tend to reaffirm the urgent need to try to differentiate descriptively in group psychology between individual and collective phenomena, as well as between identifications and transferences, on the one hand, and reality-geared perceptions, on the other. I would accordingly question the generally loose application of the term transference to either an individual or to a shared perception of the group entity in a maternal vein. For, in my view, transference as a concept pertains to an apperception in relation to a *person*, and moreover to a repetition in the present of a relatively advanced past relationship where there has been some degree of differentiation between the self and the object. The perceptions and object relations in the earliest phase of group formation, including the perception of the "mother-group," are better connoted as various kinds of identifications which, in the psychoanalytic hierarchy of object relations, precede real object ties. This is congruent with Kaplan and Roman's (1963) views on group development in therapy groups. Interestingly, too, Abraham (1973) recently claimed to have *experimental* support for her contention that there are many more primitive kinds of object relations at work in therapy groups than transferences.

It should be noted here that, in the strictest sense of the word, "identification" or "transference" represents an explanatory construct. Each pertains to inferred processes which can be utilized to explain certain kinds of social behavior. Furthermore, in scrutinizing any item of an individual's behavior in a group, one must try to differentiate, as Couch (1961) has suggested, among (1) underlying needs, (2) concealment defenses, (3) apperception of interpersonal forces, and (4) reaction to the behavioral press of overt acts of others. In this connection, group therapists must differentiate also between direct expressions of genuine needs, i.e., need for a mothering relationship, and defensive exaggerations or minimization of needs. There is also the issue of distinguishing such needs from shared fantasies which might be employed as a means of gratifying these needs.

What I termed in a previous publication the *early dependency phase* in a therapy group is characterized, in addition to the prevalence of multiple individual and group identifications, by poor reality perceptions and much magical thought, including oral fantasies. This phase is supplanted by a more advanced one in which transferences and real object ties predominate, with realistic perceptions including sexual and aggressive expressions.

I would concur with the many writers who have pointed to a probable link between our "age of anxiety" and the unprecedented recent popularity of varied experiential growth groups. The latter are sought out in people's search for intimacy, for enhanced self-esteem and sense of identity, and perhaps on a deeper level for support from a benign "mother-group." In this connection, in writing about our new human problems related to the unprecedented rate of societal change, Toffler (1970) envisioned stability zones, love networks, and time-limited supportive groups for people undergoing adaptational crises in order for them to experience, if only briefly, identification with others as well as the support of a benign group entity.

One might be justified in claiming, then, that when the small group is viewed as a helping system, not only do its members need the leader-worker and each other but also the group-as-a-group! Furthermore, in this context the crucial question is *not* how the leader-worker perceives the situation but how the group member does. These aspects have remained neglected for too long.

Summary

In this paper the concept of the "mother-group" has been subjected to special scrutiny. A historical review of the literature reveals increasing references during the last decade to group members' perceptions of the group entity in a maternal vein.

A previously stated hypothesis of mine which related individual members' identification with the group-as-a-whole to an unconscious wish to restore an earlier state of unconflicted union with the mother has been developed in greater detail and tied more specifically to a yearning for a return to the child's purely positive "need-gratifying relationship," which Anna Freud has postulated as occurring developmentally between the phases of "primary narcissism" and that of "object constancy".

In contradistinction to some writers' views of the early phase of group development as regularly containing simultaneous perceptions of a threatening "mother-group" image, it is suggested that, pending further objective observations of therapy groups, it is more likely that the leader and the other group members, rather than the group-as-a-whole, are the objects of such early fearful and hostile feelings.

In order to attain the much-desired theoretical clarity in the group process field generally and in group psychotherapy specifically, the need for attempting to differentiate between individual and collective phenomena, on the one hand, and among identifications, transferences, and reality-geared perceptions, on the other hand, is reaffirmed.

A possible link between the recent mushrooming of various kinds of experiential "growth" groups and people's need for enhanced self-esteem and support from perhaps a benign "mother-group" in this age of anxiety is suggested.

References

Abraham, A., (1973), A Model for Exploring Intra- and Interindividual Process in Groups. *Int. J. Group Psychother.*, 23:3–22.

Arsenian, J., Semrad, E. V., and Shapiro, D. (1962), An Analysis of Integral Functions in Small Groups. *Int. J. Group Psychother.*, 12:421–434.

Bion, W. R. (1960), *Experiences in Groups.* New York: Basic Books

Couch, A. S. (1961), The Psychological Determinants of Interpersonal Behavior. In: *Proceedings of the Fourteenth International Congress of Applied Psychology.* Copenhagen: Munksgaard.

Durkin, H. E., (1964), *The Group in Depth.* New York: International Universities Press.

Edgecombe, R., and Burgner, M. (1973), Some Problems in the Conceptualization of Early Object Relationships. *The Psychoanal. Study Child,* 27:283–314. New York: Quadrangle Books.

Foulkes, S. H. (1964), *Therapeutic Group Analysis.* New York: International Universities Press.

Freud, A. (1965), *Normality and Pathology in Childhood.* New York: International Universities Press.

Freud, S. (1921), *Group Psychology and the Analysis of the Ego.* London: Hogarth Press, 1948.

Gibbard, G. S., and Hartman, J. J. (1973), The Significance of Utopian Fantasies in

Small Groups. *Int. J. Group Psychother.*, 23:125–147.

Greenacre, P. (1972), Crowds and Crisis: Psychoanalytic Considerations. *The Psychoanalytic Study of the Child*, 27:136–154. New York: Quadrangle Books.

Grotjahn, M. (1972), Learning from Dropout Patients. *Int. J. Group Psychother.*, 22:287–305.

Guntrip, H. (1961), *Personality Structure and Human Interaction*. New York: International Universities Press.

Jacobson, E. (1964), *The Self and the Object World*. New York: International Universities Press.

Jaques, E. (1970), *Work, Creativity and Social Justice*. New York: International Universities Press.

Kaplan, S. and Roman, M. S. (1963), Phases of Development in Adult Therapy Groups. *Int. J. Group Psychother.*, 13:10–26.

Money-Kyrle, R. (1950), Varieties of Group Formation. In: *Psychoanalysis and the Social Sciences*, ed. G. Roheim. New York: International Universities Press.

Redl, F. (1942), Group Emotion and Leadership. *Psychiatry*, 5:573–596.

Ruiz, P. (1972), On the Perception of the "Mother-Group" in T-Groups. *Int. J. Group Psychother.*, 22:488–491.

Schafer, R. (1968), *Aspects of Internalization*. New York: International Universities Press.

Scheidlinger, S. (1955), The Concept of Identification in Group Psychotherapy. *Am. J. Psychother.*, 9:661–672.

—— (1964), Identification, The Sense of Belonging and of Identity in Small Groups. *Int. J. Group Psychother.*, 14:291–306.

Schindler, W. (1951), Family Pattern in Group Formation and Therapy. *Inter. J. Group Psychother.*, 1:100–105.

—— (1952), The Group Personality Concept in Group Psychotherapy. *Int. J. Group Psychother.*, 2:311–315.

—— (1966), The Role of the Mother in Group Psychotherapy. *Int. J. Group Psychother.*, 16:198–200.

Slater, P. E. (1966), *Microcosm*. New York: John Wiley.

Slavson, S. R. (1964), *A Textbook in Analytic Group Psychotherapy*. New York: International Universities Press.

Stone, L. (1961), *The Psychoanalytic Situation*. New York: International Universities Press.

Toffler, A. (1970), *Future Shock*. New York: Bantam Books.

Activity-Interview
Group Psychotherapy:
Theory, Principles, and Practice

MORTIMER SCHIFFER

Mortimer Schiffer was a science teacher in the 1930s when he became involved with S. R. Slavson through volunteer work. This led to a change in career and the two worked closely together over many years. Schiffer has made a number of contributions to the child group psychotherapy literature over a period spanning 1946 to 1977. He participated in the elaboration of many of the specialized treatments for children such as Activity Group Therapy, Activity-Interview Group Psychotherapy, and Play Group Therapy. He developed the Therapeutic Play Group for use in public elementary schools in 1950. Schiffer developed many group-based programs within the school system and trained staff to conduct them.

Schiffer made an important contribution with his edited volume of Slavson's principal writings (Slavson SR. Dynamics of Group Psychotherapy. New York: Aronson, 1979). His Preface to that volume provides a comprehensive summary of the origins of group psychotherapy in America.

This paper was presented at the American Group Psychotherapy Association Annual Conference in 1975.

Schiffer M: Activity-interview group psychotherapy: theory, principles and practice. *International Journal of Group Psychotherapy* 27:377–388, 1977.

Activity group therapy (AGT), an ego-level method of treatment in which interpretations of behavior are eschewed, was the progenitor of all existing, fundamental forms of group therapy with children and of the various methods of group treatment of all ages. It was first employed in 1934 at the Madeline Borg Child Guidance Institute of the Jewish Board of Guardians in New York City by its inventor, S. R. Slavson. This clinically designed method, properly utilized, remains the treatment of choice for a large majority of emotionally troubled, latency-age children (Slavson, 1943; Scheidlinger, 1947; Slavson and Schiffer, 1975). A basic principle of AGT is that defects in children's personalities and characters and attendant behavioral manifestations are attributable in the main to experience, and they can be subsequently modified by corrective experience in a therapeutically conditioned environment.

As experience with AGT broadened, it was found that some latency-age children did not respond sufficiently because they were too deeply disturbed. These children, in addition to behavioral disturbances, had symptoms of anxiety and guilt, unusual fears and other intense emotions stemming from neurotic etiology (Gabriel, 1934; Rosenthal and Nagelberg, 1956; Coolidge and Grunebaum, 1964). Many of these children would not, or could not, respond to individual analytic treatment. Other group methods had to be devised in which discussion would be employed in addition to play and simple work activities. Slavson, in 1937, evolved the theory, principles, and practices underlying Activity-Interview group psychotherapy (A-IGP) (Slavson, 1945, 1947, 1955).

A-IGP addresses itself to the internal sources of children's psychic conflicts within the limits of their emotional and intellectual capacities and their tolerance for analytic inquiry and interpretation. This is accomplished through interviews with individual children and group discussions that are carried on at opportune times during treatment sessions. Through exploration of individual and group play, fantasies, work activities, and other forms of individual and interindividual communications, both verbal and nonverbal, some of the underlying meanings of manifest behavior, attitudes, and feelings are brought to light. Explanations and interpretations are sensitively presented by the therapist when timely, and also later by the children when, heartened by initial gains through this new experience, they become motivated to seek for meanings themselves.

The therapist lays the groundwork for the group discussion during early sessions to familiarize the children. Sometime during the latter part of the first session he invites them to come together around a small table. It can be expected that some may delay sitting, whether from shyness or defiance or perhaps from a desire to test the therapist. When most are seated the therapist begins by explaining that there will be a "talking" part in each session when the children can speak about problems. He states in words to this effect: "I think you probably know that you came to the group because you had some problems in getting along, some at home, some at school, and some in both, and that you are not happy about it. Here we want to talk about it and see if we can make things better for ourselves. Who would like to start?"

If, after waiting a short time, no child responds, the therapist turns to one who would be least threatened in his estimation and asks: "Johnny, why do you think you were sent to the group?" Johnny's response may be monosyllabic or more extensive depending on the degree of his outgoingness and aggression, but in either circumstance the therapist carefully probes for elaboration by inviting others to comment on Johnny's response, to add to it, or to volunteer similar experiences of their own. Judging by events and the ease of communication that evolves, the therapist may permit discussion to flow independently. During these preliminary group discussions the therapist may make casual reference to an incident that occurred during the early part of a session which, in his estimation, has a meaningful relationship to a child's problem. It could be a remark such as: "Did anyone notice how Peter was banging the wood before and how angry he looked?" Or, "Joan and Selma seemed to be really upset about the torn picture." It is unwise in the beginning to pursue any child's disclosure in depth. At all times the therapist must be sensitive to children's feelings and their tolerance limits, which is possible only when he possesses comprehensive knowledge of each child's total problem and can correctly assess the nature and adequacies of each child's defenses.

It must be borne in mind that sessions in A-IGP cannot be administered within a rigid, strictly adhered-to format with which children can be expected to comply by seating themselves at stated times for the "talking" part of each session. Not only will their behavior and unforeseen events operate from time to time to delay, challenge, or temporarily cancel such parts of a session, but the therapist himself may decide in the light of an ongoing general colloquy in the group not to interrupt.

Psychotherapy of children encounters resistance, as with adolescents and adults, but it is significantly less than with the latter. In accordance with their psychology and constitutional predisposition children for the most part tend to act out more directly negative feelings that arise. However, the nature and meaning of the acting out behavior of children are different from that of adults. When adult patients act out, it is a form of resistance; with children it is a form of meaningful communication, seemingly inappropriate at the moment but congruous with their basic feelings.

In addition to group discussions another significant level of communication takes place between the therapist and individual children through interviews that occur playfully and sometimes adventitiously during sessions. The therapist usually initiates these, although later, in an advanced state, a child may independently seek out the therapist. An interview may start with a reflection of a child's remark or a reference to an element of his play, an incident that is occurring between children, or some other meaningful situation. Many opportunities will arise to facilitate the therapist's approach to each child: a picture or clay object being worked out, an unusual emotion that may be expressed, such as sudden anger, fear, jollity, etc. Or, in the absence of these, the therapist may merely inquire, "How are things today?" Any of these openings usually leads to dialogue which may be utilized therapeutically. It is apparent that, unlike AGT, in which the therapist remains peripheral to the group for the most part and deliberately avoids initiating activities, while maintaining a consistent, accepting neutral role, the therapist in A-IGP does initiate contact with the children.

With the passage of time, as the children come to know each other, more incidents arise of a nature to evoke strong emotions and also enable the therapist to become involved. This occurred in one instance when two girls struggled fiercely over possession of a doll. These girls had previously demonstrated much sibling rivalry in their behavior toward each other, a displacement from actual rivalries in their respective families. The therapist said simply, "You're angry with each other." This direct observation opened a floodgate of angry recriminations of child against child, which slowly ebbed in response to the suasive, meaningful inquiry of the therapist into the details of the incident and the emotional responses of the girls, and finally, also, in response to their own grudging but more reflective contributions.

There are times when cathartic expression is sufficient *without* exploring the latent or even conscious meanings. For example, a child may unconsciously divulge his angry feelings toward a parent by displaced acting out against the therapist, perhaps in generalized defiant behavior, banging or sawing a piece of wood vigorously and haphazardly without any intention of making something, wasting paper, or in other ways that represent negative transference behavior. The therapist, in passing, may say, "I guess you're pretty angry today, Mike." Note the avoidance of, "It looks like you're angry with *me* today," which actually may be the case but which would arouse guilt or defensiveness on the child's part. As in all forms of analytic therapy, adolescents and adults included, but especially so with children, there are times when abreaction is sufficient unto itself without intervention.

As children become accustomed to the therapist's investigative role in interviews and in group discussions, and as they participate more actively in learning about the less conscious meanings of their emotions and behavior, they become more relaxed, especially as they begin to feel the sanguine effects of psychotherapy. Moreover, as they feel free to express conflicted, suppressed thoughts and feelings, the children will at times become "auxiliary therapists" and offer their own appraisals of each other's behavior, thus furthering and encouraging the therapeutic process. As the scope of discussions extend, the children are enabled to deal in even greater depth with both individual and common problems, and the therapist finds it less needful to be an initiator or facilitator.

The acquisition in therapy of true psychological *insight* (not understanding) is a complex process. Through the fusion of many perceptions and thoughts and accompanied by emotional catharsis the patient eventually learns how early life experiences are related to his symptoms and behavior and how his resistances and other defense mechanisms evolved to cope with inner stresses. Obviously, pre-pubertal children lack the ideational capacities, particularly the inductive reasoning power, and the *need* for such depth-integrated insight, and consequently the motivation. Children are mostly concerned with the here-and-now of their unhappiness, frustrations, disappointments, developmental task failures, anxieties, fears, and other disabling emotions. While it is undeniably true that some of these have neurotic origins, it does not follow that the children are capable of discerning this in analytic depth. It would be exceedingly difficult and unwise, for example, were a therapist to attempt to bring his child-patient to a real understanding of the incestuous nature of his oedipal drive or to relate his selfish, grasping possessiveness to anal determinants and repetitive water play to urethral preoccupation.

The child's capacity to sense changes within himself and in his behavior that come about in therapy is known as *derivative insight*. Derivative insight is the child's consciousness of newly acquired and increased capacities to cope with situations wherein he felt lacking before, which leads to an improved self-image, a feeling of status in the group, and social success. Derivative insight does not flow from single acts or from interpretations given by the therapist, though such experiences may act as critical events integrating and strongly reinforcing gains already made in treatment. Rather, after a period of time in therapy, during which the debilitating effects of a rigidized superego have been reduced and much ego strengthening has occurred, the child reflectively begins to see himself in a new light.

As was noted earlier, most children who are treated in A-IGP, in addition to behavioral difficulties, have neurotic traits and incipient symptoms associated with the oedipal conflict. Pre-pubertal children can tolerate the expression and examination of libidinal feelings, among others, because these feelings have not yet become sexualized as a consequence of puberty and adolescence. Once the crises of adolescence come into play, resistance to the analytic therapies increases enormously.

Because of the assurance and relaxation the children acquire in the positive transference to the therapist, internalized feelings and thoughts surface through less threatening play that then becomes subject to sensitive exploration by the technique described earlier. The extraordinary cathexes attached to the emotional material are dissolved through a combination of active, motoric play, which in itself has a de-energizing effect, and through the interviews and group discussions that promote more reflection and some cognitive awareness in the child. The result is that neurotic traits are sloughed off permanently without the process of working through that is essential in the analytic treatment of adults. This is possible in latency-age children because of the uncrystallized nature of their personalities and characters and the still germinal state of their ego defenses which enables new, corrective experiences in psychotherapy to be internalized. Adolescents and adults cannot respond in this manner because their personalities, character structures, and ego defenses have become rigidified.

In all types of analytic therapy children demonstrate a readiness to "understand" themselves only after they feel they are understood.

Therefore, there is therapeutic advantage when the therapist early in treatment succeeds in conveying something meaningful to the child through interpretation. Such an experience makes the child an ally in treatment. Melanie Klein stated, "The way back to the unconscious (in the child) is easier to find." We might add: especially when the child becomes a willing guide.

Children should not be overwhelmed with interpretations beyond their capacities to comprehend them or beyond that which is psychologically utilizable by them. Moreover, the therapist needs to be mindful of the timing of interpretations in accordance with his patients' emotional readiness. Excessive interpretation overloads children (also adolescents and adults) and has no merit. In the simplest terms possible the therapist should state what is necessary and stop there. Assimilation of meanings is the child's task, and this task requires time, as do most changes that come about through therapy. The effects of therapy are really felt mostly in the intervals between treatment sessions, when the experiences have had sufficient time to become psychologically integrated.

The term "explanation" is perhaps more accurate psychologically than "interpretation" because of children's limited thought and ideational capabilities. An explanation by a therapist is more than didactic information. In practice, it may consist of a verbalized observation by the therapist, perhaps a reflection of a child's remarks with an added, leading comment or question, or an elucidation of a child's momentary feeling, attitude, or behavior by pointing to similar responses that occurred at other times.

The group process provides ample opportunities for involving several children at once so that the therapist's observations and explanations touch upon the children's life experiences and attendant problems more extensively.

> Robert places a small infant doll headfirst into a toy toilet bowl, angrily hitting it on the buttocks. He then examines its desperate state, feet sticking up in the air. Catching the eye of the observing therapist, he appears guilty. Sandy spots this play and says laughingly, "Look at that." Robert, as if his "secret" has been exposed, is silent. Therapist: "He's upside down." Robert nods. Sandy says, almost hopefully, "Maybe he'll drown." No response from Robert. Therapist: "Maybe he did something to make you angry." Robert: "Yeah." Then Sandy adds, "Babies are no good." The therapist affirms that, "Babies do get lots of attention." This was all the encouragement Robert needed. He began to speak angrily of his feelings about his infant sibling and his sense of rejection. He and Sandy spoke quite openly, now encouraged by the discovery that they shared a common source of irritation, younger siblings. The therapist listened, occasionally nodding. Toward the end he offered: "It's not easy getting used to new babies after you've been the only one. Mother and father get so busy with them they kind of forget you're around. I can see why you sometimes wish babies would go away."

The therapist's condensed "explanation" of what was obviously being communicated by the children gave further impetus to their frustration and anger, which was then expressed in an animated manner. The therapist did not contribute interpretively beyond helping Robert to "open up" the floodgates of formerly unexpressed anger toward a younger sibling. For the present this was sufficient. Time and subsequent interviews and group discussions can extend such emotive discharges into more reflective levels.

In A-IGP, the therapist also performs an important educational function in that he is a source of accurate information on matters important to his patients but about which they are uninformed, poorly informed, or even misinformed. Children are receptive to information and explanations on subjects or situations that generate common anxiety. This can be an instance, for example, where a boy reveals that he has seen for the first time a person without a penis (infant, girl, or woman), or a girl describes the reverse. Or during a group discussion a child bursts out, "Babies come out of the back. You know, the tushy." In one therapy group the therapist brought pictorial illustrations of the human body, male and female, that visualized interior organs and intrauterine fetal development. This was done to clarify the children's discussion in a prior session.

The therapist makes a point of coming into contact with all the children in A-IGP because, as in all analytic treatment, the relation between patient and therapist is fundamental. Interviews with individual children not only help them work out problems that are troubling them but also fosters emotional closeness to the therapist. Children need such contact and kindness on a personal level, in addition to the other therapeutic experiences treatment in a group may provide.

At times, children's tensions and frustrations will be manifested in acting-out behavior, producing a disorderly, even chaotic climate. This becomes attenuated either spontaneously after cathartic discharge or through the therapist's intervention that helps transmute acting out to investigation of behavior through discussion. Despite intensification of emotions that temporarily discomfit the children or make them feel guilty or anxious about the consequences of boisterous behavior, they remain in treatment because of the essential positive transference to the therapist.

Hostile and other strong feelings related to parents and siblings, suppressed out of a fear of consequences, can be safely enacted in the therapist's presence with libido-activating materials that change primitive impulses into less baleful forms. When the therapist explores the "tableau" of the children's play sensitively, nonjudgmentally, correctly touching on both manifest and underlying meanings, the cathartic advantage to the children associated with such play is magnified greatly. It is as if the therapist, in putting words to deeds (the children's play), assists them in surmounting the too constricting, over-punitive superego. Because the therapist's accepting manner and explanations give credence to the essentially symbolic play, and also demonstrate his understanding, the positive transference becomes further enhanced and more benign superego forces begin to supplant unhealthy ones. The therapist does not deny the reality of the children's intense feelings and urges, nor through manner or word lend them approval. Rather, through his verbalizations and demeanor he accepts the children's need to ventilate blocked feelings, intimating their justifiability when indicated, and suggests alternative ways of coping. Above all, the therapist conveys to all his clients the global sense that real feelings betrayed in play or impulsively shouted out in group discussions need not be disastrous.

A-IGP is eminently suitable for latency-age children with behavior problems complicated by oedipal components, unusual fears, anxiety, and such symptoms as sleeplessness, enuresis and sexual preoccupations disharmonious to a child's phase of development. If symptoms are many and intense, individual therapy may be necessary in addition to group treatment.

There is greater latitude in selecting clients for A-IGP and also in grouping them than in nonanalytic group therapy, such as AGT, in which the psychological balance of a group is a critical element. In AGT fractious situations are resolved by the built-in "checks and balances" inherent in the correct selections of clientele and their proper grouping. This is essentially therapy *by* the group. This is different from A-IGP, where, as in analytic group treatment generally, therapy is of the patient *in* a group. As has been indicated earlier, in A-IGP the therapist's interventions in the group's arguments, dissensions, and other abrasive interactions help restore order.

Despite the greater range of clients acceptable in A-IGP, there are some problem types which are counterindicated. These include children who are sadistically aggressive, who have severe behavior disorders, those with pronounced homosexual tendencies, severe sibling rivalry, or strong affect hunger, and, in general, children who tend to act out impulsively and motorically and who would be insufficiently responsive to interventions. Also excluded from A-IGP are schizophrenic, psychopathic, or brain-damaged children and those with combined psycho-organic conditions of a severe nature.

Five or six is the maximum number of children for an analytic group, a lesser number than in AGT where eight is optimal. The demands of analytic procedures and the more personal relationship needs of the patients for the therapist necessarily limit the size of the group. Groups may be homogeneous as to sex or mixed. In the latter case the therapist may be of either sex, but in the former the therapist should be of the same sex as the patients. Mixed groups have value in fostering discussions related to sex differences, conception, pregnancy, births, and related matters of interest to all children.

Group sessions are held once or twice weekly for ninety minutes to two hours. The room is similar in size and furnishings to that used for

AGT (Slavson and Schiffer, 1975). Toilet facilities should be attached to the meeting room or immediately nearby to avoid children's separation from the group. Arrangements need to be made for parents, who usually accompany their children, to wait in a lounge or other facility at some distance from the group treatment room. It is inadvisable to permit parents easy access to the therapist in the presence of the children before, during, or immediately after group sessions if situations that might complicate the therapist's role and arouse disturbance in the children are to be avoided.

The materials used in A-IGP are selected for their libido-evoking properties. They should lend themselves to fantasy enactments in play and to the expression of anal, oral, urethral, and sexual preoccupations, with the confusions, anxieties, and fears that hypercathect these developmental phases. The recommended materials are water, watercolors, crayons, paints, plasticine, objects representing family members such as dolls and hand puppets of both sexes, and a doll house with furniture. Also useful are several handpuppet heads of birds or animals that represent power and danger, e.g., lion, hawk, that children can use to express violent feelings in sublimated fashion; also, two or three face masks depicting fearsome, imaginary, fantasy creatures, e.g., witch, devil, including one benign one such as a fairy godmother.

Occasionally, children will make some simple objects out of wood, using a few tools and other materials that are available: several hammers, light saws, nails, and narrow pieces of soft wood. These facilitate the release of aggression through banging and active sawing.

Only a limited snack, cookies and milk, is offered during group sessions and preferably at times other than when children assemble for the "talking" part. It is important that food—its nature, preparation, and method of serving—*not* become a central feature, as it is in AGT where assembling for refreshments is an important event in every session. The fundamental analytic approach to A-IGP would be interfered with by elaborate repasts. Moreover, food and other indulgences offered by the therapist, including small gifts and other items, make it more difficult for children to discharge negative transference feelings toward the therapist, which is an essential part of psychotherapy.

References

Coolidge, J. C., and Grunebaum, M. (1964), Individual and Group Therapy of a Latency Age Child, *Int. J. Group Psychother.*, 14:84–96.

Gabriel, B. (1939), An Experiment in Group Treatment. *Amer. J. Orthopsychiat.*, 9:146–169.

Rosenthal, L., and Nagelberg, L. (1956), Limitations of Activity Group Therapy: A Case Presentation. *Inter. J. Group Psychother.*, 6:166–179.

Scheidlinger, S. (1947), Activity Group Therapy with Primary Behavior Disorders.

In: *The Practice of Group Therapy*, ed. S. R. Slavson. New York: International Universities Press.

Schiffer, M. (1969), *The Therapeutic Play Group*. New York: Grune & Stratton.

Slavson, S. R. (1943), *An Introduction to Group Therapy*. New York: Commonwealth Fund.

——— (1945), Differential Methods of Group Therapy in Relation to Age Levels. *Nervous Child*, 4:196–209.

——— (1947), Differential Dynamics of Activity and Interview Group Therapy. *Amer. J. Orthopsychiat.*, 17:293–302.

——— (1952), *An Introduction to Group Therapy*. New York: International Universities Press.

——— (1955), Criteria for Selection and Rejection of Patients for Various Types of Group Psychotherapy. *Int. J. Group Psychother.*, 5:3–28.

———, and Schiffer, M. ,(1975), *Group Psychotherapies for Children. A Textbook*. New York: International Universities Press.

The Working Alliance in Analytic Group Psychotherapy

HENRIETTE T. GLATZER, PH.D.

At the beginning of her career, Henrietta Glatzer worked with Helen Durkin in Brooklyn under the supervision of John Levy. Together they co-authored a paper concerning their experiences (Durkin HE, Glatzer HT, Hirsch JS. Therapy of mothers in groups. American Journal of Orthopsychiatry 14:68–76, 1944). The careers of Durkin and Glatzer have run in close parallel. Both worked in child psychotherapy with Slavson and both were Training Analysts at the Postgraduate Center for Mental Health in New York City. Glatzer has remained a leader in AGPA throughout her career. She was the first Chairperson of the Nominating Committee in 1943 and became the first woman President in 1976–1978. Her Presidential address dealt with the importance of an attitude of service to patients.

It was difficult to choose from among the many papers Glatzer has contributed. The one chosen is a late paper illustrating her mastery of the general psychodynamic literature and her adaptation of it to the group context. The concept of the "working alliance" is now solidly established as a critical component for effective individual therapy. Glatzer uses the concept to emphasize the importance of the member-to-member interaction as a principal component of the "working alliance" in therapy groups. Her writing reflects her gently human but direct and uncompromising style. Note her reaction to the use of "action techniques."

—Editor

Glatzer, Henrietta T: The working alliance in analytic group psychotherapy. *International Journal of Group Psychotherapy* 28:147–161, 1978.

Until recently the treatment alliances have not been accorded the same importance in analysis as have transference and transference neurosis, the prime interactional processes. References to them, however, have been made from the earliest days of psychoanalysis, beginning with "we make of the patient a collaborator" (Breuer and Freud; 1893-1895), and on to "effective positive transference" (Freud, 1912, 1913), "the ego alliance" (Sterba, 1934), "the auxiliary superego" (Strachey, 1934), "the analytic atmosphere" (Bibring, 1937), "the analytic pact" (Freud, 1937, 1940), and "the rational transference" (Fenichel, 1941). Freud's general concept of transference included his original notion of the treatment alliance, i.e., both the patient's capacity to establish a friendly rapport and the emergence of positive transference feelings. This led to the erroneous use of the term "positive transference" to designate the treatment alliance. Freud's formulation of the structural model of the id, ego, and superego

305

gave impetus to the development of ego psychology. The idea of the treatment alliances as something other than a special aspect of transference grew out of the central importance of autonomous ego functions in ego psychology.

After the publication of Zetzel's important paper (1956) in which she first used the term "alliance" as distinct from Freud's "analytic pact," there has been increasing attention paid to the delineation of the treatment alliances from transferences proper. They have chiefly been called therapeutic alliance, working alliance, or treatment alliance (Sandler, Dare and Holder, 1973). Although the consensus is to contrast the alliances with the irrational aspects of the transference neurosis, Kanzer (1975) feels that "there can be no precise distinction between the two, any more than is possible between health and neurosis." Moreover, he regards "the alliances more as exercises in analytically oriented psychotherapy than parameters of the traditional technique." He is concerned about the pragmatic uses of such a concept in psychoanalysis, but in a private communication expressed the opinion that the application of the working alliance to group psychotherapy is natural.

Greenson (1965, 1967), in contrast to Kanzer, feels that "the working alliance deserves to be considered a full and equal partner to the transference neurosis in the patient-therapist relationship." Interminable analysis, he writes, characterized by "copious insight and paucity of change," is due to the failure of the patient to develop a working alliance with the analyst. Greenson also notes that those patients who cannot set apart a reasonable, observing, analyzing ego from their experiencing ego will not be able to maintain a working alliance. Greenson's definition of the working alliances as "the relatively non-neurotic rational rapport which the patient has with his analyst in his capacity to work purposefully in the treatment situation" is akin to Sterba's (1934) notion that "an actual alliance is formed between the patient's reasonable ego and the analyst's analyzing ego."

The term "working alliance" as used in this paper is similar to Greenson's and refers to the healthy, realistic collaboration between the patient and the therapist and between patient and patient. The contention of this paper is that the group process stimulates the unfolding of the working alliance in all patients. The appropriate use of therapeutic interpretations, which constitutes the working alliance, is accelerated in a group in several ways. The group therapist can limit himself to appropriate interpretations because (a) the other members provide the means to effect a working alliance when he is in countertransference or makes mistakes with a patient, and (b) they also maintain the working alliance by helping the patient to regress to fantasy material and then assisting him in examining and analyzing his regressed behavior.

The group process is also useful in developing enough motivation to establish and continue the alliance in borderline, narcissistic, and impulse-ridden patients whose ego resources are usually too fragile to form the special kinds of object relations necessary to weather the stresses and frustrations of treatment.

The Group Process

Patients with poor ego functioning who are able to regress in treatment but have difficulty in observing and synthesizing reality and those patients who are fearful of even partially giving up their reality testing often respond to the inherently natural atmosphere of a group with its more realistic, straightforward, and direct procedures. The reassuring presence of other group members decreases dependence on the therapist and reduces initial anxiety about passive submission to an omnipotent figure which, in turn, makes the analyst seem more human and less frightening. It is easier for a more regressed patient to identify with his peers than it is with his therapist because the other members are not as enmeshed as the analyst in the patient's archaic transferences. The patient is, therefore, better able to accept reasonable observations from them. Challenges by them of his characterological defenses become less threatening to his narcissism as he sees others responding to the same challenges with self-scrutiny instead of hurt feelings and defensive anger as is his wont. It is not only the analyst but the other members and the group-as-a-whole who act as an auxiliary reasonable ego. Fellow members may verbalize for a patient when he finds it difficult to find words. They may free-associate, introspect, and help an inhibited patient to regress to fantasy material; at the same time they also reinforce reality by stopping the regression as they press him to examine and analyze his behavior with them. An ongoing, cohesive group has learned from the therapist to find meaning behind behavior and words and so can conceptualize for the patient the underlying connections between what he feels and how he acts. They effectively and caringly take on the therapist's analyzing role. The patient's self-esteem is raised by their friendly interest in, and speculations about, his interactions with them, and he is eventually stimulated to search for his own deeper motivations. His sense of being an active adult is reinforced when he finds that he can contribute to everyone's intrapsychic understanding by disclosures of his own irrational feelings and conflicts and the other members are able to use his unconscious material for their own benefit. As the group moves from the beginning to the middle stages, it becomes more task-oriented and the analyst's interventions become less necessary and less frequent. The more regressed patient now finds it easier to identify with his peers and to participate in the working alliance. His self-respect improves as he joins them in their explorations and evaluations of all material, including the giving and associating to dreams.

The true sign of the working alliance is when the patient actively uses the interpretation and applies it meaningfully. If he does not make use of the interpretation, he is at the mercy of his neurosis and is not identified with the therapeutic process. When he has the insight, he has to deliberately decide whether or not he is going to continue with a piece of neurotic behavior. In a well-functioning group, the members help him make the choice. They search for signs of change, and if he keeps on repeating the same neurotic pattern, they become impatient and accuse him of wasting the time of the group. The group expects a patient to become an adult working member and does not hesitate to put pressure on him to grow up and use his insights to change his behavior.

The group may also become the "incorruptible superego" (Glatzer, 1969) who will not let the patient get away with self-pity and neurotic interacting with provocative partners but will insist that he face the existence of his masochism and press him to give up his self-damaging behavior. The concept of the incorruptible superego is not similar to Strachey's idea that the analyst becomes the auxiliary superego. What Strachey calls the auxiliary *superego* is really the auxiliary *ego*, which does help the patient to begin and maintain a working relationship. The patient's superego, on the other hand, actually sabotages the alliance. The superego, particularly in depressed and guilt-ridden patients, is corruptible (Alexander, 1929) and is bribed with pain and depression to accept disguised id wishes. Depression is a form of penance, a mea culpa which is destructive to the alliance. Getting depressed after every masochistic act is another way of perpetuating the neurosis. The patient should identify with the analyst's more casual attitude toward the neurosis, but it is so easy to make the therapist into a stern superego figure. Instead of viewing therapy as a learning process in which one cannot avoid making mistakes, the patient excoriates himself and converts a learning situation into a sadomasochistic situation. The group is very tolerant of "mistakes" and helps the patient to accept his human errors and the fact that if he makes a mistake or falls into a trap, he need not endlessly atone for it.

The patient's ability to identify with the therapist's reasonable ego can strengthen both the horizontal (between members) and vertical (patient to therapist) working alliances in a group. The impact on the group member who is helping another is ego-reinforcing. He is able to perceive in others what they cannot perceive and his valid insights are accepted by the other patients and/or the therapist. When I am piecing together interlocking transference behavior in the group, I refer back by name to the members who have made insightful and productive observations and agree with them before I add any additional interpretations of my own, if they are necessary. This is not done as an artifice but as a natural reaction and respect for the accurate perceptions that members contribute to the developing insight. This interaction is probably similar to the "real relationship" which Greenson describes as "genuine and real." The group also acts as a restraining influence on the therapist when he becomes therapeutically overzealous. They become realistically jealous or angry if he becomes countertransferentially involved. When the group analyst realizes this, it is imperative that he admit it, as this acknowledgement reinforces the working alliance or "task relatedness" (Bion, 1961) of the entire group. By acknowledgment I do not mean burdening the group with self-revelations, which I feel is an error and a caricature of being authentic. On the other hand, if his expressed human appreciation and respect for other patients' appraisals of the situation is tranferentially distorted, some group members will support the analyst. They reinforce reality for the jealous or angry patient when they remind him that his contributions have also been acknowledged by the group therapist in that session or in the past and put pressure on him to question the ego-syntonic quality of his character defenses.

The temptation to justify action intervention in analytic group psychotherapy in the mistaken notion that it will set up and continue a working alliance has been my concern for some time. The intense reality of the group situation and the multiple, cross-locking transferences and resistances place greater strain on the group therapist and increase chances of countertransference. By countertransference, I mean all personal, irrational reactions which adversely affect his therapeutic technique. I feel the use of action techniques has been advocated more and more in group psychotherapy because the level of anxiety of the group therapist increases geometrically in periods of strong resistance, and oral countertransference is frequently evoked when the working alliance seems to have broken down (Glatzer, 1975). Paradoxically enough, this temptation should be lessened in a well-functioning, interacting analytic group. A group analyst does not have to take these extra measures at nurturing the nontransference reactions between the resistive patient and himself. The other members and the group-as-a-whole share with the therapist the role of becoming a "new object" for the patient. Artificial devices by the group therapist to effect "a corrective emotional experience" are an unnecessary manipulation. The group members have the means to effect this as they intuitively provide the phase-specific types of support the patient needs. It is natural for them to suggest, confront, disclose, clarify, educate, reassure, or whatever with relative ease. The group analyst, therefore, can more easily restrain his "proprietary zeal" (Freud, 1940) and restrict himself to the therapeutic task of interpreting transference and resistance. He can limit his noninterpretive efforts to maintain a working alliance to the basic human influences his personality will have on the patient as he manifests qualities of courtesy, friendliness, humane understanding, empathetic neutrality, and warm but not intrusive interest.

Examples

Perhaps the following material will illustrate some of these points. As I said earlier, the group analyst does not have to work so hard at fostering the working alliance in a well-functioning, interacting group. Even when he does get caught in countertransference, anxiety, or therapeutic overzealousness, other patients will extricate him. In the following example, sibling rivalry with one patient, Noel, was an added incentive to another patient, Melinda, to work harder at being more successful than he in expediting the analytic progress. This happened when I got bogged down by my overappreciation of Noel's catalytic role. He was an extremely bright, articulate man who was the most open in the group about revealing feelings and primitive fantasies. Melinda was a borderline woman who could sense relatively easily the underlying crosscurrents in the group. Recognition of this ability by me and the group had increased her self-esteem measurably. Competition with Noel acted as a further impetus for her to use her fine intuitive ability to unearth the repressed intragroup tension which had been stirred up the week before.

Noel came in thanking the group for having helped him so much last week with some disturbing aspects of his new affair and said he was eager to pursue it further. It was unusual for anyone in the group to try to dominate the session after he or she had had a productive hour and was not in a state of anxiety. When some man said Noel was trying again to hog the time, I commented that maybe Noel had stirred up some anxiety in the men last week and encouraged them to stay with his problem. This was so, but they were not ready to probe this area. Noel had touched on his archaic fear of women and I thought he might stimulate some of the men to examine their similar repressed fears if he continued on this topic. They went on, but, of course, the discussion grew flat and dull and went nowhere. Patty, another member, apparently jealous of my attention to Noel and apparently unconsciously encouraged by my permission to rehash, stiffened her resistance and described her "new" old problem with her boy friend and her "new" old insights about him. Since these were variations of similar superficial insights with which the group had worked many, many hours with her, I began to wonder to myself why the group was still trying to struggle with the same deeply entrenched defenses instead of picking up her resistance. But I did not interpret. In retrospect, I felt that I must have felt guilty about encouraging the group to continue with Noel's problem and wanted to be "fair" to Patty and give her equal time, so I let them persist in telling her what they had always told her and what she never seemed to synthesize—that she was still expecting more from him than he was capable of giving. This went on for a while until Melinda interrupted to say that the group was avoiding something and was going along with the camouflage problems of Noel and Patty.

She added that they both had gotten a lot of help from the group the week before but wanted special attention from me and kept looking to get my okay. The group was letting this happen, she said, to avoid some embarrassing kinds of feelings which were going on in the group. She was right. Although some people, like Patty, accused Melinda of being jealous of the attention paid to Patty and Noel, most of the others realized and agreed that the group had become boring and repetitious. Bolstered by the majority of the group, Melinda turned to Alex, a married man with strait-laced and puritanical ideas, and said, "You and Rhoda were flirting with each other last week." Alex turned crimson but poo-pooed the notion by saying that of course he liked Rhoda but only as a father since she was as young and pretty as his daughter and was so sincere about trying to work out her problems. I now recalled the subtle sexual repartee between them. Someone else remembered that Tom, another member, got upset last week when someone "joked" that Tom's always backing up Noel had homosexual overtones. Tom had indeed transferred his homosexual anxiety about his brother onto Noel and, like Alex and Rhoda, was content to let the group stay with safe material. The others were probably reacting to my seeming overinterest in Noel, and, in unconscious protest, they stopped working analytically. The group, spurred on by Melinda, now began to dig in and talk about their repressed feelings to one another and to me. The tenor of the group changed dynamically as the working alliance was restored and the deeper layers of anxiety masked by more superficial concerns were released and their transference meanings investigated.

The weakness in "basic trust" which Erikson (1950) notes in adult personalities of schizoid and depressive character is a deterrent to the formation of a working alliance. The group milieu in a multitude of ways helps reestablish such a state of trust and strengthens it so that the patient can move on to the therapeutic job of separating the observing ego from the experiencing one. Here is an illustration.

Vanessa was a schizoid and depressive patient who periodically acted out her deep suspicions of me. She came to the group one day looking agitated and glowered at me until someone asked her why she seemed so upset. She complained loudly about the awful way I had screamed at her in her individual hour and how I tyrannized her and dictated her life; in addition, she claimed I had sided unfairly with her oppressive husband in a recent argument they had had. Alice, another patient, who rarely expressed any but positive feelings to me and was usually the most reserved, the most dependent and "loyal," resonated to Vanessa's paranoid projections. Alice burst into tears as she announced that she was leaving treatment because her complete faith in me had broken down and she could no longer trust me. Even Vanessa quieted down at this unusual happening, and she and the group listened with interest to Alice's accusations of how I manipulated her just as her devious mother used to. The group urged her to tell them what had taken place. Alice explained that in her individual session before the last group meeting, I had refused to answer her request for an exact definition of the two kinds of female orgasms. She viewed this refusal as a manoeuvre on my part to force her to reveal her sexual problems in the group. Alice had always found it uncomfortable to talk about her sexual conflicts in the group, but even more so since I had added Iris, a tall, voluptuous woman with a seductive and pseudo-aggressive air. Alice was fixated on the idea that her relative disinterest in and slowness to respond to her husband's sexual approaches were due to a deficiency in her feminine internal construction. She was, therefore, basically envious of Iris's lack of sexual inhibitions. She said Iris cheapened any exchanges about sexual experiences with outrageous stories of her sexual exploits. The group agreed with her on this point, but added that could not be the real reason for her sudden decision to leave treatment.

Alice had felt forced by me the previous week to discuss her sexual inadequacies because she said it was easier to talk about sex in Iris's absence; she also felt I had intentionally stirred up her anxiety about sex in her individual hour. It was as if she were accusing me of deliberately having kept Iris away from the last group session and thus manipulating her in two ways to reveal her sexual apprehensions to the group. She sobbed as she ended her story with: "I thought I could always trust you, but you have completely destroyed my faith in you."

Vanessa, temporarily silenced, began anew to excoriate me. She now had additional evidence of my perfidy. I decided to attend to Vanessa's anxiety first and commented that I wondered if her rage at me for feeling I was partial to her husband in their quarrel might not be related to what had gone on at the previous group session when she and Burton had an altercation. (Burton was identified with her older brother whom she felt her mother favoured and who had tyrannized her in childhood.) Vanessa had become jealous of my interpretations to Burton at that session and had displaced that jealousy onto her husband and misconstrued what I had said about their quarrel. My remark now reminded two other members how Vanessa always reacted with jealousy and rage whenever I focused on Burton. They told her to quiet down and reminded her that she had always complained about me when I helped Burton in any way. They turned to Alice and together they pointed out the compulsive aspect of her insistence in wanting technical information. They emphasized that it was her feelings about the two orgasms which were important to examine.

Judd, another member, said, "You want to know about the mechanics so you can get away from the feelings." He compared it with his reluctance to have sex with his wife when she initiated it, though he physically wanted to and stalled her until the physical desire got stronger than his disinterest. He later found out that this disinterest was a cover for his underlying fear of being passively overwhelmed by her. Everyone but Vanessa reinforced reality for Alice and pursued the idea that she was afraid of something else and had projected that fear onto me. They were unanimous in observing that Alice had never been happier in her life and that should have given her greater confidence in me. They faced her with her strong overreaction. Iris told Alice that she was surprised at her insistence on the mechanics of the orgasm since it was the whole feeling and psychological tone that gave the orgasm its complete quality. This was a marked change in Iris who usually sounded like the femme fatale in the group when she regaled the group with her exotic sexual experiences. Iris had been visibly shaken when the group agreed earlier with Alice that it had been easier to talk about sexual problems in her absence. Alice looked at Iris and said, "You make me feel like a dyke because I don't have super orgasms like you. You act like the original female sexpot who makes me feel not whole." Iris this time, not in her usual abrasive manner but in a slow, thoughtful way, replied, "I wonder why I make you feel like a dyke when it never occurred to me." This clued me into the connection to Alice's negative transference to me. Alice had attended a Women's Liberation talk just before her individual hour. At that meeting, vaginal orgasms had been denounced as conjurations of old fossil Freudians to make women feel not whole. In her individual therapy session she expressed inadequacy as a women because she did not experience vaginal orgasms. She insisted that I tell her whether they really existed. When I replied that there were both kinds and tried to get at her underlying anxiety, she persisted in her demands for physiological data. Alice was an unusually intelligent and informed woman; her pseudo-stupidity was her defense against further exploration of her negative transference to me. As noted before, she could not permit herself to admit strong anger to me. At that individual session she experienced my acknowledgement of the existence of vaginal orgasm as labelling her a dyke since she did not have them. Vanessa's acting out her fantasy of me as the manipulating pre-oedipal mother resonated with Alice's disappointment in me and facilitated the emergence of the deeper layers of archaic distrust which heretofore had been concealed under her idealization of me. When the other group members showed Alice how she had set me up, Alice could accept this from them and went on to tell the group about her homosexual anxieties. Alice's transference distortions became apparent even to Vanessa and helped Vanessa to recognize the same irrational elements in her own outbursts at me. Vanessa could not feel her jealousy of my attention to Burton the previous week and smilingly admitted her exaggerations of my behavior in her individual session. The group's insistence on exploring the underlying feelings beneath Alice's angry impulsive decision to leave harnessed the working alliance in both Alice and Vanessa with palpable evidence in both of the psychodynamic process of separating the observing ego from the experiencing one.

Admission of the "lesser crime" (Bergler, 1952) is one of the weak ego's ways of defending against the punishing superego. Masochistic wishes are offensive to the superego because pain and overwhelming guilt are meant as punishment and a deterrent but instead are libidinized by the ego. Psychically the great crime is the masochistic solution of an aggressive conflict by the ego against the superego. "Crimes" that are "greater" from a conscious viewpoint can be used as a defense for "smaller" ones. The unconscious ego, accused by the superego of a specific "forbidden wish," defends itself by admission of guilt for another offense. This intransigent defense gives lip service to the working alliance but is an adroit betrayal of it. In a group, one patient's awareness of this subtle defense can be dramatically highlighted and can set off a chain of similar awarenesses in other members. Let me give an example.

Jilian returned to the group from a vacation during which she had visited her critically ill mother with whom she had always had a hostile-dependent relationship. She was feeling very guilty and depressed after the visit but was at a loss to explain her mood since she thought she had straightened out matters with her mother so she could accept her mother for what she was. She described her mother's sarcastic greeting to her and the repetitive derogatory remarks which Lilian turned into jokes so that things went along rather nicely. Paul, another member, interrupted to say that Jilian's mother was just like his mother and that he would have blasted out at her and shut her up. Jilian went on to tell how she had kept her cool until the last day when, because of her mother's stinginess, she could not get enough hot water to wash her hair and consequently yelled and screamed at everyone. All her good intentions were wiped out because now her mother could say, "Jilian comes all that distance just to yell at her poor, sick, half-blind old mother." Jilian was distraught. Martin said, "You fell for the game. I almost did the same with my mother when she accused me of being an evil influence on my younger brother, putting him up to smoking in school and being the cause of his getting caught. My first impulse was to defend myself and tell her off, but I recognized that I was still carrying the engraved image of the 'terrible' mother in me and could not see that she was an easily threatened woman who drank whenever she got anxious. She felt threatened by my brother's good visit with me and guilty that she was unable to give him as good a time." He telephoned his mother and explained that he was not trying to take his brother from her and tried to reassure her in other ways. Later, he told his brother not to highlight his weekly visits with him because it made his mother too anxious. Formerly, there would have been a family blow-up, and he would have been in a depression for weeks. This time it not only blew over quickly but some basic issues were worked on. Some group members picked up this topic and discussed their need to give parents, especially mothers, the power to make them feel impotent and depleted. Jilian still did not understand this and remained depressed.

Paul also had difficulty accepting this but jocularly admitted that he still saw his frail 82-year-old mother as ten feet tall. Paul was an impulse-ridden man whose sexual promiscuity and sexually abusive language was an unconscious defense to prove to his mother and the world that he was not as castrated by his mother as he felt his father had been. He now dismissed his mother as not his problem; he blamed his failures in business on his ambivalence about his weak, inept father who would not stand up for his rights. He said men in his business negotiations became father figures whom he could not best because he could not do that symbolically to his father. Martin, who had just gone through this in another variation, said "That's just like me. I took the blame for the lesser crime. I ignored what the group told me last week about my impossible, suffering relationship to my boss (an alcoholic) and how I made him into my unreasonable, unpredictable mother but fastened on to Iris's observation that my real problem was not knowing what kind of work I wanted to pursue so that I could start looking for another job. I beat myself up all week for the lesser crime of being indecisive when the real crime was repeating with my boss the same outraged feelings of being taken advantage of that I had felt with my mother and the world. You, Paul, do the same. You admit to the lesser crime of feeling sorry for your father and say that therefore you cannot protect yourself in business deals, instead of acknowledging the major crime of making the businessmen into the 'bad' mother so you can get screwed by them." Paul began to hear this as if for the first time. Jilian, who had thought she had not interacted neurotically with her mother, realized now through Martin's interpretation of Paul's similar psychodynamics that the last-day blow-up about the hot water and the subsequent guilt and depression when she came home was part of the old pattern. She had been blaming herself for the lesser "crime" of being mean and yelling at her mother rather than for the real crime of succumbing on the last day of her vacation to the old masochistic game with her mother. She cheered up visibly at this recognition.

Summary

Working alliance, as used in this paper, refers to the healthy, realistic collaboration between the patient and his therapist and between the patient and other group patients in working therapeutically. A brief history of the treatment alliances and the recent delineation of them from the transferences proper was given, as well as theoretical discussions and clinical examples to demonstrate how the group process accelerates the working alliance of all its members and is especially useful to borderline, narcissistic, and impulse-ridden patients who have fragile ego resources with which to form the special kind of object relationships necessary to begin and continue a working alliance.

References

Alexander, F. (1929), *Psychoanalysis of the Total Personality*. New York: Nervous and Mental Disease Publishing Co.

Bergler, E. (1952), *Super-Ego*. New York: Grune and Stratton.

Bibring, E. (1937), Therapeutic Results of Psychoanalysis. *Internat. J. Psycho-Anal.*, 18:170–189.

Bion, E. (1961), *Experiences in Groups*. London: Tavistock Publications.

Breuer, J., and Freud, S. (1893–1895), Studies on Hysteria. *Standard Edition, 2*. London: Hogarth Press, 1955.

Dickes, R. (1975), Considerations of Therapeutic and Working Alliances. *Internat. J. Psychoanal. Psychother.*, 4:1–24.

Erikson, E. (1950), *Childhood and Society*. New York: W. W. Norton.

Fenichel, O. (1941), *Problems of Psychoanalytic Technique*. Albany, N.Y.: Psychoanalytic Quarterly, Inc., pp. 27–53.

Freud, S. (1912), The Dynamics of Transference. *Standard Edition, 12*:97–108. London: Hogarth Press, 1958.

——— (1913), On Beginning the Treatment. *Standard Edition, 12*:121–144. London: Hogarth Press, 1958.

——— (1937), Analysis Terminable and Interminable. *Standard Edition*, 23:209–253. London: Hogarth Press, 1964.

——— (1940), An Outline of Psychoanalysis. *Standard Edition*, 23:141–209. London: Hogarth Press, 1964.

Glatzer, H. T. (1969), Working Through in Analytic Group Psychotherapy. *Internat. J. Group Psychother.*, 19:292–306.

——— (1975), The Leader as Supervisor and Supervisee. In: *The Leader in the Group*, ed. Z. A. Liff. New York: Jason Aronson.

Greenson, R. (1965), The Working Alliance and Transference Neurosis. *Psychoanal. Quart.*, 34:155–181.

——— (1967), *The Technique and Practice of Psychoanalysis*, Vol. 1. New York: International Universities Press.

Kanzer, M. (1975), The Therapeutic and Working Alliances. *Internat. J. Psychoanal. Psychother.*, 4:48–68.

Sandler, J., Dare, C., and Holder, A., (1973), *The Patient and the Analyst*. New York: International Universities Press.

Sterba, R. (1934), The Fate of the Ego in Analytic Therapy. *Internat. J. Psycho-Anal.*, 15:117–125.

Strachey, J. (1934), The Nature of the Therapeutic Action of Psychoanalysis. *Internat. J. Psycho-Anal.*, 15:127–159.

Zetzel, E. (1956), Current Concepts of Transference. *Internat. J. Psycho-Anal.*, 37:369–376.

A Group-Centered Approach to Group Psychotherapy

LEONARD HORWITZ, PH.D.

Leonard Horwitz has contributed extensively to the group psychoanalytic literature as well as to the organizational development of group psychotherapy. He served as AGPA President from 1984 to 1986. The Menninger Clinic, where Horwitz has been Chief of Psychology and Director of Group Psychotherapy, has a long history of interest in group dynamics and produced some of the early papers on viewing the total institution as an interactive system. From the early 1960s, the Clinic has also had a long and fruitful working acquaintanceship with J. D. Sutherland, former Director of the Tavistock Clinic in London and a colleague of Ezriel's in formulating the idea of a common group tension.

In this selection, Horwitz provides further elaboration and criticism regarding the application of the idea of the group-as-a-whole. He quotes the study by David Malan which suggested that the "pure" Tavistock approach did not provide enough support for the individual in the group and resulted in poor or negative results (see the Malan et al. reference in the paper). This selection, together with the final article by Stein, considers, from slightly different perspectives, ways of integrating theories of the group-as-a-whole without losing track of individual issues. These two articles build on the theme of integration developed by Parloff elsewhere in this volume. This represents a maturing of theoretical understanding with an acknowledgement that no single perspective is likely to be adequate for comprehending the complexities of group interaction. —Editor

Horwitz L: A group-centered approach to group psychotherapy. *International Journal of Group Psychotherapy* 27:423–439, 1977.

Every group therapist must come to terms with the individual-group dialectic, whether he does so explicitly or unwittingly. He must decide how much his orientation and interventions will be directed toward the process of the entire group and how much toward the individual patients in the group. But no matter where the therapist makes his stand, both group forces and individual personalities will actively influence the process. The therapist may choose to ignore one facet and emphasize the other, but more usually he will attempt to find some integration of the two.

Polarities of the two approaches have emerged on the group psychotherapy scene and are exemplified on the one hand by Perls' gestalt therapy and on the other by Bion's theories of basic assumption life in groups. The gestalt therapist often treats his patients in a group but he alone interacts with one individual for a significant period while the rest of the group acts only as an audience. The Bion approach, more often used in "study groups" than in therapy groups, consists of interventions which are solely and exclusively limited to the entire group. Most group therapists avoid either of these extremes and find a niche on the individual-group continuum based on the extent to which they have been trained to attend to group dynamic forces.

This paper will offer a critique of the present holistic approaches to group psychotherapy, those methods which emphasize the use of group processes in order to further the treatment of the individual. First, we will argue for the therapeutic utility of incorporating a holistic method. Next, the shortcomings of one well-known holistic approach will be examined. Finally, an approach will be presented which, it is hoped, corrects the aforementioned weaknesses without discarding the power of a group-centered or holistic method.

I. The Holistic Approaches

Holistic approaches to group psychotherapy have been associated mainly with Bion (1959), Ezriel (1973), and Whitaker and Lieberman (1964). Each of these authors has presented a somewhat different system from the others, but they have all been consistent in their effort to use the properties, processes, and dynamics of the entire group in the service of furthering the therapy of the individuals within the group. They make explicit in their systems a variety of group dynamisms which they attend to and utilize in their interventions. They concern themselves with such phenomena as resonance, mirror reactions, scapegoating, spokesman phenomena, and cohesion.

But the group phenomena mentioned above do not constitute the essential nature of the holistic approach nor does their use necessarily differentiate the holistic therapist from those with a more individualistic orientation. The latter have been variously described as intrapersonal or interpersonal in their approach and they utilize in varying degrees certain of these group phenomena. For example, it is a rare group therapist, regardless of persuasion, who does not recognize scapegoating as an important group phenomenon which influences his management and interventions. Yalom (1975), who describes himself as a cross between interpersonalist and holistic, pays considerable attention to properties of the whole group, and in fact makes the phenomenon of *cohesion* a fundamental organizing concept in his therapeutic work. Additionally, he sets forth conditions under which he will make group-wide interventions or "mass interpretations." Even Wolf and Schwartz (1962), despite their vehement polemics against the intrusion of group dynamics and the "group mystique" into group psychotherapy, seemed to move gradually toward a recognition of the need to understand group-wide processes.

It would appear that the distinction between the holistic therapist and others who use varying degrees of individualistic and group orientations is hardly worth making. But my contention is that there is a fundamental difference between the holistic therapist and others in terms of what I shall call the "group-centered hypothesis." That is, holistic therapists adopt the hypothesis that there is a *common group theme* which influences all group behavior at any given moment. This unifying factor is variously described and named by the leading holistic authors: Bion calls it the basic assumption, Ezriel the common group tension, and Whitaker and Lieberman the group focal conflict. The common feature among these writers is that over and above their interest in various specific group phenomena mentioned earlier, they make the assumption of an underlying *unity of theme* consisting of a shared conflict, usually a wish versus a fear, which binds the members and gives coherence to the process.

The most explicitly developed holistic approach is the Tavistock method, which has been most closely identified with Henry Ezriel. It has been described in detail in several articles by the author (1973), and I shall offer only a most concise summary. Ezriel contends that the common group tension grows out of a commonly shared transference and resistance reaction toward the therapist, and, furthermore, that each patient responds to these shared wishes and fears with his own characteristic defenses, symptoms, and behaviors. When the therapist has been able to diagnose the common group tension as well as the idiosyncratic responses of each individual to the group theme, he offers a comprehensive interpretation of the "group structure" at that time.

The present writer believes that there are several distinct advantages to using a group-centered hypothesis like the common group tension. Although I differ with certain important aspects of the Ezrielian method, I believe that the group-centered hypothesis offers several outstanding advantages over the non-holistic methods. In a previous paper (1971), I have elaborated these advantages and shall outline them here briefly.

1. In a group-centered approach, the therapist will tend to be less concerned about the problem of an equitable distribution of time for each patient compared with an individualistic approach insofar as each member's contribution is viewed as a contribution to the whole. As in free association in psychoanalysis, each contribution in the group helps to elaborate an aspect of a shared conflict, which in turn sheds light on every participant's problems.

2. The therapist is more likely to avoid misunderstanding and error by viewing an individual's behavior as embedded in the context of the whole group. When a group member is heard as the spokesman for a group

point of view, his behavior is often understood quite differently than when he is perceived independently of the group.

3. The universalization phenomenon with its resulting enhanced cohesion tends to be heightened in a setting where commonalities among patients are constantly being sought out and uncovered.

4. As the patient begins to appreciate that his wishes and fantasies are almost always shared in some degree by others in the group, he begins to experience the "protection by the group theme," with the result that anxiety associated with expressing unacceptable wishes becomes attenuated.

5. The holistic approach tends to intensify the therapeutically useful regression insofar as the therapist works toward increasing the contagion effect in the group by offering group-centered interventions.

These advantages, however, are only acquired at the expense of certain clear-cut weaknesses; these are exemplified in all of the holistic approaches but particularly in the Tavistock-Ezriel method. But before turning to these weaknesses, let me deal with certain objections to the holistic approach which I consider invalid.

II. Invalid Objectives to Holistic Approaches

Parloff (1968) has characterized the holistic approaches as engaging in "treatment of the group" as opposed to treatment of the individual. He described this orientation as dealing with the "group as a unit" and as regarding the group as a "composite single patient." All of these characterizations contain a partial truth but a major fallacy.

Bion (1959) did indeed prescribe dealing only with group-wide phenomena, making only group-wide interpretations, and permitting individuals to extract what they could apply to themselves from the therapist's interventions. His orientation, however, was mainly toward groups of professionals interested in studying group processes and his method does not represent a significant *therapeutic* approach. Ezriel, as well as Whitaker and Lieberman, on the other hand, adopted methods which integrated group forces with individual pathology and therefore could not be fairly characterized as *only* "treating the group as a unit." Rather, it would be more accurate to say that the group's unitary properties were used by the therapist to further the understanding and treatment of the individual. The salient point is that the objective of group psychotherapy for the holistic as well as the individualistic therapist remains the treatment of each individual.

A related objection is that the holistic point of view tends to anthropomorphize the group. Insofar as one looks upon the group as a "composite single patient," one is attributing properties to the group which more properly belong to a single individual. The error of this argument lies in the confusion between analogy and identity. The group may develop certain norms which are analogous to the superego, or it may develop a common group tension which is analogous to an intrapsychic conflict, or it may even free-associate in a manner similar to a single patient on a couch. This kind of analogical thinking has a practical value in helping the therapist move from the familiar to the less familiar provided he is aware that the phenomena in question have important differences as well as similarities. The anthropomorphizing objection automatically assumes a confusion before the group therapist or theorist has been proven guilty of it.

Another serious reservation voiced by many against the holistic point of view comes under the category of the "tyranny of the group." Its proponents argue that a method which encourages the search for underlying commonalities leads to a variety of abuses against the patient's individuality, his autonomy, his freedom of choice and action. They say that such groups tend to breed conformity, fail to recognize individual differences, and require each patient to fit into a mould. Wolf and Schwartz (1962) have been the most vocal spokesmen for this objection, and they characterize their groups as democratic in contrast to holistic groups, which are described as autocratic or even fascistic.

This characterization of the holistic point of view confounds a *recognition* of group forces with a prescription for certain group behavior. One might well argue that a group-centered hypothesis has never adequately been proven and therefore the holistic therapist is operating on an erroneous assumption. But to argue that the application of a group-centered hypothesis curbs freedom of choice is tantamount to saying that the interpretation of an unconscious motive of an individual destroys his freedom. As Shaffer and Galinsky (1974) point out in their excellent discussion of this issue, the enhanced awareness of total group forces, conscious or unconscious, can only contribute to the individual's ability to escape the potential tyranny of the group.

Finally, several writers have raised the objection that the holistic approaches tend to lead into traps of over-generalization. They say that the therapist who assumes a common group tension or a group focal conflict falls prey to squeezing his patients into a Procrustean bed since he bases his inference upon the behavior of a small number of patients (often only two or three) and generalizes to the entire group. They also make the important point that silence does not always indicate assent and therefore one is not justified in drawing conclusions about those who fail to express themselves.

This objection certainly has partial validity insofar as the holistic method invites more generalization than does its individualistic counter-parts. On the other hand, the silent patient is not exactly a tabula rasa on which anything can be writ. The therapist may not have at his disposal a patient's verbalizations, but he is able to observe a whole variety of nonverbal behaviors including his attentiveness or inattentiveness, reactions of approval or disapproval, his posture, his facial expression, and other significant nonverbal behaviors. Even more important is the fact that the therapist acquires over a period of time a fund of knowledge about each patient's conflicts, attitudes, and reaction patterns so that on those occasions where speculation is indeed being made, he is not manufacturing his inferences out of whole cloth.

III. Objections to the Tavistock Method

As indicated earlier, the holistic point of view embraces some outstanding advantages to a therapist who is attempting to integrate group forces with individual psychology. But a group-centered or holistic approach also opens the door to serious shortcomings which require careful examination. For this purpose, we shall be assessing one major holistic approach, the Tavistock-Ezriel method, described earlier.

Therapist Participation Excessively Restricted

Ezriel asserts that the therapist should refrain from any participation until he has understood the common group tension as well as the idiosyncratic individual reactions of each patient. The task is made even more complicated by the requirement that the therapist understand the particular impulse-defense-anxiety configuration in each of his patients, which Ezriel refers to as the "desired-required-calamitous" relationships. Furthermore, the therapist is restricted in his role to making only transference interpretations.

Although there may be some difficulty in distinguishing between Ezriel's stylistic preferences and the dictates of a holistic point of view, one is struck by the restrictions imposed on the therapist's role, reminiscent of the rule of abstinence in psychoanalysis with the individual patient. In accordance with this role the therapist becomes a prisoner of his method. He is not permitted to engage in the variety of interventions which might help patients to deal with excessive anxiety, perhaps even the threat of serious decompensation; the therapist is not able to act as a catalyst to promote interaction and participation; he is not permitted to interrupt resistant-avoidant behavior until he sees the whole picture.

This effort to transpose a classical psychoanalytic individual situation to a group setting seems unduly frustrating for the patient. In psychoanalysis the patient has the therapist's exclusive attention for an hour at each session, a basic underlying gratification inherent in the process. Although there are certain inherent gratifications involved in group, there is the fundamental frustration of being one among several. Even if the two situations, psychoanalysis and group therapy, were indeed comparable, it is a well-documented observation (Horwitz, 1974) that the patients who are able to tolerate classical analysis are limited indeed, and one would have to be extremely selective in the kinds of patients one would admit to such a frustrating group.

But the most solid evidence for the weakness of the Tavistock-Ezriel approach is the research by Malan et al. (1976) in which a representative sample of patients was studied two to twelve years after completing thei r group psychotherapy at the Tavistock Clinic. The results were less than encouraging for the majority of the patients studied. The common complaint, repetitively voiced by patient after patient, was the low profile maintained by the therapist, leading to a frequent perception of the therapist as unduly detached. Furthermore, many felt that the therapist had little or no concern about them as individuals. The authors conclusion was that the attempt to transpose an individual psychoanalytic method to the group situation is unwarranted and that modifications are necessary to overcome patients feelings of excessive frustration and impersonal treatment. In terms of a criticism of the method represented by Ezriel, the danger appears to be one of the therapist waiting too long to formulate a complete, definitive, all-inclusive interpretation and thus unduly frustrating his patients.

Malan et al. (1976) summarize their conclusions as follows: ". . . it does seem possible that therapists ought to feel less constrained by what they have learned in their classical psychoanalytic training—and should feel free to offer greater warmth and encouragement, greater participation in the group interactions, and individual sessions when the need arises, without the fear that such interventions will result in disruption of the group or interference with the group transference relationship" (p. 1315).

Individual Needs Ignored

An objection related to, but different from, the therapist's overly limited participation, pertains to the quality of the therapist's interventions. He is often seen by his patients as providing input only insofar as he is describing the behavior of the whole group. According to the Ezriel method, comments about individual patients are given exclusively within the context of a group-centered intervention. The paradigm used is that the whole group is dealing with a particular kind of conflict (the common group tension) and only after such a framework is established does the therapist go around the room delineating individual and idiosyncratic reactions to the shared conflict.

Even though interpretations are indeed individualized, the obvious impact on large numbers of patients, at least in retrospect, is that the therapist rarely addresses a personalized or individual comment to them. In the Malan et al. (1976) study, they tended to experience the therapist and group as ignoring their need for individualized attention and concern. Many of the patients in the Malan study might just as well have been treated in a Bion study group, where interventions are solely addressed to the group as an entity, since the overall impact was that the therapist never spoke to them personally but only to the group as a whole. In other words, there is some evidence that the technique of intervening solely and exclusively within an explicitly stated common group framework has the psychological effect on the patient that his individual needs are being underplayed or even ignored in favor of some vague group ideology.

Omniscience of Therapist

Another objection related to the therapist's infrequent interventions, and to his highly comprehensive (and lengthy) statements which integrate and presumably explain everything, is that the method tends to infantilize the members by contributing to the already existing transference disposition that the therapist is all-knowing. One objective of psychotherapy is to help a patient overcome his dependency wishes and to view himself as a capable, self-sufficient adult. Group psychotherapy has the special virtue of providing members with the opportunity to have a real experience of offering help and understanding to peers. This experience in itself provides a growth opportunity and contributes to enhanced self-esteem for each patient.

The therapist's long periods of silent observation followed by oracular pronouncements contribute to the regressive dependency of the patient. The patient as a therapist-surrogate in the constructive healthy sense is not exploited fully in the Tavistock model (Bacal, 1975). It is not unlike the effect of the gestalt therapist, whose method is active, managerial, and intrusive; he clearly and explicitly conveys that the therapist, not the patient group, has the requisite understanding, skill, and wisdom to provide help.

Neglect of Peer Transference

Most group therapists accept the formulation that three kinds of transference develop in a group: toward the therapist, peers, and the whole group. Ezriel's writings suggest that the latter two forms are considered displacements from the really essential therapist transference. He cautions that the therapist must be ever alert to transference manifestations that are being diluted by references away from him, i.e., toward persons outside the group or even within the group. He goes on to say that only interpretations coming directly from the therapist, and pertaining to the therapist transference, have a mutative effect.

Various formulations have been proposed regarding the relationship between therapist and peer transference. Stein and Kibel (1975) take the position that peer transference is a defense against the underlying therapist transference. While their basic understanding is similar to Ezriel's, their technical suggestions are quite different since they propose that the therapist must work first with the defensively displaced peer transference *before* he interprets its significance vis-à-vis the therapist. Ezriel tends to view peer interaction as generally involving the therapist in some way (like struggles to be the favored sibling) and therefore he does not propose a sequential ordering of interpretation.

Bacal (1975) agrees with the others in entertaining all of the above possibilities but also proposes that peer transference may be a significant phenomenon in its own right at certain times. In fact, says he, the therapist transference may sometimes be a defense against peer transferences. Bacal goes on to propose the concept of "transference structuring" which may either be basically therapist-oriented or peer-oriented. I would add the third alternative of a combined therapist-peer structuring. A valid criticism of the Ezriel method is its neglect of peer relationships in favor of the therapist transference. The latter may dominate the scene, qualitatively and quantitatively but it is a dubious assumption that it entirely preempts peer relationships.

IV. A New Group-Centered Approach

The author's experience with the Tavistock-Ezriel method has led him to appreciate the usefulness of group-centered interventions while recognizing the restriction the method places on the therapist's input and activity. As for the patient in a Tavistock group, he frequently experiences himself as only a spokesman for and subordinate to a group theme and not as a separate, autonomous individual who speaks for himself. The paradigm of interpretation presented by Ezriel is essentially *deductive*: the contributions by several members are permitted to develop with little or no comment from the therapist until the group theme emerges. Individualized comments are only made after the common group tension has become clear and been interpreted.

The method proposed here is that an *inductive* paradigm be used: A member's contribution should first be dealt with and responded to in terms of his individual, idiosyncratic, characterological features. As the contributions increase, and preferably within a single session, the therapist may generalize from the individual instances and formulate comments of a groupwide nature. Usually these interventions will stimulate other members to respond with their dominant affective reactions, which in turn will further elaborate the group theme.

A cautionary note in applying this inductive approach: No single rule of technique covers all therapeutic instances. We are not proposing to substitute one rigid formula for another. Rather, we are proposing an approach which may very well be constituted more by exception than rule. A common group theme does not always emerge within a single session, so that a group-centered interpretation may not be made. Also, we must sometimes allow for the possibility that a group-centered hypothesis is not functioning and the therapist may therefore be operating on a more individualistic basis. In other words, the technique must never force itself upon the presented material. The tail of the technical principle should not wag the dog of the material presented. We concur with the observation by Foulkes (1969) that a group therapist must always permit himself to experience surprise, to welcome the novel and unexpected.

******

Specific details of a case vignette have been omitted.

******

The major point regarding technique illustrated in this session is *the focus upon individuals, by the group and by the therapist, before a holistic interpretation is made.* Thus, Kate's inability to stay out of the "peacemaker" role was explored at the beginning in terms of some vague dissatisfaction with what she was getting from the family, and, by a slight inferential leap, from the group. After Dave, a new member, made clear his frustrated dependency wishes in the group, the members were able to help him see his growing feelings of isolation from the group, especially in the light of another member's (Judy) growing feeling of integration within the group. This observation helped to clarify further the nature of Kate's frustration within the group: the fact that a few patients in the last session had reported on progress related to their treatment.

When the group returned to further exploration of Dave's dissatisfaction, the theme of wanting "divine guidance" from the therapist was more clearly evident. It was handled partly by the group's explaining how Dave's withdrawal from seeking help in the group (not discussing his recent marital failure, for example) was the result of his expecting frustration of his demands. The similarity between him and Kate in their excessive expectations of themselves in helping others was also mentioned.

Only after these two patients had had an opportunity to explore their current feelings and preoccupations in detail and only after the therapist had interpreted the underlying motivations of their behavior, did the therapist introduce a holistic interpretation. The common thread running through both patients' reports was generalized to the group: Strong wishes for the therapist to remove their distress magically were producing withdrawal, depressive, and compensatory behavior both within the group and in their lives outside.

The generalization that the whole group was to some extent involved in the same conflict was based only in part on the material presented in this summary. It also derived in part from a previous session in which another member had all but pleaded with the therapist for an answer regarding the advisability of termination and his turning away sullenly because the solution had not been given.

The holistic interpretation is designed to stimulate further those affects and memories already being stirred through empathy and identification with fellow members. That the general groupwide comment served this purpose is suggested by the content elicited from Judy. Like the other two patients, Judy was dealing with her own strong wishes to be another child in the family by using reaction formation, the parental role she was assuming (like Kate's peacemaking role) had the anxiety and excessiveness which suggested that it was partly a reversal into its opposite. Thus, all of the members mentioned were struggling with dependency needs in their own idiosyncratic ways.

Summary

A holistic approach to group psychotherapy consists essentially of using a group-centered hypothesis which assumes that a group is dominated at any given moment by an underlying conflict common to all members. This assumption affords numerous advantages to the therapist in understanding and interpreting the behavior of the group. Commonalities among members are highlighted, resulting in greater cohesion, protection or support by the group theme, and enhancement of understanding for every member from the contribution of each individual. The shortcoming of a major holistic approach, the method used at the Tavistock Clinic and associated mainly with Ezriel, is that it tends to be too restrictive and gives the impression to the patient that his individuality is secondary to the group process. Another holistic approach is described and illustrated which, unlike the deductive Tavistock approach, is inductive in the sense that individualized work is emphasized first before a more generalized groupwide interpretation is offered.

REFERENCES

Bacal, H. A. (1975), A Therapist, Peer, and Group Transference Approach: Transference Structuring as a Guide to Intervention in Group Psychotherapy. Unpublished paper.

Bion, W. R. (1959), *Experiences in Groups*. New York: Basic Books.

Durkin, H. E. (1964), *The Group in Depth*. New York: International Universities Press.

Ezriel, H. (1973), Psychoanalytic Group Therapy. In: *Group Therapy: 1973, An Overview*, ed. L. R. Wolberg and E. K. Schwartz. New York: Intercontinental Medical Book Corp., pp. 183–210.

Foulkes, S. H. (1969), Personal communication.

Horwitz, L. (1971), Group Centered Interventions in Therapy Groups. *Comprehensive Group Studies*, 2:311–331.

Horwitz, L. (1974), *Clinical Prediction in Psychotherapy*. New York: Jason Aronson.

Malan, D. H., Balfour, F. H. G., Hood, V. G., and Shooter, A. (1976), Group Psychotherapy: A Long-Term Follow-up Study. *Archives of General Psychiatry*, 33:1303–1315.

Parloff, M. B. (1968), Analytic Group Psychotherapy. In: *Modern Psychoanalysis*, ed. J. Marmor. New York: Basic Books.

Scheidlinger, S. (1974), On the Concept of the "Mother Group." *International Journal of Group Psychotherapy*, 24:417–428.

Shaffer, J. B. P., and Galinsky, M. D. (1974), *Models of Group Therapy and Sensitivity Training*. Englewood Cliffs, N. J.: Prentice-Hall.

Stein, A., and Kibel, H. (1975), *Relationship of Peer and Therapist Transference in the Holistic Approach: A Group Dynamic-Peer Interaction Approach*. Unpublished paper.

Whitaker, D S., and Lieberman, M. D. (1964), *Psychotherapy Through the Group Process*. New York: Atherton Press.

Wolf, A., and Schwartz, E K (1962), *Psychoanalysis in Groups*. New York: Grune & Stratton.

Yalom, I. D. (1975), *The Theory and Practice of Group Psychotherapy*. New York: Basic Books.

Indications for Concurrent (Combined and Conjoint) Individual and Group Psychotherapy

AARON STEIN, M.D.

Aaron Stein (1913–1983) was a highly regarded teacher of group psychotherapy at the Mount Sinai School of Medicine in New York, where he founded the Division of Adult Group Psychotherapy. Stein began his career in collaboration with Louis Wender at Hillside Hospital. He thus provides a direct link between the early exploratory years of group psychotherapy and current practice. Stein combined Wender's common sense focus on current problems with particular attention to the power of the group. He was exploring group level ideas before encountering the notions of the British school of the group-as-a-whole.

Stein has had a powerful influence on the field of group psychotherapy through his teaching activities. He was a hearty and charming man who enjoyed life and transmitted his zest and enthusiasm to those around him. Several commemorative lectures and presentations attest to his legacy. One of these is the Aaron Stein Memorial Lecture at AGPA Annual Meetings, which customarily takes the form of a creative arts presentation in recognition of Stein's great love for the theater, an arena similar in many respects to group psychotherapy.

This selection is one of the last articles written by Stein. The theme of concurrent therapy is one that had interested him for some time. His ability to translate theory into clinical application is evident, a quality greatly valued by his students. A more comprehensive look at Stein's ideas is found in a posthumous paper prepared by Howard Kibel (Stein A, Kibel HD: A group dynamic-peer interaction approach to group psychotherapy. International Journal of Group Psychotherapy 34:315–333, 1984).
— Editor

Stein, A: Indications for concurrent (combined and conjoint) individual and group psychotherapy. In LR Wolberg, ML Aronson (Eds.), *Group and Family Therapy, 1981.* New York: Brunner/Mazel, 1981.

Concurrent individual and group psychotherapy, including both combined and conjoint therapy, is a complicated and difficult form of treatment. The experience gained with it during the past 20 years has clearly demonstrated that it is a most useful type of therapy, especially with more severely ill patients for whom either individual or group therapy alone is most difficult. The dynamic and technical considerations involved will be reviewed and specific indications and contraindications for concurrent group and individual psychotherapy will be discussed.

Two types of concurrent therapy are currently utilized: *combined* and *conjoint* individual and group psychotherapy. Combined treatment refers to the simultaneous use of individual and group psychotherapy with the same therapist conducting both. Conjoint individual and group psychotherapy refers to the use of these modalities with different therapists cooperating while separately conducting the individual and group psychotherapy. Obviously these similar but different approaches raise important technical issues which will be discussed later.

Review of the Literature

The earlier literature dealing with concurrent individual and group psychotherapy was reviewed in a previous article (12). Two recent articles by Bieber (1) and Scheidlinger (10) review the more recent literature.

In the '50s many workers who described the use of concurrent individual and group psychotherapy were careful to indicate that the use of the group modality did not interfere with utilization of the transference to the therapist in the individual analytic therapy (1, 10, 12). They also indicated that the use of concurrent individual and group therapy did not adversely affect the group therapy. The reasons for these cautions stem from controversies in the literature at the time. There were group therapists (12) who felt that the use of group psychotherapy interfered with the development of the transference neurosis in individual therapy and that, therefore, group therapy should not be used with patients requiring intensive individual analytic therapy. Other group therapists, some American (12) and several British (10, 12) advocated the exclusive use of group treatment for most patients and viewed the introduction of individual sessions as dilution of the potent transferences in the group and as a resistance to the group treatment medium.

The workers who, in the '50s and '60s, began to use concurrent individual and group psychotherapy indicated their reasons as follows: Individual treatment had reached a plateau, and increased resistance due to transference to the therapist and to the characterological defenses of the patient was evident; transference manifestations, especially negative ones related to the therapist, were not expressed. Other resistances and defenses could not be effectively exposed and dealt with, and interpretations were resisted and negated. Therapeutically necessary interactions, nonverbal and verbal, were blocked. It was felt that the concurrent use of group psychotherapy would overcome these difficulties by increasing the opportunities for increased transference manifestations, including the negative ones, and for dealing with the formidable resistances of characterological defenses.

The technical problems involved were described and discussed by many of the writers cited above. It was agreed by most workers that frequently the type of individual most usefully treated with concurrent individual and group psychotherapy was a severely ill patient who developed a primitive type of transference to the therapist. This point will be discussed in detail later on.

Theoretical and Dynamic Considerations

The theoretical and dynamic considerations involved in utilization of concurrent individual and group psychotherapy can usefully be summarized as follows:

There are differences in the manifestations of the transference in individual and group psychotherapy. These were discussed in an earlier article of mine (12): "In intensive individual analytic psychotherapy conditions are set up to focus unconscious (regressive infantile) transference drives upon the therapist so as to make these conscious and available for interpretation in the therapeutic work. In direct contrast to this, the conditions existing in group psychotherapy, including the presence of a number of patients, tend to inhibit the transference to the leader (without, however, altering it) and to deflect it on to the patient numbers, who (utilizing identification and projection), interact, that is act out the deflected transference manifestations from the leader toward each other in a realistic fashion during the group session . . ." (p. 420).

In the same paper I pointed out: "This perhaps oversimplified statement would seem to indicate that at least in relation to the transference to the leader the concurrent use of intensive individual analytic therapy and group psychotherapy could set up conditions in which the patient would respond in two different and opposing fashions . . ." (p. 420). Today one would add to the last statement the caution: . . . unless care is taken by the therapist to analyze, interpret and integrate the transference manifestations in both forms of treatments so as to facilitate the therapeutic work. A further admonition would be to the effect that, in certain patients with primitive transference drives directed towards the therapist (resulting from regressive maturational difficulties), the uncovering interpretation and integration of the primitive defenses and transference manifestations must proceed slowly and carefully.

Freud (3) attributed the ties between the members of the group to libidinal forces. Each member enters the group with an unconscious fantasy of forming some sort of exclusive relationship with the leader. Although the leader remains a potential source of fantasized libidinal gratification, the presence of other group members makes him or her an unattainable object for exclusive gratification. The necessity of sharing the leader as a libidinal object leads to inevitable frustration of unconscious wishes and ambivalence toward the leader.

As a result the relationship to the leader undergoes a regressive change, through the mechanism of introjection, from object choice to identification. Freud suggested that the members of the group then tend to overvalue the leader and put him/her in the place of their ego ideal and, through this common identification with the same object, develop strong ties with each other. From this it is apparent that the transference manifestations toward the leader are also shared by the group members and that the group members unite to control and divert these transference attitudes towards each other. This, as well as the presence of a number of members in the group, alters the way in which transference to the leader is manifested in the group. The transference manifestations directed toward the leader are inhibited and are deflected towards the other members of the group.

These changes in the transference manifestation to the leader are particularly important in fostering member-to-member interaction in group psychotherapy. The inhibition and deflection of the transference manifestations from the leader to the members lead to an increase in intragroup tension among the members. This intragroup tension stimulates and to a large extent determines at any given moment the intensity and nature of the intermember transference manifestations.

As a result of their continued frustration by the leader, the group members' ambivalence increases and the member-to-member interaction then proceeds through a number of phases. In the first phase, the members are still seeking and hoping to obtain gratification from the leader— attention, support, nurturing, etc.; this is the phase of dependence on the leader. As their frustration and ambivalence increase they unite and are resistant to the leader's efforts and go through another phase in which they defy and rebel against the leader. During this phase of rebellion the members help each other to express forbidden libidinal and aggressive wishes.

They then turn towards each other, in the next phase of the group interaction, and attempt to obtain from each other the gratification they could not obtain from the leader. During this phase, frequent and intense member-to-member transference interactions occur and the members interact in the ways that are characteristic for them; this peer or member-to-member interaction is the means by which unconscious transference manifestations are expressed and exposed in the group.

In this way the group members collaborate to express common unconscious affects and drives—those that they share both as a result of the similar nature of their conflicts and of their mutual ambivalence to the leader. While in one aspect of peer interaction they help each other to obtain gratification for their transference wishes, they also compete for dominance and leadership in the group. It is during this peer or member-to-member interaction phase that the group-as-a-whole responses develop with each member contributing to these in his/her own characteristic fashion in collaboration with the others. This is the time when opportunities for the most effective therapeutic interventions occur.

It is apparent that the interactions in the group are the result of complicated and constantly shifting object relations and transference manifestations occurring between the leader and the members and between the members themselves. First, the leader is seen as an object or even as a part object whose attributes can provide exclusive gratification for the fantasized unconscious wishes of the group members. Later, these wishes are frustrated and the object choice regresses to identification with a narcissistically idealized and ambivalent image of the leader. As the group interaction proceeds through the phases described above, the group members resist and defy the leader, rebel against his/her restrictions and turn to each other as objects for possible gratification of transference wishes. Since the members do respond at first, partial gratification of their unconscious childish wishes occurs. This is hopefully worked through in the therapy.

The group itself is also set up as an object which in the fantasy of the group will satisfy a "nonconflictual, need-gratifying relationship with the mother" (10)—the group becomes "the mother group." While this relationship might provide therapeutic support, it also serves as a resistance, especially to working through in termination. The attitude or method of functioning of the leader of the therapy group is the most important, indeed the crucial factor, facilitating member-to-member interaction in the group therapy.

The leader must maintain a group centered attitude, limit his interaction with individual members and continue to resist and frustrate individual members' persistent efforts to interact with him and thus gratify unconscious transference wishes. In this way the leader facilitates the development of intragroup tension and member-to-member interaction. All the reactions and interactions going on are called to the attention of the entire group. The careful maintenance of this group-centered approach frustrates the individual members' desire for exclusive gratification from the leader and sets in motion the phases of the group's interactional pattern as already described. This initial unconscious transference response of one member to another constitutes an "acting out" of the member-to-member interaction. It occurs in a very real fashion in the group session. Again, the importance of this is that it is the means by which the transference manifestations are exposed and made available for therapeutic discussion and interpretation.

This member-to-member interaction, resulting from the frustration of the transference to the leader, serves as a source of resistance in several ways. First, since the members do respond to each other's transference roles in characteristic ways—they find at least partial gratification for their frustrated transference wishes. Second, as noted above, they will collaborate in the group-as-a-whole responses to try to obtain further gratification of the leader, and these group-as-a-whole responses further act as resistances to the therapeutic work of the group. These are Bion's "basic assumptions," or the "focal conflicts," "group tensions," or "group concerns" noted by various authors. Finally, the transference to the group as a whole, as the "good mother group," provides a source of comfort and support, but it also serves as a resistance. Awareness that these factors lead to resistance enables the therapist to deal with them and work them through at the proper time.

As noted, each member collaborates and contributes to the development of the intergroup tension in a way that is specifically characteristic for him. This means that he participates in the member-to-member interaction in accordance with his own characterological traits, the habitual attitudes and reactions that are part of his personality and that are for the most part ego-syntonic. Accordingly, characterological traits and particularly pathological character traits, including the tendency to split objects and affects, are apparent much more quickly and clearly in group psychotherapy and are thus more readily available for therapeutic scrutiny. These character traits are the first and most immediately apparent defenses against self-investigation. They are the first line of defense and are usually ego-syntonic (2, 9).

Indications for Use

The above theoretical and dynamic considerations apply to group psychotherapy, both when it is used alone and also when it is used concurrently with individual therapy. Indications and contraindications for the use of group psychotherapy have been described elsewhere (11) and will only be indicated briefly here:

> The indications for group psychotherapy based on theoretical and clinical grounds arising from the nature of the relationships in the group interaction may be summarized as follows: Most "psychosomatic" cases, most character disorders including masochistic characters, rigid and schizoid personalities, borderline and certain chronic psychotics and neurotics with underlying characterological or borderline defects. All of these are suitable for group psychotherapy and for some the treatment of choice is group psychotherapy.
>
> Another very specific use of group psychotherapy in relation to many of these patients is to help them enter into a psychotherapeutic relationship as a preparation for individual treatment or in helping them resolve a therapeutic relationship in preparation for leaving individual treatment. In this respect, the use of combined group and individual psychotherapy broadens the indications for the utilization of group psychotherapy (11).

Turning now to the contraindications for group psychotherapy:

> In the patient whose personality and ego strength are relatively intact, unconscious conflict leads to neurotic symptoms and these require intensive individual psychotherapy or psychoanalysis so that the transference may be developed and utilized in uncovering and treating the unconscious conflicts. The transference neuroses and the less severe characterological disorders fall into this group and for these group psychotherapy is generally contraindicated (11).

To undertake group psychotherapy, a patient must be able to withstand: 1) a minimal amount of frustration; 2) a certain amount of regressive identification with others; and 3) the emotional tensions arising from the group interactions. Narcissistic and borderline patients with defective ego boundaries who are unable to withstand minimal tensions—these might be categorized under the heading of oral narcissistic character—need the support of a close relationship to the individual therapist and are not suitable for group psychotherapy alone, but can be treated with combined therapy.

This type of patient needs the support and gratification to be obtained from the uninterpreted transference of the individual treatment and, at the same time, needs the opportunity provided by the group treatment to defend himself against and dilute the intense, primitive transference to the therapist. The use of both forms of treatment blocks development of the anxiety provoking "transference neurosis" in individual treatment and provides a more realistic figure with whom to identify and more effective reality testing and ego supporting mechanisms in the relationship and interaction of the group treatment. However, even with this type of case, careful selection is necessary; for some of these patients, group treatment alone is still the treatment of choice.

Recently, reports have begun to appear in the literature regarding the treatment of borderline patients with group therapy alone and with concurrent individual and group therapy.

Modifications of technique using the group-as-a-whole approach have been successful in enabling these patients to become aware of and begin to deal with their primitive transference manifestations, split and partial object relationships, and preoedipal unconscious infantile conflicts (5, 6, 7).

The use of combined and conjoint individual and group psychotherapy should be considered in two major instances: 1) when the difficulties in the transference to the individual therapist interfere with progress in the patient's therapy; and 2) when the patient's characterological defenses are so resistive that therapy cannot proceed effectively.

With regard to the first of these considerations, difficulty with the transference to the therapist in individual therapy can become a very strong obstacle to the therapeutic progress with certain types of patients. The transference manifestations may shift from more mature levels to more primitive ones with the emergence of primitive defenses such as "splitting," projective identification and part object relationships. This occurs when the patient tends to develop too aggressive, too erotic or too dependent a relationship to the therapist or where the patient would find a close relationship to the therapist too threatening and too anxiety provoking, or where it would lead to acting out and leaving the treatment. Patients with borderline conditions or pseudoaffective types of schizophrenia tend to develop very intense relationships with the individual therapist, with whom they need a close supportive relationship. This often needs to be diluted or deflected by the relationships in the therapy group.

The same thing is true of severe character disorders, masochistic, passive aggressive and other patients who find it too difficult within the limits of their severe psychological defenses to develop a useful relationship with the individual therapist. Putting them in a group at the same time helps the therapy move along. Finally, for patients with oral narcissistic traits who tend to develop intense, clinging, ambivalent relationships with the therapist in individual therapy, the use of combined therapy often facilitates dealing with the transference in both forms of therapy.

Scheidlinger (10) comments on this as follows:

> By introducing simultaneous group treatment. the patient's rigid narcissistic paranoid withdrawing or dependent transference patterns become subject to the group's scrutiny and confrontation. The therapist may at first need to use the individual therapy sessions to support the patient in view of the group's attacking his tenaciously defended perceptions. Subsequently the inevitable negative reactions to the other group members (siblings) are likely to be displaced onto the therapist, where they belong. At the same time the positive transference ties to the group peers and perception of the group entity in a positive maternal role can serve as a support on the painful road to the analysis of the patient's angry perceptions of early objects in both individual and group treatment. Individual sessions can be used flexibly at times to offer ego support and at other times for analytic exploration and working through. Group meetings as well are likely to serve varied functions at different stages of treatment. These include experimental frustrations or gratification of transference wishes, direct verbal expression and confrontation of transference feelings coupled with reality testing and resolution.

The second major consideration has to do with the nature of the patient's defenses, particularly his characterological defenses. Some of this has already been noted, namely that in borderline patients, patients with severe characterological disturbances, characterologic defenses may impede the work of the treatment. Deflecting or diluting this by putting the patient in a group helps him to deal with the difficulties in the one-to-one relationship, while at the same time, the individual therapy provides the necessary support. Of particular importance is the use of combined therapy with patients whose rigid character structure does not permit them to become aware of underlying emotional reactions. Placing them in individual therapy alone results in a tedious, long, drawn-out process. Combining this with group psychotherapy, where they can see and hear others' emotional reactions and interactions, greatly facilitates the therapy (4). For such rigidly defended patients, combined or conjoint therapy is a treatment of choice.

Scheidlinger points out (10):

> When the group member's narcissistic defenses of grandiosity, aloofness and arrogance persist over a period of time the other members are bound to confront and later to undertake efforts to demand relevant self-scrutiny and modification of the unacceptable conflict.. . . The frequent painful sequelae of such interactions are likely to involve the therapist in both the group and individual sessions as supporter, confronter, interpreter as the situation may demand. The group setting has special value for helping patients reveal, become aware of, and deal with problems related to sexual identity and the relationship to members of the opposite sex and to problems of schizoid withdrawal. Similarly, difficulties in relation to competition and authority and the characteristic patterns and defenses of dealing with these are quickly and readily apparent in the group setting and can be worked with therapeutically there and worked through more thoroughly in the individual sessions.

In conclusion, another major consideration for concurrent individual and group psychotherapy has already been mentioned and will merely be repeated here for the sake of completeness. This is preparing a patient to enter intensive individual therapy and helping a patient begin to leave individual therapy. The borderline patient or the rigidly defended patient in the supportive climate of the group may become aware of the need for further exploration and working through of conflicts related to unconscious infantile drives. A group experience helps such a patient see other group members as role models for the acceptance of irrational feelings as well as the need for self-exploration. Similarly, when it is necessary for a patient to terminate individual therapy, the support of the group and the confrontation of the group in helping the patient deal with his unresolved transference to the individual therapist are most useful in helping him work through the necessary separation.

Countertransference Attitudes

The countertransference manifestations of the therapist can greatly influence his choice of combined or conjoint individual and group psychotherapy. This needs careful scrutiny on the therapist's part when he decides to put a patient into combined therapy. It is incumbent on the therapist to separate his own needs from the needs of the patient.

An individual therapist will tend to think of group psychotherapy for a patient when his countertransference needs are not being met in the individual therapy, such as his need for recognition as a parental or authority figure, or his need for more emotional nurturing or response from the patient. Countertransference needs can also appear in response to negative, hostile transference manifestations of the patient in individual therapy. The therapist may also find it hard to face the constant scrutiny and demands of the patient in individual therapy. He may think of group therapy when he finds the patient to be too frustrating in individual therapy.

On the other hand, the therapist may find it difficult to deal with patient's needs for fusion and symbiosis and may wish to join with him in holding onto the relationship in individual therapy in too intense and too emotional a fashion. He may then at least consider the possibility that group psychotherapy could have a beneficial effect upon dealing with the patient's transference and help to begin the process of separation. Another countertransference manifestation which may lead the therapist to recommend group therapy prematurely is when the working through process becomes too frustrating and too difficult.

Ormont (8) discusses at considerable length countertransference difficulties in the use particularly of conjoint therapy.

Technical Considerations

Determining at what point the patient should be introduced into a second form of treatment is of crucial importance. Whether the patient has begun in group therapy and then individual therapy is added or the other way around, a period of time is necessary for the patient to work through the acute problems that brought him to treatment, to establish enough self-esteem to withstand the frustrations of the other form of treatment and to establish some sort of a working relationship or alliance with the therapist in either form of treatment so that he can enter into the second form of treatment. Various other technical considerations are involved such as the type of group, the stage at which the group has arrived and, similarly, the stage which the individual treatment has reached.

In concurrent individual and group therapy, the interaction of the group session is most useful in eliciting and resolving resistances, especially characterological differences and in eliciting and exposing a variety of multiple transference manifestations—to the therapist, to the other members and to the entire group. These transference manifestations are both of the oedipal and preoedipal types, "neurotic" and the primitive types. The group sessions also provide an opportunity for the patient to try out various types of role behavior, activity–passivity, leader–follower, and various new approaches. These can then become subject to therapeutic scrutiny in the group.

In the individual sessions a more detailed analysis and working out of the transference and resistive manifestations is possible. Here the various types of transference and resistance can be studied, analyzed, integrated and the long process of working through can be accomplished. Both the group session and the individual session may at times be used to provide ego support and some partial gratifications for the patient.

The use of individual and group therapy, whether in the combined or conjoint form, can intensify the difference in the transference manifestations in the two forms of therapy. This can take a variety of forms, for example, patients can hold on to the therapist in individual therapy as the good parent and manifest hostility and aggressive attitudes towards him in group therapy. They will often not utilize the material from the group in individual therapy and will not utilize the material from the individual sessions in the group sessions. Patients can assume certain roles in the individual therapy and completely different ones in group therapy. Split object relation manifestations can be increased by the use of the combined or conjoint individual and group psychotherapy with the therapist being seen as a partial good object with related affects or as a partial bad object.

Despite these difficulties, the use of both combined and conjoint individual and group psychotherapy can have beneficial effects. The difference in the transference manifestations to the two forms can be much more quickly observed. Negative, and to a lesser extent, positive attitudes which did not appear in one form or the other of therapy become apparent as the two forms of therapy are utilized .

Once these differences in the transference manifestations and the characterologic roles and the object relations are exposed they become available for therapeutic scrutiny. The various resistances exposed can then be pointed out to the patient and analyzed to further the therapeutic work.

The Relationship between the Therapists

Obviously, in order for the use of two therapies to be helpful, the therapists must be aware of the difficulties of combining individual and group psychotherapy as noted above. This is particularly true in conjoint therapy with different therapists carrying out each form of therapy. Here communications between the two therapists must be adequate in order to help the therapy move along. Regular communication at frequent enough intervals with an agreed upon sharing of information from each form of therapy is the best way to handle it. If the two therapists know each other and their styles of working and their theoretical frameworks are along the same lines, the process of communication between them is greatly facilitated. This is particularly true if they know each other well enough to discuss transference manifestations as they appear in the therapy and also countertransference manifestations. If this can be done effectively, the work of utilizing the two forms of therapy can be greatly facilitated.

Obvious difficulties in sharing information will occur. Neither therapist may want to expose himself to the other in these transference–countertransference manifestations.

Frequently the best place to use combined individual and group therapy or conjoint individual and group therapy is in a hospital setting or in a clinic or agency setting where the staff members communicate together in the course of their work. Here they get to know each other and some of the difficulties in exposing themselves and their work are less pronounced than in private practice. However, increasingly both combined and conjoint individual and group therapy have been used in private practice. Again, the most important factor is that the two therapists should know each other and trust each other and should have similar points of view that will enable them to understand the communications and to work together.

The use of these two forms of therapies helps the therapist become aware of the differences in the patient's reactions much more quickly than if he is working in one form alone. In conjoint psychotherapy working collaboratively with a colleague who shares the same point of view and with whom one can communicate makes the process a most stimulating and interesting one.

Case Illustrations

B.V., a business executive, married and in his late 40s, was referred for group therapy by his individual analyst because of persistent marital and family difficulties. He had been in intensive analytic treatment for several years. It helped in lessening some of his depressive and anxiety symptoms, but had seemingly come to a standstill in relation to the marital and family problems as well as various psychosomatic complaints. His own family history was a complicated one. His father left his mother when he was a very young child. The mother wandered around with him trying to get settled, and in the course of this, married unsuccessfully several times. He had a submissive but very ambivalent relationship with the mother. He had been involved in teaching until he began his business career in which he was very successful. His present marriage was the second for both himself and his wife, and there were several children from both marriages. The occasion for his entering analysis was the pregnancy and birth of a daughter to his present wife. She was an extremely bright woman who had been analyzed and was getting her graduate degree in mental health sciences. She was also cold, intellectual, manipulative and guilt provoking.

Constant quarrels over finances and the children led to sexual, marital and family difficulties.

After several individual sessions, the patient entered a group and at first participated well, though in an intellectual and analytic way. He presented a placating, submissive attitude toward the women, mingled with a derogatory and dominating manner. Towards the men he was ingratiating at times but quite competitive, and he rapidly became the leader in the group. It was difficult for the group to believe the accounts of his quarrels with his wife in which he acted like a guilty little boy. However, he was finally confronted with this and his ambivalent attitudes towards women, his competitive attitudes towards men. This began when he had enraged a rather quiet woman in the group by a derogatory remark he made and she angrily turned on him.

At first, the group therapist and the individual analyst kept in touch, but the individual analyst, a reserved and analytic person like the patient's wife, decided to terminate the patient's individual treatment. The present therapist began to see the patient individually once a week. In the individual sessions, the patient's guilt, anger and competitiveness were pointed out and the need to work these out in the group was reiterated. After several violently angry outbursts at the therapist and at the group, his guilt and anger in relation to passive oral and aggressive conflicts were expressed. He then became more assertive in relation to his wife and family and his sexual relationship with his wife improved. At the same time there was a lessening of the psychosomatic symptoms.

This case illustrates: 1) the exposure and resolution of negative transference attitudes in the group; 2) exposure and uncovering of character defenses in the group; and 3) uncovering and exploration of preoedipal passive aggressive and dependent conflicts.

K.M., a mental health professional, single and in her late 30s, was referred for combined therapy by her previous individual therapist with complaints of persistent episodes of depression and difficult interpersonal relationships at work and socially. There was a family history of mental illness and both parents had been depressed and alcoholic. The patient had had many years of individual therapy with some improvement, but always reached a static plateau. She was submissive and cooperative in individual therapy, showed little affect and tended to intellectualize and analyze. In interpersonal relations she described excessively passive and masochistic relationships with men. This was repeated in her transference attitude to the male therapist. She was overtly friendly but distant with women and covertly very competitive and slightly paranoid.

After a period of several months she was placed in a group. There for a long time she was quiet for the most part, seemed depressed and preoccupied, and participated very little. A look of sadness and anxiety caused the group members to treat her very carefully and to avoid confrontation until the group therapist pointed this out. They began then persistently to question her withdrawal. She began to respond, at first apologetically, and then with masochistic outbursts, saying, "What's the use of talking—nobody listens or cares!" This provoked anger and attacks from the other members. After a long period of this type of masochistic provocation, the persistent confrontation of the group released an outburst of violent anger that left her shaking and crying. She then revealed her hidden envy and competitiveness with women and her provocative rages at men, including the therapist. She was able to relate this to her relationship with her withdrawn father and her critical mother. In individual therapy her passive–masochistic defenses gave way to a less guarded and more emotional participation.

Transference attitudes to the therapist were elicited and worked through as well as her characterological defense of engaging in provocative and masochistic power struggles and then withdrawing. She was promoted at work, took more leadership there and was able to develop an ongoing relationship with a man for the first time.

This case illustrates the use of combined therapy: 1) in the exposure and resolution of transference masochistic patterns in the group; 2) in the use of the group sessions to reveal and resolve character defenses; and 3) in the use of the individual session to analyze and work through the transference and characterological defenses in relation to passive, oral and aggressive conflicts.

Summary

Twenty years of experience with concurrent individual and group psychotherapy (both the combined and conjoint forms) has established this form of treatment as a useful treatment approach with specific indications and therapeutic advantages. It is specifically indicated and is probably the treatment of choice for borderline patients, most severe character disorders and rigid personalities. Combined therapy with these patients and also with some severe neurotics facilitates working out severe transference distortions, severe character defenses and certain specific patterns of pathological interpersonal relationships.

The literature was reviewed and the reasons for the utilization of the combined concurrent form of treatment were traced. The specific advantages of the concurrent form of treatment include: the clear demonstration of ego-syntonic character pathology within the group, the opportunity to rapidly expose multiple transferences including split and punitive types of transferences manifestations; the diminution of resistances to treatment as a result of confrontation by peers; provision of ego support without concomitant countertherapeutic dependency and regression, and the enhancement of analytic working through.

Specific indications for concurrent therapy were described, particularly in relation to facilitating the resolution of transference, character resistance and interpersonal psychopathology. Technical considerations in the utilization of this forms of therapy were described. Contraindications to the employment of concurrent therapy were also described. Case examples were presented, illustrating the advantages of the concurrent form of individual and group therapy.

References

1. Bieber, T.B.: Combined individual and group psychotherapy. In. Kaplan H.S.. & Sadock, B.l.. (Eds.). *Comprehensive Group Psychotherapy*. Baltmore, Williams & Wilkins, 1971.
2. Fenichel. O.: *The Psychoanalytic Theory of Neuroses*. New York, W.W. Norton, 1945, pp. 537–540.
3. Freud. S. (1921): Group psychotherapy and the analysis of the ego. *Standard Edition*, 18: 67–143. London, Hogarth Press, 1955.
4. Glatzer, H.T.: Treatment of oral character neuroses in group psychotherapy. In. Sager, C.F., & Kaplan, H.S., (Eds.). *Progress in Group and Family Therapy*. New York, Brunner/Mazel, 1972, pp. 54–65.
5 . Horwitz, L.: Group psychotherapy of the borderline patient. In. Hartocollis, P., (Ed.), *Borderline Personality Disorders*. New York, International Universities Press, 1977.
6. Kernberg, O.F.: *Object Relations Theory and Clinical Psychoanalysis*. New York, Aronson, 1976.
7. Kibel, H.D.: The rationale for the use of group psychotherapy for borderline patients on a shorterm unit. *Int. J. Group Psychotherapy*, 28: 339–358, 1978.
8. Ormont, L., & Strean. H.: *The Practice of Conjoint Therapy: Combining Individual and Group Treatment*. New York, Human Sciences Press, 1978.
9. Reich, W.: *Character Analysis* (3rd ed.) New York. Noonday Press, 1949, pp. 3–111.
10. Scheidlinger, S., & Porter, K.: Group psychotherapy combined with individual psychotherapy. In: Karasu, T.B., & Bellak, L., (Eds.), *Specialized Techniques in Individual Psychotherapy*. New York, Brunner/Mazel, 1980.
11. Stein, A.: Indication for group psychotherapy and the selection of patients. *J. Hillside Hospital*, 12: 145–155, July-October 1963.
12. Stein. A.: The nature of transference in combined therapy. *Int. J. Group Psychotherapy*, 14:413–424, 1964.
13. Symposium on Combined Individual & Group Psychotherapy. *Int. J. Group Psychotherapy*, 14:403–454, 1964.

INDEX

Index